The Catecholamines in Psychiatric and Neurologic Disorders

The Catecholamines in Psychiatric and Neurologic Disorders

Edited by
C. Raymond Lake, M.D., Ph.D.
Professor of Psychiatry and Pharmacology
Uniformed Services University
of the Health Sciences
F. Edward Hébert School of Medicine
Bethesda, Maryland

Michael G. Ziegler, M.D.
Assistant Professor of Medicine
University of California, San Diego,
School of Medicine
San Diego, California

With 31 Contributing Authors

Foreword by Julius Axelrod, Ph.D.

BUTTERWORTH PUBLISHERS
Boston · London
Sydney · Wellington · Durban · Toronto

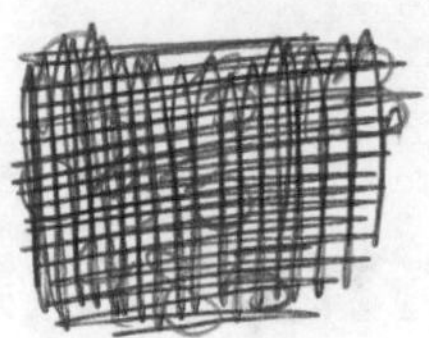

Every effort has been made to ensure that the drug dosage schedules within this text are accurate and conform to standards accepted at time of publication. However, as treatment recommendations vary in light of continuing research and clinical experience, the reader is advised to verify drug dosage schedules herein with information found on product information sheets. This is especially true in cases of new or infrequently used drugs.

Cover illustration adapted from Weideking C, Lake CR, Ziegler M, et al. Psychosom Med *1977; 39:143–8.*

Library of Congress Cataloging in Publication Data

Main entry under title:
The Catecholamines in psychiatric and neurologic disorders.

Includes index.
1. Neuropsychiatry. 2. Catecholamines.
3. Catecholamines—Metabolism—Disorders.
I. Lake, C. Raymond, II. Ziegler, Michael G.
[DNLM: 1. Catecholamines—physiology. 2. Mental Disorders—metabolism. 3. Nervous System Diseases—metabolism. WK 725 C3578]
RC343.C33 1985 616.8 84–19960
ISBN 0–409–95184–6

Butterworth Publishers
80 Montvale Avenue
Stoneham, MA 02180

10 9 8 7 6 5 4 3 2 1

Printed in the United States of America.

Contents

I. Stress

II. Neuropsychiatric Disorders

Contributing Authors

Andrew S. Baum, Ph.D.
Associate Professor of Medical Psychology, Uniformed Services University of the Health Sciences, Bethesda, Maryland

Gerald L. Brown, M.D.
Staff Investigator, Unit of Childhood Mental Illness, Biological Psychiatry Branch, National Institute of Mental Health, Bethesda, Maryland

Michael H. Ebert, M.D.
Professor and Chairman, Department of Psychiatry, and Professor, Department of Pharmacology, Vanderbilt University School of Medicine, Nashville, Tennessee

John A. Ewing, M.D.
Professor Emeritus of Psychiatry and Founding Director, Center for Alcohol Studies, University of North Carolina School of Medicine, Chapel Hill, North Carolina

Irl Extein, M.D.
Medical Director, Psychiatric Institute of Delray, Delray Beach, Florida

Giora Feuerstein, M.D.
Chief, Neurobiology Research Division, Research Associate Professor, Department of Neurology, and Research Assistant Professor, Department of Pharmacology, Uniformed Services University of the Health Sciences, Bethesda, Maryland

Robert J. Gatchel, Ph.D.
Professor of Psychology, University of Texas Health Sciences Center at Dallas, Dallas, Texas

Howard A. Gross, M.D.
Medical Director, Eating Disorders Unit, St. Clare's Hospital, Denville, New Jersey

Neil E. Grunberg, Ph.D.
Assistant Professor of Medical Psychology, Uniformed Services University of the Health Sciences, Bethesda, Maryland

Henry H. Holcomb, M.D.
Staff Psychiatrist, Section on Clinical Brain Imaging, Laboratory of Psychology and Psychopathology, National Institute of Mental Health, Bethesda, Maryland

Elaine Hull, Ph.D.
Associate Professor of Psychology, State University of New York at Buffalo, Amherst, New York

Walter H. Kaye, M.D.
Staff Psychiatrist, Section of Experimental Therapeutics, Laboratory of Clinical Science, National Institute of Mental Health, Bethesda, Maryland

Joel E. Kleinman, M.D., Ph.D.
Staff Psychiatrist, Adult Psychiatry Branch, National Institute of Mental Health, Bethesda, Maryland, and Division of Special Mental Health, Intramural Research Program, St. Elizabeth's Hospital, Washington, DC

C. Raymond Lake, M.D., Ph.D.
Professor of Psychiatry and Pharmacology, Uniformed Services University of the Health Sciences, Bethesda, Maryland

Ulf Lundberg, Ph.D.
Senior Research Associate, Department of Psychology, Karolinska Institutet, Stockholm, Sweden

Ali Jose Milano, M.D.
Professor de Farmacologica, Universidad de los Andes, Merida, Venezuela

Dennis L. Murphy, M.D.
Chief, Laboratory of Clinical Sciences, National Institute of Mental Health, Bethesda, Maryland

Robert D. Myers, Ph.D.
Professor of Psychiatry and Pharmacology, Center for Alcohol Studies, University of North Carolina School of Medicine, Chapel Hill, North Carolina

William Z. Potter, M.D., Ph.D.
Chief, Section on Clinical Psychopharmacology, Laboratory of Clinical Science, National Institute of Mental Health, Bethesda, Maryland

Judith L. Rapoport, M.D.
Chief, Unit on Child Mental Illness, National Institute of Mental Health, Bethesda, Maryland

Audrey Reid, B.S.
Biochemist, Department of Psychiatry, Uniformed Services University of the Health Sciences, Bethesda, Maryland

Richard J. Ross, M.D., Ph.D.
Assistant Professor of Psychiatry, University of Pennsylvania School of Medicine, and Staff Psychiatrist, Veteran's Administration Hospital, Philadelphia, Pennsylvania

Larry J. Siever, M.D.
Director, Outpatient Psychiatry Clinic, Veterans Administration Medical Center, Bronx, New York, and Associate Professor of Psychiatry, Mount Sinai School of Medicine, New York, New York

Jerome E. Singer, Ph.D.
Professor and Chairman, Department of Medical Psychology, Uniformed Services University of the Health Sciences, Bethesda, Maryland

Mary Elizabeth Smith, M.D.
Department of Pediatrics, Rainbow Baby and Children's Hospital, Cleveland, Ohio

David E. Sternberg, M.D.
Medical Director, Falkirk Hospital, Central Valley, New York and Lecturer in Psychiatry, Yale University School of Medicine, New Haven, Connecticut

Paul F. Teychenne, M.D.
Consultant Neurologist, Neuropsychiatric Institute, The Prince Henry Hospital, Sydney, Australia

Thomas W. Uhde, M.D.
3 West Chief, and Chief, Anxiety and Affective Disorders Unit, Clinical Research Unit, Section of Psychobiology, Biological Psychiatry Branch, National Institute of Mental Health, Bethesda, Maryland

Robert J. Ursano, M.D.
Associate Professor of Psychiatry, Uniformed Services University of the Health Sciences, Bethesda, Maryland

Richard Jed Wyatt, M.D.
Chief, Neuropsychiatry Branch, National Institute of Mental Health, Bethesda, Maryland

Alan Zametkin, M.D.
Staff Psychiatrist, Child Psychiatry Branch, National Institute of Mental Health, Bethesda, Maryland

Anthony P. Zavadil III, M.D.
Fellow, Endocrine-Metabolics Section, Department of Medicine, Walter Reed Army Medical Center, Washington, DC

Michael G. Ziegler, M.D.
Assistant Professor of Medicine, University of California, San Diego, School of Medicine, San Diego, California

Foreword

Catecholamines were first identified as body constituents more than 80 years ago with the isolation and characterization of epinephrine as the pressor substance of the adrenal medulla. The determination of a functional role of catecholamines progressed slowly for the next half century. In the 1920s Loewi and Cannon showed that catecholamine-like compounds are released from nerves. About 20 years later von Euler demonstrated that norepinephrine is the neurotransmitter in sympathetic nerves. Beginning in the middle 1950s rapid advances in our knowledge of catecholamines took place as a result of several developments. A relatively simple method for measuring catecholamines in the brain and other tissues by fluorescent spectroscopy was developed. Reserpine, a drug introduced for the treatment of hypertension and schizophrenia, was found to deplete serotonin and catecholamines from the brain. The laboratory in which I worked demonstrated that sympathetic nerves can be labeled with radioactive norepinephrine. In the early 1960s, Falck and Hillarp devised methods for visualizing catecholamines in nerves by a histofluorometric procedure.

My interest in catecholamines was first stimulated by a paper written in 1956 by the psychiatrists Osmond and Hoffer, who reported that the ingestion of adrenochrome can cause hallucinations. They proposed that schizophrenia might be due to aberrant metabolism of epinephrine to adrenochrome. Little was known about the metabolism of epinephrine or other catecholamines at that time. Because of my previous work on the metabolism of amphetamines and ephedrine, which are sympathomimetic amines which resemble catecholamines in their actions and chemical structure, and because of the provocative adrenochrome hypothesis for schizophrenia, I decided to find out how catecholamines are metabolized in the body. I spent several months trying to show that epinephrine can be converted to adrenochrome in the adrenal medulla, but my efforts yielded disappointing results.

The first clue regarding a pathway for the metabolism of catecholamines came from Armstrong and co-workers, who observed that patients with epinephrine-forming tumors (pheochromocytomas) excreted large amounts of a compound which they identified as 3-methoxy-4-hydroxymandelic acid (VMA). From the structure of this compound it became apparent that epinephrine and norepinephrine could be methylated and deaminated in the body. Within a few weeks I found an enzyme that methylated catecholamines, and it was soon confirmed that catecholamines are metabolized in the body by

O-methylation and deamination. The O-methyl amines, which we named metanephrine, normetanephrine, and 3-methoxytyramine, were also found to be present in the brain and excreted in the urine. Soon afterward, Irving Kopin and I identified 3-methoxy-4-hydroxyphenylglycol (MHPG) as a major metabolite of norepinephrine and epinephrine. As described in this volume, MHPG was thought for some time to be a useful marker for brain norepinephrine activity. After an extensive search no evidence for the formation of adrenochrome from epinephrine was found. With the elucidation of the metabolic pathways for catecholamines, Seymour Kety and co-workers found no difference in the metabolism of catecholamines between normal and schizophrenic subjects.

^{3}H-norepinephrine and ^{3}H-epinephrine became productive tools for studying the fate of catecholamines in the body and the effect of adrenergic drugs on the disposition of these amines. Unlike the case of acetylcholine, it was soon observed that enzymes were not involved in the rapid inactivation of catecholamines. Using ^{3}H-norepinephrine, we established that the major mechanism for inactivation of norepinephrine occurred by reuptake into sympathetic nerves. In a cat in which the sympathetic nerves were destroyed unilaterally by removal of the superior cervical ganglia, ^{3}H-norepinephrine was shown to be taken up in the innervated but not the denervated tissues. This simple experiment told us a great deal about the rapid inactivation of norepinephrine and provided a stimulus for future work. In additional studies using radioautography and electron microscopy, my colleagues and I demonstrated that ^{3}H-norepinephrine is taken up in sympathetic nerves and then stored in dense core vesicles. The process of uptake and storage of norepinephrine explained the action of many drugs. We showed that cocaine and antidepressant drugs blocked the reuptake of ^{3}H-norepinephrine by sympathetic nerves. Amphetamine was also found to block reuptake as well as to release catecholamines.

As our understanding of the metabolism of catecholamines and the effects of drugs on the inactivation and release of norepinephrine was evolving, the catecholamine hypothesis was postulated by psychiatrists to explain affective disorders. This hypothesis proposed that clinical depression is caused by decreased availability of catecholamines in the brain and is relieved by drugs that increase catecholamine levels at the adrenergic receptor. This hypothesis stemmed from the observation that tricyclic drugs and monoamine oxidase inhibitors prevent the inactivation of norepinephrine and also alleviate depression and that reserpine, a drug which depletes catecholamines, can induce depression. Although the catecholamine hypothesis has not been entirely substantiated, it has served as a valuable framework for studying affective disorders.

Techniques for characterizing and measuring adrenergic receptors, first developed about a decade ago, led to a deeper understanding of the functional significance of catecholamines. The burgeoning of receptor research was made possible by the synthesis of agonists and antagonists of catecholamines that have high specific radioactivity. With the use of radioactive ligands and pharmacologic tests, four adrenergic receptors (β_1, β_2, α_1, α_2) and two dopamine receptors (D_1, D_2) were established. The availability of adrenergic ligands explained the action of such therapeutic drugs as β-adrenergic blockers and α-adrenergic antagonists and agonists which are used for the treatment of hypertension. It also provided a useful tool for developing safer and more effective antihypertensive drugs. The recognition that antipsychotic drugs can block dopamine receptors led to an important conceptual advance in our understanding of schizophrenia and stimulated productive research toward understanding and treating this complex disease.

A considerable portion of this volume is devoted to methods for measuring the plasma levels of epinephrine and norepinephrine under various physiological states and in several pathological conditions. It took many years of intensive investigation to devise sufficiently sensitive, specific, and reproducible methods for the assay of catecholamines in plasma. The first reliable methods used were radioenzymatic assays; more recently, high-pressure liquid chromatographic methods were introduced. A critical ingredient in the radioenzymatic assay for catecholamines in plasma is ^{3}H-S-adenosylmethionine. In 1960 Don Brown and I synthesized radioactive S-adenosylmethionine enzymatically with a partially purified enzyme from rabbit liver, adenosine triphosphate and ^{14}C-methylmethionine. With the synthesis of radioactive S-adenosylmethionine, several methyltransferase enzymes were soon discovered including histamine N-methyltransferase, phenylethanolamine-N-methyltransferase, the melatonin-forming enzyme hydroxyindole-O-methyltransferase and a nonspecific N-methyltransferase. The purification and characterization of catechol-O-methyltransferase and phenylethanolamine N-methyltransferase and the availability of radioactive S adenosylmethionine made it possible to assay plasma levels of catecholamines.

One of the more dramatic demonstrations of the value of basic research in catecholamines was the development of an effective therapeutic agent for Parkinson's disease. In 1959 Carlson found that administration of reserpine to rats markedly reduced the dopamine content of the caudate nucleus and caused Parkinson-like tremors. Our laboratory at that time showed that catecholamines cannot cross the blood-brain barrier. The tremors were relieved when dopa, a dopamine precursor that can cross the blood-brain barrier, was administered. These animal experiments prompted Hornykiewicz to examine the levels of dopamine in the brains of patients who had died of Parkinson's disease. Hardly any dopamine was found to be present in the caudate nucleus of these patients. These observations led Cotzias to conduct experiments showing that the prolonged administration of high doses of L-dopa relieves the symptoms of Parkinson's disease.

Over the past several years, many powerful new technologies have been introduced in catecholamine research. Numerous neurotransmitters, including amino acids and peptides, have been recognized. These advances set the stage for investigators to ask more sophisticated and penetrating questions regarding the role of catecholamines in normal and pathological states. The papers published in this volume reflect the many basic and clinical developments taking place in the field of catecholamine research.

Julius Axelrod
National Institute of Mental Health

Preface

Central and peripheral catecholaminergic neurotransmission regulates many bodily functions. For example, one or more of the catecholamines (CA) are important in the modulation of blood pressure, responses to stress and exercise, body movements, memory, learning, mood, emotion, thought processing, appetite, and the mediation of psychotropic drug action. The study of CA has been approached from several directions. Animal research employing sophisticated histochemical and fluorescent antibody techniques has provided detailed anatomic and physiologic information about CA processes in the central and peripheral nervous systems, but since these techniques require tissue for analysis, parallel human studies have been impossible. Fortunately, advances in human CA assay methodology in the 1970s, including the development of complex radioenzymatic and high-pressure liquid chromatographic techniques which can measure CA in human plasma, have greatly increased our understanding of how the CA regulate movement and behavior. While early fluorimetric techniques could barely detect the change in plasma norepinephrine that occurs when people stand, these newer techniques are exquisitely sensitive. Our newfound ability to measure catecholamines and their metabolites in blood, urine, and cerebrospinal fluid has allowed us to make some basic observations: a brief period of exercise can increase plasma CA tenfold; CA regulate their own release through autoreceptors; the kidneys secrete CA.

Plasma norepinephrine (NE) levels from supine, resting subjects reflect basal sympathetic activity while sympathetic responsivity can be evaluated by comparing these basal levels with the NE values in plasma after a standardized five minute stand. An intact sympathetic nervous system responds to the stand with a doubling of its activity, which is paralleled by a 100 percent increase in circulating NE. A wider application of this approach involves examining these neurotransmitter mechanisms in various patient groups. For example, NE plasma measurements are now used in the diagnosis and treatment of neurologic patients with orthostatic hypotension. In addition, studying CA in schizophrenic patients may advance our understanding of this disease by helping to define homogeneous subgroups. Already there is consistent evidence that paranoid schizophrenics share CA abnormalities. Even if we cannot establish this as a cause-and-effect relationship, the identification of a reliable marker entirely secondary to the disease would be extremely valuable.

Investigating the mechanisms of action of drugs effective in the treatment of psychiatric conditions, especially schizophrenia and major affective disorders, has provided important information about abnormalities associated with the behavioral pathology. These drugs have major effects on CA metabolism, thus implicating abnormal catecholaminergic neurotransmission in the etiology of these disorders. Most recently, attention has focused on the sensitivity of CA receptors in affective disorders and the changes induced by antidepressant drugs which appear to normalize disturbed CA receptor sensitivity as mood improves.

New information that has accumulated about CA has led us to redefine our concepts of how they function in the body. The powerful techniques that have brought us this information are available for use in research and clinical settings. The goal of this volume is to bring together the most recent data published about the CA in neurologic and psychiatric disorders and instruct the reader in how best to use these new techniques.

The book is divided into five sections: I, Stress; II, Neuropsychiatric Disorders; III, Pediatric Disorders; IV, Affective Disorders; and V, Schizophrenia. The opening chapter discusses the historical background of CA research, the development and application of technology currently available to measure CA, and the establishment of normal values, a necessary step in the determination of abnormal CA neurotransmission. Because CA measurement techniques are now so sensitive that they can pick up minute biological variation, sampling procedures are very important. This first chapter outlines how to obtain samples for measuring CA, discussing how procedures as simple as venipuncture and standing can have a profound influence on CA levels. The chapter also discusses how to stress subjects in a mild and reproducible fashion to measure the responsivity of CA systems. Section I then describes how physical stress (Chapter 2), emotional stress (Chapter 3), anxiety and minor medical illnesses (Chapter 4) alter CA in humans.

Section II discusses CA findings in selected neuropsychiatric disorders. Chapter 5 provides a general review of CA abnormalities and discusses current neuroanatomical interrelationships among central nervous system (CNS) CA pathways in a variety of neurologic diseases, including patients with Parkinsonism and Huntington's chorea. Subsequent chapters (6, 7, 8, 9) detail specific abnormalities in illnesses in which CA metabolism has been more thoroughly studied. All diseases that cause postural hypotension lead to abnormal CA responses to standing, so CA levels are very helpful in pinpointing the correct diagnosis and instituting proper therapy. Chapter 6 explains how to differentiate two distinct types of neurologically based orthostatic hypotension by measuring plasma NE levels. In alcoholism and in anorexia nervosa (Chapters 7 and 8) there is compelling evidence of central abnormalities in CA metabolism which are involved in the pathophysiology of these disorders.

Section III consists of two chapters which deal with CA metabolism in neuropsychiatric disorders in children. CA have been implicated in the etiology of many childhood disorders, which are reviewed in this section. Since drugs that help alleviate hyperactivity in children release endogenous CA in the CNS, the role of the CA in hyperactivity is thoroughly discussed.

Sections IV and V review studies assessing sympathetic nervous system function and central CA neurotransmitter activity in depression and schizophrenia. In general terms, depression can be viewed as a disease involving deficient CA tone and schizophrenia as a disease of excessive CA activity. Chapters 11–15 detail CA synthesis, storage, release rate, and receptor sensitivity in these disorders. It is here where the new analytic techniques discussed at the beginning of this text promise to yield essential information about these important but poorly understood diseases.

In summary, although the CA have been the object of intense study since 1890 in animals and in tissue preparations, no appropriate animal model depicts most of the neurologic and psychiatric diseases in which CA are involved. Increasingly sensitive techniques that allow us to study CA metabolism in these patients have brought us conceptual advances in understanding these disorders and practical advances in using CA measurements to help treat these diseases. Assays of the CA, their enzymes, and metabolites are currently important in the management of many illnesses. This book provides background information about how the CA are involved in these diseases and practical information about how to use CA measurements to evaluate neurologic and psychiatric patients.

CRL
MGZ

1

Techniques for the Assessment and Interpretation of Catecholamine Measurements in Neuropsychiatric Patients

C. Raymond Lake
Michael G. Ziegler

Catecholamines (CA) are a group of compounds widely recognized for their sympathomimetic properties. The most intensely researched are epinephrine (E), norepinephrine (NE), and dopamine (DA), which have a similar structure consisting of a benzene ring, adjacent ring hydroxyl groups at positions 3 and 4, and a carbon side chain containing an amine group (Figure 1.1). One of the earliest references to CA, the structures of which were unknown at the time, was made in 1895 by Oliver and Schafer [78] who noted that an adrenal gland extract caused a pressor response in recipient animals. Two years later this pressor substance was identified as N-methyl-3,4-dihydroxyphenylethanolamine or E, also called adrenaline [1]. The similarities between the pressor effects of E and the stimulation of the sympathetic nerves, reported in 1901 [71], led 4 years later to the proposal that the neurotransmitter of the sympathetic nervous system (SNS) was an "E-like" substance [26]. It was not until 1946, however, that von Euler [35,36] isolated this substance, NE, which had been synthesized in 1904 [96], and identified it as the primary neurotransmitter of the SNS.

DA, first synthesized in 1910 [4], was shown by Blaschko [6] in 1939 to be an intermediate compound in the synthesis of NE and E, and currently is known to function as a central nervous system (CNS) neurotransmitter. DA may be involved in some types of schizophrenia (see Chapter 15), in major affective disorders (see Chapter 13), and certainly is important in blood pressure and neuroendocrine regulation. Peripheral actions are less clearly established.

By 1950 a fluorometric assay technique had been developed which attempted to estimate CA in the range found in human plasma [73]. There have been many subsequent developments in CA methodology, not all of which are reviewed in this chapter. The reader interested in a more detailed account of developments

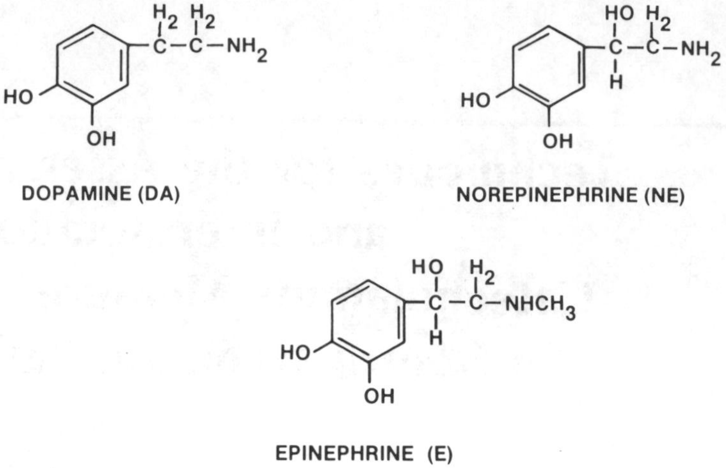

Figure 1.1 Chemical structures of the three most common biogenic catecholamines: dopamine, norepinephrine, and epinephrine.

in CA methodology should consult references 49 and 53. Our goals are to briefly discuss current assay techniques, metabolism and function, and to review the state-of-the-art techniques for SNS evaluation in normal subjects and patients suffering from various neuropsychiatric disorders.

One principal area of interest is the diagnostic utility of plasma CA measurements in the clinical evaluation of many diseases which have similar clinical pictures but different etiologies. For example, neurologic disorders of the CNS and peripheral neuropathies can produce the same autonomic symptoms, but their plasma NE levels are different (see Chapter 6). Supraventricular tachycardias can be caused by CA or by an intrinsic cardiac defect. CA levels can also help predict the success of β-blocker therapy. Many current theories of etiology of the functional psychoses involve CA (see Chapters 13 through 15).

An indication of the increasing interest in CA is the number of articles on the topic in the medical literature. CA articles listed in the *Index Medicus* have increased nearly fivefold since 1960, a trend that appears to be continuing into the 1980s with more than 1045 papers published in the first half of 1984 (Figure 1.2). Since 1960, more than 35,000 articles about CA have been published with interest initially focused on E, then, beginning in the late 1960s, on NE and more recently, on DA.

CATECHOLAMINE ASSAY TECHNIQUES

Interest in measuring CA dates to the late 1800s but it took approximately 75 years to develop assays sufficiently sensitive and specific to reliably estimate plasma

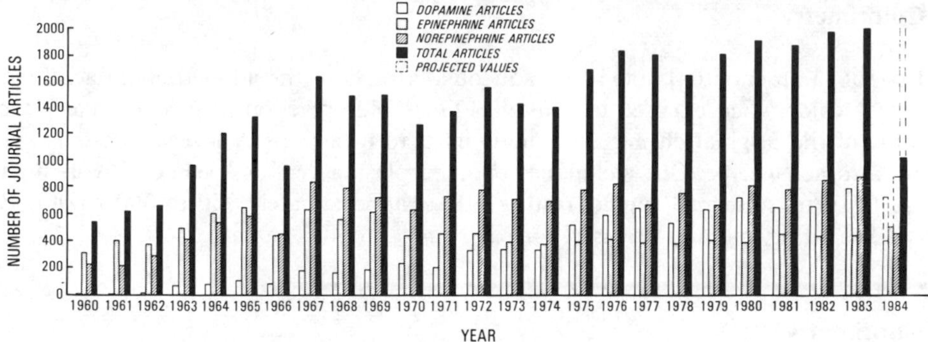

Figure 1.2 Number of catecholamine articles published each year in journals indexed by *Index Medicus* from 1960 through mid-1984.

levels. Some of the major areas in which advancements in the development of CA assays were made include the following:

Sensitivity. Because the CA are present in plasma in picogram quantities, only an extremely sensitive assay can detect them.

Specificity. CA (NE, E, and DA) are chemically similar to amines, amino acids, and fluorescent compounds that can be falsely measured as CA.

Interfering compounds. Human plasma contains proteins that bind CA, cations and purines that inhibit their enzymatic conversion, and lipids that interfere with their extraction.

Stability. CA are labile at physiologic pH and room temperature and are easily oxidized.

In vitro CA formation. CA in vivo are metabolized to glucuronides and sulfated compounds. When samples are stored at acidic pH to prevent oxidation, these CA conjugates can be hydrolyzed back to the parent CA and increase apparent blood levels of the free (nonconjugated) compounds.

Protein binding. CA are capable of binding to proteins, and the bound component may be measured by some assays but not by others.

A chronologic summary of some of the developments of CA measurement methodology follows.

Bioassays

The first CA assays were based on a measurable physiologic response to the application of CA. The simplest of these measured increase in blood pressure after injection of a compound. However, because a variety of substances besides CA can raise or lower blood pressure, this technique is nonspecific.

Colorimetry

In 1856, Vulpian [104] noted that aqueous extracts of the adrenal gland acquired a rosy color when exposed to sunlight. This color reaction formed the basis for some of the original chemical methods used to measure CA levels. These assays are also nonspecific. One technique reported plasma venous levels of CA as high as 10 μg/ml. (Normal supine, resting NE is approximately 250 to 300 pg/ml, E is 30 to 50 pg/ml, and DA is reported from 50 to 400 pg/ml.)

Fluorimetry

The CA phenolic group fluoresces with an excitation maximum at 285 nm and emission maximum at 325 nm. Fluorescence can be enhanced by chemical derivitization with trihydroxyindole or ethylenediamine. Anton and Sayre [2] thoroughly evaluated the variables involved in the fluorometric assay and concluded that only DA would interfere markedly with the assay for NE and E. Assays based on their technique accurately measure large increases in CA levels following stress but, typically, give artifactually high supine, resting (baseline) levels of CA. The method of Renzini et al [88] provides more accurate measurements of plasma CA levels following both stress and at rest. Miura et al's [74] adaptation of this assay compares favorably with radioenzymatic techniques. However, in other articles by this group [74], basal CA levels measured by their fluorescent technique were quite low.

The COMT Radioenzymatic Assay

The enzyme catechol-O-methyltransferase (COMT) transfers a methyl group from S-adenosylmethionine (SAM) to the 3 or 4 hydroxyl position of catechols. In 1958, Axelrod and Tomchick [3] published a method to purify rat liver COMT, showed that divalent cations stimulated enzymatic activity, and demonstrated the wide range of catechols methylated by this enzyme. Ten years later, Engelman et al [28] developed a double isotopic method for converting catechols to their ^{14}C-labeled derivatives. The ^{14}C-labeled E and NE are converted by oxidation to radiolabeled vanillin, which is extracted into toluene and counted by liquid scintillation spectroscopy. The sensitivity of this assay was much greater than that of currently available fluorescent or bioassay techniques, but was limited by the specific activity of the ^{14}C-SAM used as a tracer methyl donor.

E is converted to metanephrine and NE to normetanephrine by COMT. Engleman and Portnoy [27] separated these compounds by thin-layer chromatography before converting them to vanillin. The assay's sensitivity is enhanced by use of ^{3}H-SAM* [79].

* Components of this assay are packaged and offered for sale by Upjohn as Cat-A-Kit.

COMT will methylate most catechols including both the small catechol molecules and large molecules such as dobutamine. This is a disadvantage if the methylated products are not separated, but when the assay is combined with the appropriate separation techniques, a variety of CA can be measured [22]. In the COMT assay for CA, plasma samples can either be analyzed directly, or after plasma proteins are precipitated with perchloric acid. The sample is incubated with the enzyme COMT, the methyl donor ^{3}H-SAM, ethyleneglycol-bis-(β-aminoethyl ether)-N,N^1,-tetraacetic acid (EGTA) to bind inhibiting calcium, and magnesium to stimulate enzyme activity. During incubation in a buffer solution, radiolabeled O-methylated derivatives are formed, which are then extracted into a lipid solvent. The labeled amines are back-extracted into an acid layer and then separated by thin-layer chromatography. The β-hydroxylated compounds can be oxidized to ^{3}H-vanillin, which is extracted into toluene and counted by scintillation spectroscopy. Non-β-hydroxylated substituents such as DA must be extracted into a slightly more polar solution, which gives higher blank levels.

Interpretation of results from the COMT assay requires awareness of the biochemistry of the assays. Because calcium and other inhibitors of COMT activity are present in plasma in variable amounts, plasma from different sources may need to be individually standardized. Many catechol drugs, such as isoproterenol, isoetharine, dobutamine, and apomorphine, can competitively inhibit the assay. Derivatives of the antihypertensive drug α-methyldopa, such as α-methyldopamine, can also interfere. Aluminum is a potent inhibitor of the COMT enzyme, and patients with renal failure may have high blood levels of aluminum. Because the samples are separated by thin-layer chromatography, very high levels of one compound may cause some "cross-over" contamination into the chromatographic band of another compound, thus artifactually elevating levels of the adjacent compound. This elevation can be corrected by subtracting the cross-over. Despite problems with this assay, the COMT technique is less disturbed by interfering substances than the old fluorometric methods and is sufficiently sensitive and reliable to provide useful information about plasma CA in most circumstances. In fact, variability within the assay itself is usually less than variability caused by different sample collection techniques, a subject discussed in the section, Techniques for Sympathetic Nervous System Evaluation, later in this chapter.

The PNMT Radioenzymatic Assay

In the body, phenylethanolamine-N-methyltransferase (PNMT) converts NE into E by transfer of a methyl group from SAM to the primary amine of NE [47,69]. The enzyme can be partially purified from bovine adrenal glands. In the test tube radiolabeled ^{3}H-SAM is used as a methyl donor to convert NE to radiolabeled E, which can be isolated and counted by scintillation spectroscopy. The enzyme is fairly specific for β-hydroxylated phenylethylamines and does not appreciably label DA or further metabolize E. The PNMT technique is the most reliable assay available for measuring plasma NE levels and can accommodate large numbers of samples easily [69]. Some laboratories have experienced difficulty in adequately purifying PNMT, so the technique has been used less widely than the COMT method.

The PNMT assay has several other advantages over the COMT-based radioenzymatic technique. The PNMT assay is more specific for NE than is the COMT technique because PNMT has much greater substrate specificity than does COMT. Because PNMT is not inhibited by aluminum, CA can be preconcentrated on alumina prior to assay and the assay can be made extremely sensitive when large volumes of plasma (1–20 ml) are concentrated on alumina and eluted into 0.1 ml of 0.1 to 0.3 N HC1. The same preconcentration step eliminates inhibiting substances and allows the assay to be easily standardized for tissue or plasma samples without fear that standardization will vary widely from sample to sample. Henry et al's [47] technique for purifying radiolabeled E from other radioactive contaminants without using chromatography makes the PNMT method one of the most rapid NE assay systems available.

The PNMT assay is performed by shaking the plasma sample with alumina to adsorb CA and then washing the alumina and eluting CA with a small volume of acid. The acid eluate is incubated with PNMT and ^{3}H-SAM to form ^{3}H-E from the NE. The ^{3}H-E is then adsorbed onto alumina, which is washed three times to remove contaminating ^{3}H-SAM. The ^{3}H-E is eluted from the alumina and any remaining ^{3}H-SAM is precipitated prior to scintillation counting of the ^{3}H-E product [69].

Liquid Chromatographic Assay Techniques

Modern liquid chromatographic techniques, called high-pressure or high-performance liquid chromatography (HPLC), separate CA or metabolites and internal standards into sharp peaks. After separation, CA can be detected by native fluorescence, by fluorescence of their chemical derivatives, or by electrochemical detection. The resolving power of this technique makes it desirable for research applications.

Separation Techniques

Early HPLC separations used cation exchange materials that were relatively inexpensive and offered separation efficiencies of 1,000 plates per meter. Newer 5- to 10-μm reverse-phase and cation exchange materials increase the efficiency to greater than 25,000 plates per meter and allow shorter columns, which shorten the time needed to perform the same analysis. Reverse-phase columns can be used directly, but have most frequently been modified using "soap" chromatography with the addition of sodium octylsulfate or sodium heptylsulfonate to the mobile phase. The hydrophobic, anionic detergents are strongly adsorbed to the stationary phase, in effect transforming it into a cation exchange column. This transformation creates a versatile column suitable for the separation of neutral and anionic substances as well as CA.

Fluorescence Detection

Once CA are separated by HPLC, a sensitive detection system is necessary to quantify the small amounts present in human plasma. Natural fluorescence of the amines requires several nanograms for detection. Derivatized fluorescence techniques can greatly enhance the sensitivity of detection. CA can be derivatized by trihydroxyindole, ethylenediamine, ninhydrin, fluorescamine, or O-phthalaldehyde to greatly enhance their fluorescence. Derivatization may be done precolumn or postcolumn, the latter having recently been automated. Yui and Kawai [114] compared the sensitivity of these detection techniques and concluded that postcolumn derivitization with trihydroxyindole is the most sensitive and specific detection system.

Electrochemical Detection

CA are unstable in solution because they oxidize easily, a characteristic used to advantage in electrochemical detection in which the solution containing CA is passed by a carbon electrode with an electrical potential in the range of +600 mV. The CA are oxidized to orthoquinones, and the resulting electric current passing across the electrode is proportional to the amount of CA present. The electrochemical potential of the CA group is similar to that of uric acid, which is present in 10,000-fold higher concentrations than the biogenic amines. For these reasons, the amines need to be separated prior to electrochemical detection by isolation on alumina and then separation by HPLC. This process can provide detection limits in the range of 25 pg/ml [114], which makes the system, when performing optimally, applicable to the measurement of human plasma CA levels. Because all CA are detected with equal sensitivity, this technique is more applicable to research than is fluorescence or derivitization, which are variably sensitive to NE, E, and DA.

Gas Chromatography

CA are polar, nonvolatile, and unstable molecules, and thus are unsuitable for use in gas chromatographic procedures. However, they are small enough to allow volatile derivatives to be made by chemical techniques. These derivatives can be separated by gas chromatography. As with any chromatographic technique, CA must be detected after separation, which is accomplished by flame ionization detection, electron capture, or mass spectroscopy. Flame ionization is not sufficiently sensitive to detect the low concentrations of CA in plasma. Electron capture is approximately 2000 times more sensitive but lacks specificity. Mass spectroscopy has a sensitivity similar to that of electron capture detection but is much more specific. Gas chromatography with mass spectroscopy (GCMS) is extremely accurate because it can be standardized by deuterated CA, which differ slightly in molecular weight from the compounds being measured. Because of this, GCMS provides a reference standard against other less rigorous procedures and has been used, for example, to verify the accuracy of the PNMT radioenzymatic assay [117]. However, the technique is so time-consuming and expensive that it is not suitable for routine CA assays.

TECHNIQUES FOR SYMPATHETIC NERVOUS SYSTEM EVALUATION

Plasma Norepinephrine Levels as an Index of Sympathetic Nervous System Function

Measurement of supine plasma NE levels facilitates assessment of SNS tone; calculation of the increment in NE produced by standing for five minutes enables evaluation of the ability of the SNS to respond to orthostatic change. These procedures are valuable diagnostic tools and are discussed in this and subsequent chapters.

The evidence that plasma NE levels reflect SNS activity in human beings is substantial but largely indirect. In the mid-1800s, Bernard [5] found vasodilation after sectioning of the sympathetic chain, and Brown-Séquard [10] reported vasoconstriction on stimulation of the sympathetic chain. Although adrenalectomy does not markedly alter NE levels in urine, it does reduce E sharply, indicating that the adrenal glands produce almost all of the body's E [7]. Patients with Raynaud's disease who have had surgical sympathectomy have a decrease in venous levels of NE in the treated limb [76]. Diabetic patients with autonomic neuropathy [119] and patients with SNS disorders such as familial dysautonomia [119], idiopathic orthostatic hypotension [118], and Shy-Drager syndrome [118] demonstrate low plasma NE levels, an absence of NE release on standing, or both. A variety of stimuli that cause SNS activation in animals, such as exercise and environmental stress, also increase NE in humans [21,40,58,69]. Amphetamine and tyramine, drugs known to release NE from sympathetic nerve endings and to prevent its reuptake in animals, cause increases in circulating NE levels in humans [85,90].

The most direct evidence linking plasma NE levels to SNS activity is reported by Wallin et al [11,97,105], who made direct electrical recordings of sympathetic activity from muscle branches of the peroneal nerve in 22 healthy persons. Plasma NE correlated positively with levels of electrical sympathetic activity ($r = 0.81$, $p < 0.01$), which suggested to the authors that the overflow of NE from sympathetic junctions in muscle contributes significantly to plasma NE levels at rest. These data indicate that SNS electrical activity is reflected by plasma NE levels. NE in plasma represents the portion of NE released from SNS nerve terminals that diffuses from the synaptic cleft into the circulation. Most NE is taken up actively across the presynaptic membrane or into other cells or is metabolized by deamination, O-methylation, or conjugation. Released NE has been calculated to reach the circulation at a rate of 360 ng/m^2/min with a simultaneous clearance rate of 1.32 liters/m^2/min[30]. The initial, rapid phase half-life of NE in plasma is accepted to be approximately 2 to 2.5 minutes. Current methodology to more precisely measure apparent release (spillover) and clearance rates in human beings is discussed in this section.

Normal Plasma Catecholamine Values and Some Variables Affecting Them

Because many laboratories now measure CA using primarily the COMT, PNMT, or HPLC methods, it is relevant to compare results from normal persons measured by these different techniques. Table 1.1 indicates mean values from the literature of NE and E from approximately 800 normal subjects, supine and standing, measured by various laboratories (excluding our own) using the three techniques [40, 41,59,60]. Although the literature indicates that there is little difference between methods (see Table 1.1), data from our laboratory show that NE values from 146 volunteers measured by the PNMT technique (267 ± 13 pg/ml and 513 ± 28 pg/ml, supine and standing [N = 122], respectively) were significantly higher ($p < 0.01$ and $p < 0.05$) than NE values of 79 volunteers measured by the COMT technique (218 ± 12 pg/ml and 411 ± 29 pg/ml, supine and standing [N-35]) (Table 1.2). None of the persons were assayed by both techniques, the most accurate way of examining assay differences. However, the PNMT assay may give higher values because it requires alumina adsorption of CA from plasma, during which

Table 1.1 Plasma Catecholamines in Normotensive Control Subjects: Results from a Literature Survey*

	PNMT	*COMT*	*HPLC*
Supine			
NE (pg/ml)	272 ± 20	228 ± 30	240 ± 13
E (pg/ml)	—	48 ± 8	45 ± 3
Number of subjects	304	430	66
Mean age	38	39	28
Number of studies/number of laboratories	8/7	19/15	2/2
Standing			
NE (pg/ml)	467 ± 40	413 ± 47	533 ± 42
E (pg/ml)	—	60 ± 7	—
Number of subjects	243	213	7
Mean Age	38	39	28
Number of studies/number of laboratories	5/4	8/6	1/1

PNMT = phenylethanolamine-N-methyltransferase radioenzymatic assay method; COMT = catechol-O-methyltransferase radioenzymatic assay method; HPLC = high-pressure liquid chromatography; NE = norepinephrine; E = epinephrine.

* Data shown as mean ± standard error of the mean (SEM).

NOTE: This table excludes data taken from authors' laboratories.

SOURCE: Adapted from Goldstein and Lake [40,41].

Table 1.2 Effects of Postural Change, Stress, and Assay Technique on Catecholamine Values from Normal Control Subjects

	PNMT		COMT		
Posture	*N*	*NE (pg/ml)*	*N*	*NE (pg/ml)*	E
Supine	146	267 ± 13	79	218 ± 12[a]	22 ± 2
Reclining in lounge chair	—	—	72	261 ± 13[b]	23 ± 3
Sitting	11	401 ± 37[c,d]	56	400 ± 19[e]	28 ± 2
Cold pressor (sitting)	12	528 ± 76[c]	—	—	—
Tilted	9	405 ± 30[c,d]	—	—	—
Standing	122	513 ± 28[c]	35	411 ± 29[f]	46 ± 10[c]
Hand grip (standing)	64	749 ± 67[d]	12	792 ± 137[d]	78 ± 40[c]

PNMT = phenylethanolamine-N-methyltransferase radioenzymatic assay method; COMT = catechol-O-methyltransferase; N = number of subjects; NE = norepinephrine; E = epinephrine.

[a] $p < 0.01$ compared with Lake PNMT (two-tail t test).

[b] $p < 0.01$ compared with supine.

[c] $p < 0.01$ compared with supine (paired t test).

[d] $p < 0.01$ compared with standing.

[e] $p < 0.001$ compared with reclining lounge chair (paired t test).

[f] $p < 0.05$.

NOTE: These data were taken from the authors' laboratories.

step some protein-bound NE may bind to alumina and be measured in addition to the free NE. The HPLC technique gives a mean supine NE value between, but not significantly different from, the two radioenzymatic assays (see Table 1.1).

In our laboratory, the PNMT interassay (between assays) coefficient of variation (CV) is 8%; the intraassay (within an assay) CV is 6%. For our COMT assay, the interassay CV for NE is 7%, and the intraassay CV is 5%; for E the CVs are 11% and 10%, respectively. Thus samples for any one study should be assayed by the same assay technique and preferably in the same batch.

Accurate longitudinal studies are possible because a person's plasma NE remains constant throughout a study lasting weeks to months. This laboratory recently measured supine CA levels by the COMT assay in normal volunteers sampled at five time points: baseline (0 min), 5 minutes, one hour, 1 day, and 1 week. Standing and hand-grip levels were assayed only at baseline and one week. There were no differences in either NE or E values between any of the time points [59]. In a separate group, blood was drawn twice from each person on two occasions separated by 2 weeks for NE measurements by the PNMT method. Results demonstrated no mean differences in either the supine or standing values [69]. Although plasma NE increases with age, the slope is not steep [59,118,120]. The circulating level of NE in the resting, supine state appears stable over months to a year or more and is certainly so over days to weeks. Not only are baseline levels consistent, but standing and quantitative isometric hand-grip measurements reveal a consistent elevation in the same person over time. Similarly, E values are consistent over time. These data allow an individual's SNS function to be studied longitudinally.

Because a multitude of other external, internal, physical, and mental factors (Table 1.3) affect plasma NE levels (see Chapters 2 through 4), it is important to follow a standardized procedure developed for obtaining samples for CA measurement [58,69]. For plasma NE levels to reflect SNS activity, NE release, diffusion into the blood, reuptake, and clearance must be in "steady-state." The first step

Table 1.3 Some Factors That Can Influence Human Plasma Norepinephrine Values

Environment of subject (external stimuli)
Tobacco smoking
Caffeine consumption
Medications, including
- Diuretics (hydrochlorothiazide, furosemide)
- Vasodilators (nitroglycerine, diazoxide, hydralazine)
- β antagonists (propranolol)
- Central α agonists (clonidine)
- Depleters of CA (reserpine)
- Antidepressants (MAO-I, tricyclics)
- Marijuana
- CNS stimulants (amphetamine)
- Anorexiants (fenfluramine)
- DA agonists (bromocriptine)
- Neuroleptics (chlorpromazine)

Diet (carbohydrate intake)
Sodium intake (low-salt diet)
Volume depletion
Time of day
Age
Hospitalized versus outpatient status
Familiarity with the clinical environment (blood drawing)
Venipuncture versus indwelling cannula
Anxiety and psychologic stress
Posture
Exercise
Physical conditioning
Various illnesses (depression, mania, thyroid disease, congestive heart failure, pulmonary and renal hypertension, etc.)
Blood sample processing
Assay methodology

CA = catecholamines; MAO-I = monoamine oxidase inhibitors; CNS = central nervous system; DA = dopamine.

to achieve steady-state is to have the subject lie supine and relax. Blood should be taken while the subject is supine at least 20 minutes after venipuncture for the insertion of an indwelling catheter because blood taken immediately after venipuncture contains higher NE levels than blood withdrawn 20 minutes later [58,69]. The NE in such a blood sample reflects basal SNS function, other variables being controlled [58,69,105,118]. Pulse rate parallels the fall in NE ($r = 0.58$; $p < 0.05$) that occurs over the 20 minutes and is a useful objective measure of subject relaxation [69]. NE levels do not change for at least three more hours [69]. Standing erect for 5 minutes causes a doubling in plasma NE levels that remains constant for at least an additional 5 minutes [69] and allows assessment of SNS responsivity to the upright posture [58,69,118]. Stepwise increases in plasma NE levels are produced by stepwise increments toward the upright (see Table 1.2). Plasma NE levels in subjects fully reclining in lounge chairs are higher ($p < 0.01$) than levels of subjects fully supine. Sitting up or a head-up tilt of 60 degrees causes similar and significant increases in NE levels ($p < 0.01$) above supine values. Further activation of the SNS is induced by any of several physically stressful procedures (see Table 1.2). An isometric hand grip for 5 minutes at 30% of maximal ability in standing subjects markedly stimulates SNS activity as reflected by large increments in circulating NE [55,69]. This maneuver is conveniently done immediately after the 5-minute standing sample is taken. Placing a hand in ice water for 4 minutes also activates the SNS but variation between individuals is greater than for the hand-grip exercise, possibly because of individual variations in sensitivity to cold, pain, or both [69]. Training in a physical fitness program can decrease the amount of SNS activation for a set work load [83], but as fitness increases, the maximum NE levels attainable during maximum exertion with isotonic exercise can be doubled. Training does not alter supine resting NE levels.

In studies conducted in this laboratory, plasma E levels also increase significantly when the subject stands up and on isometric hand grip [59,60] (see Table 1.2). However, in 19 studies from the literature, mean supine plasma E levels were higher than those found in this laboratory [40,41,59,60] ($p < 0.05$). Eight of the 19 studies also measured standing levels and found a nonsignificant increase in plasma E when subjects stood (see Table 1.1) [60]. This laboratory's mean standing E value is the same as that from other laboratories so that our increase in E with standing is due to our lower supine levels.

Environmental stimuli should be minimal for most compatible results across subjects; an adjustable hospital bed in a quiet private room with relaxing background music is ideal. On standing, adjust the bed height to below knee level and instruct the subject to stand with his back to the bed so that he can be easily laid supine in case syncope occurs. Plasma NE levels appear to be lower in healthy volunteers and hypertensive subjects living in the hospital than in outpatients matched for age and severity of patient hypertension [58]. Groups in which plasma NE levels are compared should share the same medical environment. Furthermore, a familiar medical environment will, theoretically, cause less anxiety and/or lower NE values than unfamiliar surroundings and techniques such as venipuncture. Laboratory personnel and medical and nursing students may not be an ideal control group as they are often comfortable in a medical setting and their CA levels may be lower than the levels of unfamiliar subjects.

Caffeine-containing foods and beverages and nicotine should be avoided for at least 12 hours before sampling because they increase plasma NE levels [19,89]. Drugs reported to change NE levels, which include some neuroleptics such as chlorpromazine but not haloperidol, should be avoided for at least 2 weeks before blood sampling [15]. CNS stimulants such as amphetamines [90], diuretics [66,68], vasodilators [16,17,77], tricyclic antidepressants [32,62,91,103], monoamine oxidase inhibitors (MAO-I) [75,85], reserpine [16], guanethidine [16], fenfluramine [17,67], bromocriptine [109,121], and clonidine [18] should also be avoided. Diet, especially carbohydrate [20,70] and salt intake [39], may also alter plasma NE levels. Bananas, a rich source of biogenic amines, cause a substantial increase in conjugated DA and NE in human beings [20]. Table 1.3 lists factors which can influence human plasma NE levels.

Whether the time of day influences NE levels is controversial. NE is higher in cerebrospinal fluid (CSF) [125] and plasma [51] when subjects are awake but this may be due to typically increased daytime mental and physical activity and upright posture. There is an ultradian rhythm for plasma NE in rats, monkeys, and human beings with a periodicity of 107 minutes [72]. Age-matched control groups are important in experimental design because plasma NE increases with age ($r = 0.54$; $p < 0.01$) [40,41,58,120].

The relative instability of CA, especially at high pH and warm temperatures, mandates careful collection, processing, and storage of blood samples. Some reports [66] claim that blood CA levels deteriorate at room temperature within a few minutes, while others [84] conclude that they are stable for hours. We find that CA are stable in blood handled with the following precautions: Tubes containing whole blood should be chilled immediately on ice; heparin, acid-citrate-dextrose, disodium-ethylenediaminetetraacetic acid (EDTA), or EGTA can be used in the initial collection tubes to prevent clotting and retard CA breakdown; the red cells should be separated in a refrigerated centrifuge and the plasma transferred to polypropylene or polyethylene storage tubes and frozen within 60 minutes of the time of drawing; antioxidants such as glutathione should be added to the storage tubes to decrease oxidation of the plasma CA; the plasma should be stored at −70° C until assayed for CA. Plasma NE stored at this temperature does not markedly deteriorate for at least a year. If the plasma proteins are precipitated with 0.3 N perchloric acid prior to freezing, the NE is stable at only −20°C.

Apparent Clearance and Release Rates of Norepinephrine

When plasma levels of NE are used to evaluate SNS activity in a particular individual, it is assumed that the clearance rate of NE from plasma is constant and that plasma levels represent the rate of entry of NE into the circulation from sympathetic terminals. Although this is usually a valid assumption, some conditions alter clearance of NE and require evaluation by one of two infusion techniques which can measure more precisely the rates of release and clearance. In one technique, NE is infused at a rate which increases plasma levels but does not change hemodynamic measurements. Blood is sampled to measure plateau levels of NE and NE decay rates to determine the rate of NE clearance [45]. A technically simpler method for evaluating NE clearance rates is to infuse radiolabeled NE and then to measure the disappearance rate of radioactivity by alumina adsorption of the ^{3}H-NE in sequential blood samples [31,32]. However, the results from these two techniques are dissimilar in some respects. Tritiated NE infusions take longer to reach a plateau level than do nonlabeled NE and indicate that NE clearance decreases with age [33], but studies using nonlabeled NE find that age does not affect the rate of NE clearance [45]. Despite the discrepancies in studies, some clinically useful information on the rate of NE clearance has emerged. The tricyclic antidepressant amitriptyline, which blocks NE uptake in vitro, lengthens the half-life of circulating NE in human beings [32]. The half-life of circulating NE is prolonged in patients with deterioration of the peripheral sympathetic nerves [30,31], and its half-life appears shortened in some depressed patients [34].

When plasma NE levels are adjusted for NE's rate of clearance, the NE apparent release rate or spillover into plasma can be calculated. This rate is one step closer to a real measure of SNS activity than measurement of the isolated plasma level of NE. It does not, however, measure the true index of SNS activity (i.e., the intrasynaptic concentration of NE released from nerve terminals), but there are no techniques currently available that do. Because the infusion of ^{3}H-NE is considerably more complex and time-consuming than is the measurement of isolated NE levels, if the rate of NE clearance is normal, the NE levels method may be adequate for SNS evaluation.

CONJUGATED CATECHOLAMINES

CA and other phenolic compounds are metabolized by conjugation with sulfate or glucuronide. In human beings, glucuronidation of CA is a minor phenomenon but there is extensive sulfation of these compounds. The enzyme phenolsulfotransferase conjugates all of the endogenous CA but is most active with DA. The CA sulfates are rapidly excreted in the urine; nonetheless, plasma levels of these conjugated CA are considerably higher than levels of the endogenous free substrate. Of total (free plus conjugated) DA, 98% circulates as the sulfate; of NE, 68%; and of E, 83% [106]. There is wide variability between levels of circulating conjugated CA across subjects, probably explained by an inherited variability in the levels of the enzyme phenolsulfotransferase. Renal function (because the conjugated CA are excreted by the kidney) and the rate of production of the CA themselves also affect the levels of conjugated CA. Kuchel et al [56] suggest that people with very low levels of phenolsulfotransferase can have excessive CA activity because of deficient conjugation and thus inactivation of the CA.

The conjugated CA have biologic activity as evidenced by the convulsive effects of DA sulfate when it is injected into the cerebral ventricles [12]. Sulfate conjugation of CA may be an important route of metabolism, a readily available supply pool of the free CA in humans, or both [92,106]. Circulating DA sulfate may serve as a rapid source for all free CA because dopamine β-hydroxylase (DBH) apparently can hydroxylate circulating DA sulfate, causing the CA to cleave to yield free NE [13,14,106]. Conjugated DA may be elevated in some subgroups of hypertensive patients [57]. Although the role of sulfation and sulfated CA is not clearly defined, these compounds are potentially important metabolites or precursors and are currently being studied.

Three techniques have been used for analysis of the content of conjugated CA in blood and urine: HPLC with electrochemical detection, and acid and enzymatic hydrolysis of the conjugates with assay of the liberated CA.

THE NEUROLOGIC BASIS FOR CHANGES IN PLASMA CATECHOLAMINES

Epinephrine

Human adrenal medullary tissue CA content is 80% E and 20% NE. Catheterized blood samples of adrenal medullary effluent have 64% E and 36% NE concentrations. A 40 pg/ml increment in plasma E concentration can have measurable physiologic consequences on glucose homeostasis and circulatory mechanisms, but a 400 pg/ml increase in plasma NE has little hemodynamic effect, indicating that the adrenal medulla acts primarily through E. The SNS is anatomically and functionally organized to discharge diffusely, usually causing a greater rise in plasma NE than E. However, in some circumstances, the adrenal medulla receives considerably more stimulation than sympathetic nerve terminals, thereby increasing circulatory E proportionally more than NE. For example, during anxiety-producing situations such as public speaking [21] and conditions such as insulin-induced hypoglycemia [81], there is a relatively larger rise in plasma E than in NE. The burst of E elicits tachycardia, systolic hypertension, glucose intolerance, and feelings of anxiety and tremulousness. It is also possible to elicit a selective stimulation of the adrenal medulla in human beings by enhancing central cholinergic tone with the centrally active drug physostigmine [52]. If peripheral responses to physostigmine have first been blocked, there is a very large acetylecholine-mediated rise in plasma E and a small parallel increase in plasma NE, representing the output of these two CA from the adrenal medulla.

Norepinephrine

The peripheral sympathetic nerves originate primarily in autonomic ganglia that are located in two paravertebral chains on either side of and parallel to the spinal cord. The postganglionic nerves leaving these ganglia release NE as their neurotransmitter (Fig. 1.3). Preganglionic nerves originate in the intermediolateral columns

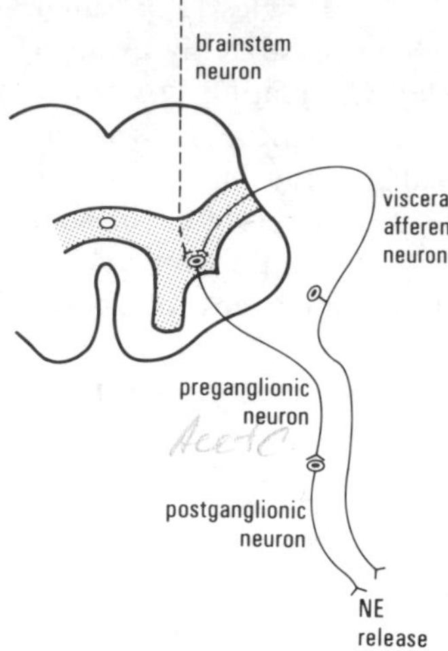

Figure 1.3 Sympathetic nerve pathways in the spinal cord. The preganglionic neuron originates in the intermediolateral horn of the spinal cord and releases acetylcholine on the postganglionic noradrenergic neuron. The preganglionic nerve receives input from visceral afferent nerves and from brainstem neurons. Stimulation of visceral afferent nerves can activate a reflex loop, which stimulates norepinephrine (NE) release. Brainstem nerves modulate this reflex and can inhibit or stimulate NE release.

of the spinal cord from the eighth cervical to the second or third lumbar segment and release acetylcholine onto the noradrenergic nerves. Preganglionic nerves have a variety of inputs from the brain and periphery. Peripheral afferent nerves, which register pain and pressure, enter the spinal cord and innervate preganglionic autonomic neurons as well as send their messages of pain to the brain. This forms an autonomic reflex loop, which stimulates SNS activity. The autonomic reflex activity is modulated by influences from the brain, especially by brainstem neurons which have terminals on the preganglionic autonomic neurons and which modulate the autonomic reflexes (see Figure 1.3).

As seen in Figure 1.4, normal plasma NE levels in this group of control subjects are approximately 300 pg/ml (PNMT assay technique) while recumbent. They roughly double on standing as brainstem neurons convey signals from the baroreceptors to autonomic nerves to help maintain a normal blood pressure. When blood volume is low, the decreased blood pressure is sensed by the baroreceptors and plasma NE levels respond in an exaggerated fashion to standing. Nerve lesions that alter SNS activity produce predictable changes in plasma NE levels, which can be helpful in diagnosing the source of the neurologic defect [58,118,119]. Many of the specific diseases that affect circulating NE levels are discussed in subsequent chapters, but we discuss here the general mechanisms by which nerve damage alters NE levels.

Lesions of Postganglionic Nerves

The postganglionic sympathetic nerves deteriorate in any disease that causes a generalized neuropathy, such as diabetes mellitus, alcoholism, and uremia. Occasionally, postganglionic autonomic nerves are selectively destroyed by an unknown mechanism. When there is a peripheral autonomic neuropathy, patients lose control

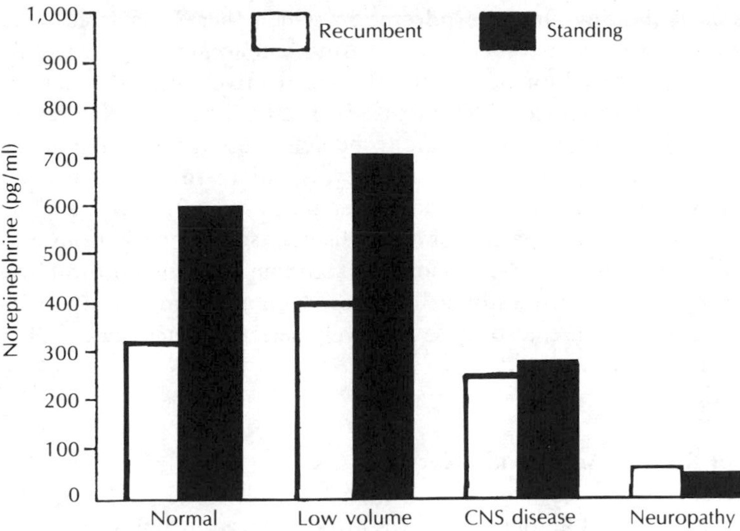

Figure 1.4 Plasma norepinephrine (NE) levels in four groups of subjects recumbent and standing. Normal subjects have NE levels of approximately 300 pg/ml, which double after standing 5 minutes (PNMT method). Normal subjects who received furosemide and a low sodium diet have increased NE levels while recumbent and standing. Patients with the Shy-Drager syndrome, a central nervous system (CNS) disease that destroys central control of autonomic nerves, have normal NE levels while recumbent, but NE fails to increase when they stand. Patients wih neuropathy of the peripheral sympathetic nerves have low NE levels that do not increase with standing.

of bowel, bladder, and sexual function and develop postural hypotension. These patients have low circulating levels of NE while at rest because they lack the peripheral sympathetic nerves to make or release NE (see Figure 1.4). When they stand, there is no change in their NE levels and they develop postural hypotension. Low, unchanging levels of NE are characteristic of peripheral neuropathy and do not occur in response to CNS diseases [118]. Partial autonomic neuropathies are frequently present in diabetics who have had the disease for 10 to 15 years. These patients have a depressed level of plasma NE while recumbent and a diminished to absent response to standing. However, these NE levels are not as low as those seen in total peripheral autonomic neuropathy.

Defects of Spinal Preganglionic Autonomic Nerves

Any generalized pathologic process of the spinal cord can cause some deterioration of autonomic preganglionic nerves (see Chapter 6). This disease process is most clearly seen in the Shy-Drager syndrome in which there is isolated deterioration of the spinal intermediolateral cells innervating autonomic ganglia. In this disease, peripheral nerves, which manufacture NE, are relatively intact, so supine plasma levels of NE are normal (see CNS disease in Figure 1.4) [118]. However, because these postganglionic nerves are unable to be activated owing to lesions of preganglionic autonomic neurons, plasma NE levels fail to increase on standing and postural hypotension develops. Partial degeneration of spinal preganglionic autonomic neurons occurs in a variety of other diseases such as parkinsonism, in which there is a slightly diminished NE response to standing and mild postural hypotension (see Chapter 5). Some of the storage diseases, such as mannosidosis, Hurler's syndrome, or Fabry's disease, also cause relatively selective deterioration of the spinal preganglionic neurons.

Defects of Rostral Autonomic Nerves

The involuntary spinal autonomic nerves are organized in reflex arcs in a manner analogous to the voluntary motor fibers. Following spinal cord transection, voluntary motor fibers are first flaccid and then become spastic with an exaggerated response to afferent stimuli. This response also happens to the involuntary (autonomic) fibers, which remain in a state of spinal shock from 1 to 6 weeks after spinal cord transection and then develop spastic autonomic reflexes. Without stimulation, these simple autonomic reflexes are quiescent but they can react in an inappropriately unrestrained fashion in response to various afferent stimuli, a phenomenon termed autonomic dysreflexia that is present in 80% of patients with high spinal cord transection. After spinal cord transection, sympathetic nerve activity is not integrated with baroreceptor function. As a result, resting NE levels can be normal or slightly low but are often very erratic, even when the patient is not undergoing an episode of autonomic dysreflexia. E levels are usually more than twice normal. Stimulation from pain or distention of the urinary bladder causes a reflex increase in NE levels in patients with high spinal cord transection. Plasma CA levels may spike to very high levels, usually in association with muscle spasm, urination, pain, or bladder distention. Episodes of exaggerated SNS activity cause hypertension and cardiac arrhythmias. During these episodes, plasma NE levels are extremely high (greater than 1000 pg/ml) as vasoconstriction below the level of the spinal cord lesion elevates blood pressure to dangerous levels.

The sympathetic nerves that release NE are part of the nervous system with preganglionic nerves originating in the intermediolateral column of the spinal cord and terminating on postganglionic nerves that secrete NE (see Figure 1.3). Preganglionic nerves are innervated by both peripheral afferent and rostral neurons and comprise a simple reflex arc. Although lesions of any of these groups of nerves may cause similar clinical manifestations, each type can produce characteristic patterns of plasma NE levels, which can be useful both diagnostically and also in helping us understand such pathologic processes as autonomic dysreflexia (Table 1.4; see Figure 1.4 and Chapter 6).

Table 1.4 Disease States and Norepinephrine Levels*

Disease (reference)	*CSF NE (pg/ml)* Control	*CSF NE (pg/ml)* Disease	*Plasma NE (pg/ml)* Control	*Plasma NE (pg/ml)* Disease
Parkinsonism				
Williams, 1978 [108]	374 ± 36	215 ± 34†	351 ± 63	233 ± 50†
Teychenne et al 1980 [99]	209 ± 25	137 ± 25†	371 ± 42	189 ± 22†
Parkinsonism plus L-dopa				
Teychenne et al 1977 [100]	209 ± 25		371 ± 42	320 ± 58
Alcohol withdrawal				
Hawley et al 1981 [46]	138 ± 16	192 ± 22	—	—
Alcoholic seizures				
Teychenne et al 1977 [100]	439 ± 40	545 ± 87	—	—
Idiopathic epilepsy				
Teychenne et al 1977 [100]	439 ± 40	555 ± 18	—	—
Hiramatsu et al 1982 [48]	111 ± 13	333 ± 85	—	—
Huntington's chorea				
Ziegler et al 1980 [115]	239 ± 17	171 ± 18†	—	—
Amyotrophic lateral sclerosis				
Ziegler et al 1980 [124]	251 ± 14	365 ± 44†	309 ± 19	455 ± 59†
Hypertension				
Eide et al 1979 [25]	167 ± 71	298 ± 60†	—	—
Lake et al 1981 [61]	310 ± 20	390 ± 15†	220 ± 30	190 ± 40
Goldstein 1981 [40]	—	—	231 ± 4	285 ± 4†
Cerebral vasospasm				
Shigeno 1982 [93]	75 ± 1	246 ± 49†	—	—
Mania				
Post et al 1978 [86]	229 ± 32	477 ± 60†	—	—
Lake et al 1982 [63]	—	—	274 ± 29	581 ± 124†
Depression				
Post et al 1978 [86]	229 ± 32	187 ± 18	—	—
Lake et al 1982 [63]		—	274 ± 29	447 ± 81†
Schizophrenia				
Lake et al 1980 [64]	91 ± 6	125 ± 11†	201 ± 24	208 ± 18

CSF = cerebrospinal fluid, NE = norepinephrine.
* Values are expressed as mean ± standard error of the mean (SEM).
† $p < 0.05$.

MEASUREMENTS OF CATECHOLAMINES AND THEIR METABOLITES IN CEREBROSPINAL FLUID

CA function as neurotransmitters in specific nerve tracts in the brain and are intimately associated with the regulation of many critical body functions. Disruption of normal function in one or more of these CA tracts is known or hypothesized to be associated with several neurologic and psychiatric symptoms and disorders including Parkinson's disease, syncope, hypotension, hypertension, schizophrenia, mania, and depression. Because these are among the most prevalent disorders in our society and the causes of some of them remain unknown, indices of central CA activity have been avidly sought. In human beings, direct examination of proposed metabolic abnormalities is important, not only to confirm or reject any primary or secondary role of CA dysregulation in the disorder, but to provide a means of differentiating subgroups of patients with similar clinical syndromes. This is particularly important in psychiatry and neurology because there are few complete animal models of the major diseases being studied, and because species differences are extremely important in the study of brain function [24].

The anatomic and physiologic isolation of the CNS from the rest of the body serves a protective function but makes diagnostic evaluation difficult. Brain tissue is rarely obtainable from living human subjects and study of autopsy material is difficult. Studies which measure levels of CA metabolites in urine have not proved as satisfactory as initially hoped. Urinary levels of 3-methoxy-4-hydroxyphenylglycol (MHPG), the principal metabolite of NE in the human brain, were thought to reflect CNS NE metabolism, but as little as 20% of urinary MHPG is actually derived from the CNS in humans [8]. Thus urinary MHPG is not a valid index of brain NE neurotransmission.

The CSF bathes the brain and spinal cord, and its contents tend to reflect the activities of the adjacent nervous system tissue [64,66,101,110,116,123–126]. DA neuronal systems are relatively discretely localized in basal ganglia and in the mesolimbic and tuberoinfundibular systems [102]. The nigrostriatal system contains the greatest concentration with the majority of DA nerve endings in the caudate nucleus, which forms the lateral wall of the lateral ventricle [24]. Assessment of CNS DA activity involves the measurement of CSF levels of homovanillic acid (HVA), the acidic metabolite of DA, because the assay procedures for CSF DA itself have not been adequately developed or applied. HVA in CSF appears to be an index of CNS DA release because systemically administered DA or HVA does not increase CSF HVA levels whereas stimulation of CNS DA neurons causes substantial increases in CSF HVA [111,112]. The spinal cord does not appear to contribute DA to the spinal CSF as it does NE because the rostrocaudal CSF HVA concentration gradient is sharp, with the highest levels found in lateral ventricular CSF. Also, CSF HVA levels are low or absent below the site of spinal canal blockage [111,112]. The HVA is removed by an active acid transport system from CSF to the systemic circulation. Probenecid inhibits this system and causes the accumulation of HVA but not the neutral metabolite of NE, MHPG [23]. The probenecid technique involves giving probenecid, 100 mg/kg of body weight, orally over 24 hours following an initial lumbar puncture (LP). With the HVA levels measured from a second LP, DA turnover can be estimated [23,24]. This procedure has some drawbacks: probenecid in these doses can cause nausea and vomiting and a marked increase in CSF NE levels [65] and two LPs in 24 hours constitute at least a moderate stress. Stable isotope studies hold some promise for future CNS DA neurotransmitter investigations [24].

Specific areas in the human CNS that are heavily innervated with noradrenergic neurons include the locus coeruleus (LC), the midbrain nuclei, which provide the principal NE nerve tract projections to the cerebral cortex, the limbic system, and the intermediolateral columns of the spinal cord [95]. The LC contains approximately half the brain's noradrenergic neurons [98] and generates approximately 70% of the NE content in the primate brain [50]. The LC and its initial projections are in close anatomic proximity to the cerebral ventricles. These noradrenergic areas are thought to modulate arousal, emotion and mood and to affect thought processes, behavior [87,101], and blood pressure [61,122].

The major metabolites of NE are VMA and MHPG. MHPG is the major metabolite of NE in the brain of several species including the rat, the human, and the rhesus macaque. MHPG and VMA are detectable in nanogram amounts in all ventricles, cistern, and subarachnoid spaces. The concentrations of MHPG and VMA in the lateral ventricle and lumbar space are in the range of 10 to 15 ng/ml and 1 to 2 ng/ml respectively. MHPG and VMA concentrations increase by as much as 50 to 100% in the third and fourth ventricles, a considerably greater rise than occurs in the lateral ventricles [44]. This increase may reflect the higher concentration of NE found in hypothalamic and brainstem structures. In contrast to the acidic metabolites of DA, the concentration gradient of MHPG decreases less sharply from the ventricles to the lumbar space [126]. The rostral increase in MHPG is only on the order of 12% for the first 17 ml of CSF removed from an LP needle, so unpaired samples would not show this difference between CSF from the lower and upper lumbar levels because of variance between subjects (Figure 1.5) [126]. CSF NE and MHPG correlated positively ($r = 0.76$; $p < 0.05$) in a 5-ml aliquot of CSF from the 33rd to the 38th ml out of the LP needle [126].

Measurement of NE itself in CSF may be the most direct means currently available for assessing central noradrenergic activity in human beings. Intravenous infusions of radiolabeled NE in monkeys cause peak CSF levels of the label amounting to only 2% of peak plasma concentrations, indicating that CSF levels of NE are not contaminated by plasma NE to any significant extent. Although there is a positive correlation between NE levels in CSF and plasma ($r = 0.78$; $p < 0.001$), acute increases in peripheral NE levels from a pheochromocytoma are not reflected in CSF levels, which leads to the conclusion that the vast majority of NE in CSF is of central origin [123].

NE was measured in human CSF in the 1960s with only moderate success because levels were generally at the lower limits of detection of the fluorometric methods then in use [120]. More recently, a radioenzymatic assay using PNMT was compared with GCMS on split samples of CSF, and the two methods were found to correlate with a coefficient of 0.95 [120]. The PNMT radioenzymatic technique was found to be reliable and sufficiently sensitive: in only two of 155 CSF samples was the content of NE less than that needed to yield five times as many counts per minute as the blank (double the counts per minute of blank is usually considered sufficient). With this method, which is considerably easier than GCMS, NE in CSF samples can be conveniently measured to a sensitivity (counts

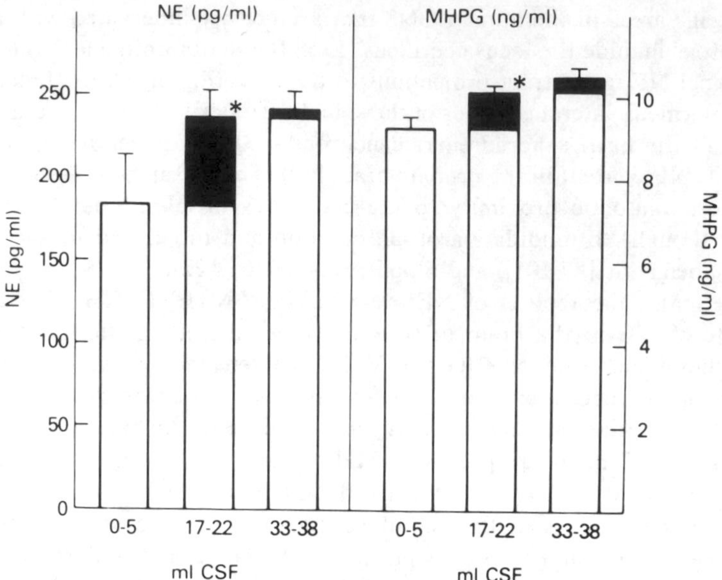

Figure 1.5 Levels of norepinephrine (NE) and its principal brain metabolite 3-methoxy-4-hydroxyphenylglycol (MHPG) in human cerebrospinal fluid (CSF). CSF was removed by lumbar puncture (LP) in recumbent subjects and NE and MHPG were measured in the first 5 ml removed and in two subsequent 5-ml aliquots. Both NE and MHPG content in CSF significantly increased between ml 0–5 and ml 17–22, but did not significantly increase further with subsequent removal of CSF up to ml 33–38. * = significant increases ($p < .002$) by paired t test.

per minute at least double that of blank) of approximately 30 pg/ml of CSF [120].

There is also a decreasing rostrocaudal gradient for NE in a series of 5-ml aliquots of CSF removed from the LP needle (see Figure 1.5) [120]. There is a 25 to 30% increase in NE from the first 5-ml aliquot (ml 0–5) to the 5 ml from ml 17 to 22 out of the LP needle. There is no further significant increase in CSF NE content once 17 ml of CSF has been removed even up to an aliquot of CSF at ml 33 to 38 (see Figure 1.5) [126]. NE present in the initial 5-ml aliquot out of the LP needle probably comes from the spinal cord [127]. An average human being has 140 ml of CSF of which approximately 110 ml is in the skull and 30 ml is in the spinal subarachnoid space [107]. Because no further significant increase in NE occurs in CSF withdrawn from 17 to 38 ml, there is apparently no CSF gradient for NE between high spinal cord and cerebral ventricles.

Before clinical applications can be attempted, normal values must be established and those variables that affect CSF NE levels identified. Establishing normal values from healthy control subjects is difficult because few normal volunteers want to undergo LP. With considerable advertising by the National Institutes of

Health, at least four control groups were generated with a combined total of 66 subjects for studies in collaboration with this laboratory. Each group served as controls for a different study involving patients with a particular neurologic or psychiatric disease. Often, interested spouses or unaffected relatives wished to volunteer as providers of control samples of CSF to help in the interpretation of those data derived from the analyses of the CSF CA from the patients. Another potential source of control CSF samples is from neurologic patients who undergo diagnostic LP but are found to have no identifiable organic lesion. Patients with tension headache or cranial arteriovenous malformations have been accepted as "neurologic" control subjects [115,123]. Various diseases are certainly related to abnormal CSF CA levels and must be screened for when evaluating a subject for use as a control [40,46,58,61,64,115,118,119]. Some of these are shown in Table 1.4 and discussed later in this and subsequent chapters.

Many of the same variables that should be consistent for analyzing plasma CA levels should also be controlled when comparing CSF CA levels between individuals or groups. To minimize the stress of the LP procedure, the patient should be in a quiet environment, preferably in his or her own private room. Drugs, such as those previously noted, should have been discontinued for time periods appropriate to their half-lives and lipid solubilities. Tobacco- and caffeine-containing foods and beverages should be discontinued for only 12 hours before the LP because, in heavy users, some withdrawal anxiety may complicate results if subjects abstain for longer periods of time. Monoamine content of the diet has not been shown to alter CSF NE levels in human beings; we found no differences in CSF content of NE between low and high monoamine diets [120]. A low-salt diet increases CSF NE in dogs [9].

The LP should be performed at the same time of day because there is a circadian rhythm in CSF content of NE in human beings and in the rhesus monkey (Figure 1.6) [82,120]. Generally, between 8 AM (0800) and 9 AM (0900) has been the most convenient time for LPs because patients are usually kept at strict bed rest and have no oral intake (NPO) from midnight until the LP is completed. From Figure 1.6, it is evident that comparing CSF NE data taken at 8 AM and at 3 PM (1500) is illogical. In this laboratory and in the literature, most control data have been generated from LPs done between 8 AM and 9 AM. Similar to plasma NE levels, CSF NE does appear to increase slightly but significantly with age but does not differ between the sexes [124].

The physical aspects of performing an LP have been thoroughly reviewed [38,80,111,113]. The skill with which the LP needle is inserted is a critical factor because pain is assumed to alter CA neurotransmission in the brain although this has not been formally tested. The degree of a patient's familiarity with the LP procedure or clinical procedures in general is worth determining. More relevant is the assessment of each subject's distress and anxiety during the LP. This information can aid in data interpretation in a situation of a traumatic tap and aberrant CSF CA levels.

Posture may not affect CSF NE as much as plasma NE levels but this has not been studied thoroughly. Two postures are commonly used for LP: the lateral

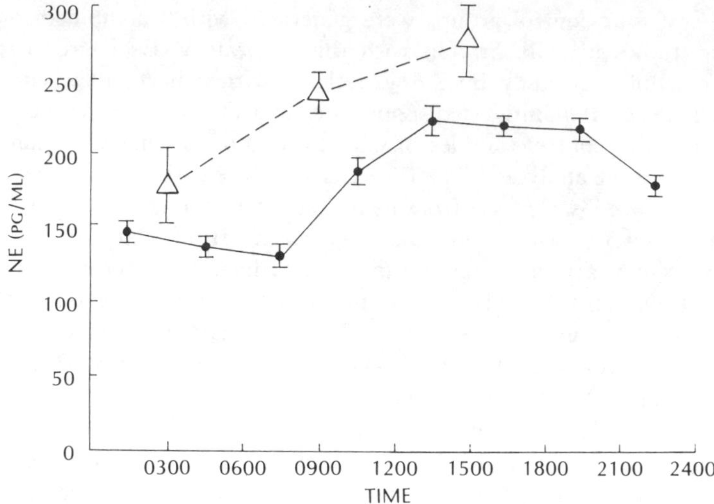

Figure 1.6 Norepinephrine (NE) levels in cerebrospinal fluid (CSF) of human beings (△) and monkeys (●) during the 24-hour day. CSF NE levels are lowest at night and peak in the early afternoon.

knee-chest (left lateral decubitus) and the sitting position. Preliminary data indicate no differences between positions when other variables are controlled (Table 1.5: compare groups 2 and 5B with 4). Both posture and activity are conveniently controlled by performing LPs at 8 AM with strict bed rest and NPO from midnight. When suitable control subjects are selected and environmental variables standardized, several additional potential sample processing variables must also be considered.

Once the CSF samples for CA assay are obtained from the LP, variable subsequent handling can cause significant artifact. The five different control groups shown in Table 1.5 allow some examination of various ways of processing the CSF samples from the time the CSF is collected until it is frozen, stored, and subsequently assayed for CA. Groups 2, 4, and 5B already had ascorbic acid in the tubes in which the CSF was initially collected from the LP needle (a.a. immediate) and had these CSF samples frozen on dry ice within 30 seconds (DI immediate) and stored at −70° C until assayed. The CSF NE content in these three groups are the highest and are not significantly different from one another despite the fact that the LP studies were conducted by different physicians in different control groups. In groups 1, 3, and 5A the samples were put only in wet (regular) ice immediately and were not frozen until some 30 minutes later. The mean NE content of groups 1, 3, and 5A is 187 pg/ml, significantly lower than that of groups 2, 4, and 5B (373 pg/ml) ($t = 2.8$; $p < 0.01$). Group 3 had the greatest variation in time taken to add ascorbic acid and to freeze the samples and had the lowest mean NE level (see Table 1.5). From these preliminary data, we conclude that the antioxidant should already be in the tubes for CSF collection before the LP

Table 1.5 Summary of Variables Affecting Cerebrospinal Fluid Norepinephrine Levels in Normal Control Groups

Group	*1*	*2*	*3*	*4*	*5A**	*5B*
N	21	18	29	10	9	
Age in years (range)	41 ± 4 (20–73)	34 ± 3 (19–58)	29 ± 2 (16–64)	45 ± 3 (31–56)	42 ± 5 (20–64)	
Description	Neurologic controls†	NHV	NHV	NHV	NHV	
Posture	LLD	LLD	LLD	Sitting	LLD	
Preservative‡	a.a. immediate	a.a. immediate	a.a. by 90 min	a.a. immediate	a.a by 30 min	a.a. immediate
Aliquot of CSF (ml)	12–16	12–16	12–16	12–16	12–20 pool	
Freezing	WI immediate; DI by 30 min	DI immediate	WI immediate; frozen at −70° C by 30–60 min	DI immediate	WI immediate; frozen at −70° C by 30 min	DI immediate
NE (pg/ml)	229 ± 20	373 ± 38	91 ± 6	337 ± 34	242 ± 72	408 ± 61

N = number of subjects; NHV = normal, healthy volunteer (no significant medical or psychiatric disorder); LLD = left lateral decubitus; CSF = cerebrospinal fluid; a.a. = ascorbic acid, 10 mg; WI = wet ice; DI = dry ice; NE = norepinephrine.

* The groups designated as 5A and 5B consist of the same 9 subjects from whom the 8-ml aliquot from ml 12 to 20 was mixed, split into two 4-ml aliquots, and handled as shown above.

† The neurologic controls were patients at the neurologic clinic with complaints such as headache for which no organic cause could be determined or patients with disorders such as cerebral arteriovenous malformations.

‡ To impede oxidation of norepinephrine.

and dry ice should be on hand to freeze the CSF samples on collection from the LP needle.

As with plasma values, assay methodology should be consistent in comparing CSF NE levels. Up to now, the majority of CSF NE values have been determined with the PNMT technique [117]. Ascorbic acid inhibits COMT and in CSF samples from Rhesus monkeys, tubes containing ascorbic acid gave NE values less than half of that from tubes without (Lake CR and Kraemer G, unpublished data, 1984). Because there are so many variables that can alter CSF NE values, a concurrent control group is very important.

CEREBROSPINAL FLUID CATECHOLAMINES IN SOME NEUROPSYCHIATRIC DISEASES

Although there are larger amounts of CSF DA than of CSF E (of which there is very little), the COMT-based radioenzymatic assay is less sensitive for DA than NE or E because of higher DA blanks. DA levels in CSF, unless increased by a drug such as L-dopa, are barely detectable by the COMT assay. However, a recently developed assay using HPLC with fluorometric detection is more sensitive than the COMT assay and can measure DA levels that are lower than normal [48]. It will be difficult to determine the importance of CSF DA in disease states until its basic neurochemistry has been examined (i.e., its circadian rhythm, gradient, response to various drugs such as amphetamine, relationship to age, blood pressure, and diet). Because NE has been examined in CSF in a variety of neurologic disorders (see Table 1.4 and Figure 1.4) we better understand both the diseases and the CNS metabolism of NE.

Destruction of central DA neurons is the major pathology of parkinsonism, but there are alterations in brain NE neurons as well. Parkinsonian patients usually have slightly low blood pressure and mild postural hypotension when they stand. CSF NE is lower in parkinsonian patients than in control subjects and levels of NE in CSF are increased above control values after treatment with L-dopa [99, 100,108]. The concentration of CSF NE in untreated parkinsonism correlates with the severity of parkinsonian tremor. L-dopa tends to increase CSF NE but does not relieve tremor as much as other drugs, such as bromocriptine, which diminish CSF NE [121].

Huntington's chorea is characterized by chorea, myoclonus, and dystonia, which result from progressive brain atrophy. The concentration of many substances associated with neurotransmission are decreased in Huntington's chorea, including γ-aminobutyric acid (GABA), glutamic acid decarboxylase, choline acetyltransferase, angiotensin-converting enzyme, and substance P [29]. The cerebral atrophy of Huntington's chorea also penetrates to NE-innervated areas causing low CSF NE levels (see Table 1.4). Plasma NE is diminished as well, along with its synthetic enzyme, DBH [94].

Amyotrophic lateral sclerosis (ALS) is a progressive, paralyzing disease characterized by degeneration of pyramidal tract fibers and anterior horn cells in the spinal cord. Patients with ALS have abnormally low levels of HVA, a metabolite of DA. Surprisingly, these patients have markedly increased levels of CSF NE. Their increased plasma NE, which probably reflects increased SNS tone, causes a rigid, monophasic pattern of blood flow through their arteries and a high incidence of nonatherosclerotic angiopathy along with an elevated blood pressure [115].

Seizures may result from various metabolic or anatomic abnormalities. It is therefore difficult to draw broad conclusions about a clinical phenomenon that is caused by so many disorders and so poorly understood. Some studies find CSF NE is slightly but not significantly elevated in seizure disorders [100,111]. One report shows low CSF DA and high CSF NE in epileptic patients [48]. Alcohol withdrawal seizures are a common and more clinically definable phenomenon. Patients with alcohol withdrawal seizures also have slightly but not significantly higher CSF NE levels than control subjects [100]. Patients in alcohol withdrawal who are not having seizures have higher CSF NE than comparable subjects [46,111]. Because NE itself does not cause seizures and has some stabilizing effect in the brain, the CSF NE elevation is probably a secondary phenomenon.

Following bleeding into the cerebral ventricles, the irritant effect of blood is often associated with cerebral vasospasm. CSF NE was measured because spasm of the arteries may also be caused by exposure to NE. Results indicate that cisternal CSF NE is considerably higher in patients undergoing vasospasm than in subjects who are not [93]. The concentration of NE in the CSF does not reach high enough levels to constrict cerebral arteries, but may reflect enhanced release of NE in the arteries [93].

Both central and peripheral NE are involved in the control of blood pressure. As noted previously, parkinsonian patients have low CSF NE levels and low blood pressure, and patients with ALS have high CSF NE levels and high blood pressure. NE is increased in CSF of patients with essential hypertension [25,61]. Further analysis of this phenomenon in a large number of patients undergoing LP for various neurologic disorders found that CSF NE correlates positively with blood pressure over a wide range of pressures and that this correlation is strongest in patients less than 40 years of age [122]. The evidence points toward a central noradrenergic abnormality in essential hypertension. When NE levels are elevated in the peripheral circulation from a pheochromocytoma, blood pressure is increased but CSF NE remains low [117].

CNS CA neurotransmitter functions are postulated to be dysregulated in some of the psychotic disorders such as schizophrenia [64] and major affective disorders [43,86]. Elevated levels of NE and DA are implicated in both of these conditions (see Chapters 11, 13 through 15). NE is elevated in CSF of schizophrenic patients [42,64], especially in the paranoid subgroup [64], and in several post-mortem studies NE in specific brain nuclei is also high in contrast to control brains [37,54] (see Chapter 14). CSF NE is significantly elevated in manic patients, but depressed patients appear to have normal NE levels in one study [86] (see Chapter 11).

Additional details of these and other disorders and the relationships and applicability of CA measurements are discussed in later chapters.

The authors wish to thank Drs. Mike Ebert, Ron Polinski, Jim Wood, Bob Post, Jim Ballanger, Fred Goodwin, Dave Sternberg, and Dan van Kammen for providing CSF and Dr. Sheryle Alagna, Kathy Moriarty, Rhona Bosin, Laurie Taylor-Donald, Audrey Reid, Sakunah Sadrud-Din, and Rosemarie Quirk for their assistance.

REFERENCES

1. Abel JJ, Crawford AC. On the blood-pressure-raising constituent of the suprarenal capsules. Bull Johns Hopkins Hosp 8:151–157, 1897.
2. Anton AH, Sayre DF. A study of the factors affecting the aluminum oxide-trihydroxy-indole procedure for the analysis of catecholamines. J Pharmacol Exp Ther 138:360–375, 1962.
3. Axelrod J, Tomchick R. Enzymatic O-methylation of epinephrine and other catechols. J Biol Chem 223:702–705, 1958.
4. Barger G, Ewins AJ. Some phenolic derivatives of beta-phenylethylamine. J Chem Soc 97:2253–2261, 1910.
5. Bernard C. Experimental research on the vascular and heat producing nerves of the great sympathetic. C R Acad Sci 40:1–32, 1862.
6. Blaschko H. The specific action of L-dopa decarboxylase. J Physiol (Lond.) 96:50P–51P, 1939.
7. Blessing WW, Sved AF, Reis DJ. Destruction of noradrenergic neurons in rabbit brainstem elevates plasma vasopressin causing hypertension. Science 217:661–663, 1982.
8. Blombery PA, Kopin IJ, Gordon EK, Markey SP, Ebert MH. Conversion of MHPG to vanillylmandelic acid. Arch Gen Psychiatry 37:1095–1098, 1973.
9. Brosnihan KB, Szilagyi JE, Ferrario CM. Effect of chronic sodium depletion on cerebrospinal fluid and plasma catecholamines. Hypertension 3:233–239, 1981.
10. Brown-Séquard CE. On the results of the section and the galvanization (electrical stimulation) of the great sympathetic nerve at the neck. Gaz Med (Paris) pp. 1–9, 1854.
11. Burke D, Sundlof G, Wallin BG. Postural effects on muscle nerve sympathetic activity in man. J Physiol (Lond) 272:399–414, 1977.
12. Buu NT, Duhaime J, Kuchel O, Genest J. The convulsive effects of dopamine sulfate conjugates in rat brain. Life Sci 29:2311–2316, 1981.
13. Buu NT, Kuchel O. The direct conversion of dopamine 3-O-sulfate to norepinephrine by dopamine beta-hydroxylase. Life Sci 24:783–789, 1979.
14. Buu NT, Nair G, Kuchel O, Genest J. The extra-adrenal synthesis of epinephrine in rats. Possible involvement of dopamine sulfate. J Lab Clin Med 98:527–535, 1981.
15. Castellani S, Ziegler MG, van Kammen DP, Alexander PE, Siris SG, Lake CR. Plasma norepinephrine and dopamine-beta-hydroxylase activity in schizophrenia. Arch Gen Psychiatry 39:1145–1149, 1982.
16. Chernow B, Lake CR, Coleman MD, Ziegler MG. Effect of antihypertensive therapy on sympathetic nervous system activity in patients with essential hypertension. Fed Proc 43:72–77, 1984.
17. Chernow B, Lake CR, Cook D, Coyle J, Hughes P, Coleman M, Ziegler MG. Fenfluramine lowers plasma norepinephrine in overweight subjects. Int J Clin Pharmacol Res 3:233–237, 1983.

18. Chernow B, Lake CR, Ziegler MG, Zaloga GP, Coleman MD. The effect of clonidine on sympathetic nervous system activity in essential hypertension. Int J Clin Pharmacol Res 3:9–15, 1983.
19. Cryer PE, Haymond MW, Santiago JV, Shah DD. Norepinephrine and epinephrine release and adrenergic mediation of smoking-associated hemodynamic and metabolic events. N Engl J Med 295:573–577, 1976.
20. Davidson L, Vandongen R, Beilin LJ. Effect of eating bananas on plasma free and sulfate-conjugated catecholamines. Life Sci 29:1773–1778, 1981.
21. Dimsdale JE, Moss J. Plasma catecholamines in stress and exercise. JAMA 243:340–342, 1980.
22. Durrett LR, Ziegler MG. A sensitive radioenzymatic assay for catechol drugs. J Neurosci Res 5:587–598, 1980.
23. Ebert MH, Kartzinel R, Cowdry RW, Goodwin FK. Cerebrospinal Fluid Amine Metabolites and the Probenecid Test. In Neurobiology of Cerebrospinal Fluid, JH Wood (ed), 97–112. New York: Plenum Press, 1980.
24. Ebert MH, Perlow MJ. Utility of Cerebrospinal Fluid Measurements in Studies of Brain Monoamines. In Structure and Function of Monoamine Enzymes: Proceedings of a Conference Held in Steamboat Springs, CO, E Usdin, N Weiner and MBH Youdim (eds), 963–984. New York: Marcel Dekker, 1977.
25. Eide I, Kollach R, DeQuattro V, Miano L, Dugger R, Van der Meuler J. Raised cerebrospinal fluid norepinephrine in some patients with primary hypertension. Hypertension 1:255–259, 1979.
26. Elliot TR. The action of adrenaline. J Physiol (Lond) 32:401–467, 1905.
27. Engelman K, Portnoy B. Sensitive double-isotope derivative assay for norepinephrine and epinephrine. Circ Res 26:53–57, 1970.
28. Engelman K, Portnoy B, Sjoerdsma A. Plasma catecholamine concentrations in patients with hypertension. Circ Res 27 (Suppl 1):I141–I146, 1970.
29. Enna SJ, Ziegler MG, Lake CR, Wood JH, Brooks BR, Butler IJ. Cerebrospinal Fluid Gamma-Aminobutyric Acid: Correlation with Cerebrospinal Fluid and Blood Constituents and Alterations in Neurological Disorders. In Neurobiology of Cerebrospinal Fluid, JH Wood (ed), 189–196. New York: Plenum Press, 1980.
30. Esler M, Jackman G, Bobik A, Leonard P, Kelleher D, Skews H, Jennings G, Korner P. Norepinephrine kinetics in essential hypertension: Defective neuronal uptake of norepinephrine in some patients. Hypertension 3:149–156, 1981.
31. Esler M, Jackman G, Leonard P, Bobik A, Skews H, Jennings G, Kelleher D, Korner P. Determination of noradrenaline uptake, spillover to plasma and plasma concentration in patients with essential hypertension. Clin Sci 59:311s–313s, 1980.
32. Esler M, Jackman G, Leonard P, Skews H, Bobik A, Korner P. Effect of norepinephrine uptake blockers on norepinephrine kinetics. Clin Pharmacol Ther 29:12–20, 1981.
33. Esler M, Skews H, Leonard P, Jackman G, Bobik A, Korner P. Age-dependence of noradrenaline kinetics in normal subjects. Clin Sci 60:217–219, 1981.
34. Esler M, Turbott J, Schwartz R, Leonard P, Bobik A, Skews H, Jackman G. The peripheral kinetics of norepinephrine in depressive illness. Arch Gen Psychiatry 39:295–300, 1982.
35. Euler US von. A specific sympathomimetic ergone in adrenergic nerve fibres (sympathin) and its relations to adrenaline and nor-adrenaline. Acta Physiol Scand 12:73–97, 1946.
36. Euler US von. Identification of the sympathomimetic ergone in adrenergic nerves

of cattle (Sympathin N) with laevo-noradrenaline. Acta Physiol Scand 16:63–74, 1948.

37. Farley IJ, Price KS, McCullough E, Deck JHN, Hordynski W, Hornykiewicz O. Norepinephrine in chronic paranoid schizophrenia: above-normal levels in limbic forebrain. Science 200:456–458, 1978.
38. Fishman RA. Cerebrospinal Fluid. In Clinical Neurology, AB Baker and LH Baker (eds), 1–40. Hagerstown, Md: Harper & Row, 1977.
39. Fujita T, Henry WL, Bartter FC, Lake CR, DeLea CS. Factors influencing blood pressure in salt sensitive patients with hypertension. Am J Med 69:334–344, 1980.
40. Goldstein DS. Plasma norepinephrine in essential hypertension: a study of the studies. Hypertension 3:48–52, 1981.
41. Goldstein DS, Lake CR. Plasma norepinephrine and epinephrine levels in essential hypertension. Fed Proc 43:57–61, 1984.
42. Gomes UCR, Shanley BC, Potgeiter L, Roux JT. Noradrenergic overactivity in chronic schizophrenia: Evidence based on cerebrospinal fluid noradrenaline and cyclic nucleotide concentrations. Br J Psychiatry 137:346–351, 1980.
43. Goodwin FK, Post RM, Dunner DL, Gordon EK. Cerebrospinal fluid amine metabolites in affective illness. Am J Psychiatry 130:73–79, 1973.
44. Gordon E, Perlow M, Olivier J, Ebert M, Kopin I. Origins of catecholamine metabolites in monkey cerebrospinal fluid. J Neurochem 25:347–349, 1975.
45. Grimm M, Weidmann P, Keusch G, Meier A, Gluck Z. Norepinephrine clearance and pressor effect in normal and hypertensive man. Klin Wochenschr 58:1175–1181, 1980.
46. Hawley RJ, Major LF, Schulman EA, Lake CR. CSF levels of norepinephrine during alcohol withdrawal. Arch Neurol 38:289–292, 1981.
47. Henry DP, Luft FC, Weinberger MH, Fineberg NS, Grim CE. Norepinephrine in urine and plasma following provocative maneuvers in normal and hypertensive subjects. Hypertension 2:20–28, 1980.
48. Hiramatsu M, Fujimoto N, Mori A. Catecholamine levels in cerebrospinal fluid of epileptics. Neurochem Res 10:1299–1305, 1982.
49. Holly JMP, Makin HLJ. The estimation of catecholamines in human plasma. Anal Biochem 128:257–274, 1983.
50. Huang YH, Redmond DE Jr, Snyder DR, Maas JW. In vivo location and destruction of the locus coeruleus in stumptail macaque. Brain Res 100:157–162, 1975.
51. Kato T, Hashimoto Y, Nagatsu T, Shinoda T, Okada T, Takeuchi T, Umezawa H. 24-Hour rhythm of human plasma noradrenaline and the effect of fusaric acid, a dopamine beta-hydroxylase inhibitor. Neuropsychobiology 6:61–65, 1980.
52. Kennedy B, Janowsky D, Risch S, Ziegler M. Central cholinergic stimulation causes adrenal epinephrine release. J Clin Invest 74:972–975, 1984.
53. Kleine TO. New developments for the determination of neurotransmitters and their metabolites in urine, blood plasma, cerebrospinal fluid and nervous tissue. J Clin Chem Clin Biochem 19:1085–1094, 1981.
54. Kleinman JE, Bridge P, Karoum F, Speciale S, Staub R, Zalcman S, Gillin JC, Wyatt RJ. Catecholamines and Metabolites in the Brains of Psychotics and Normals: Post-Mortem Studies. In Catecholamines: Basic and Clinical Frontiers (vol. 2), E Usdin, IJ Kopin, and J Barchas (eds), 1845–1847. New York: Pergamon Press, 1979.
55. Kozlowski S, Brezezinsha Z, Nazar K, Kozlowski W, Franczyk M. Plasma catecholamines during sustained isometric exercise. Clin Sci Mol Med 45:723–731, 1973.
56. Kuchel O, Buu NT, Hamet P, Larochelle P, Bourque M, Genest J. Essential hyperten-

sion with low conjugated catecholamines imitates pheochromocytoma. Hypertension 3:347–355, 1981.

57. Kuchel O, Buu NT, Unger T, Lis M, Genest J. Free and conjugated plasma and urinary dopamine in human hypertension. J Clin Endocrinol Metab 48:425–429, 1983.
58. Lake CR. Relationship of sympathetic nervous system tone and blood pressure. Nephron 23:84–90, 1979.
59. Lake CR, Chernow B, Feuerstein G, Goldstein D, Zeigler MG. The sympathetic nervous system in man: Its evaluation and the measurement of plasma NE. In Norepinephrine, MG Ziegler and CR Lake (eds), 1–26. Baltimore: Williams and Wilkins, 1984.
60. Lake CR, Chernow B, Goldstein D, Glass DG, Coleman M, Ziegler MG. Plasma catecholamine levels in normal subjects and in patients with secondary hypertension. Fed Proc, 43:52–56, 1984.
61. Lake CR, Gullner HG, Polinski RJ, Ebert MH, Ziegler MG, Bartter FC. Essential hypertension: central and peripheral norepinephrine. Science 211:955–957, 1981.
62. Lake CR, Mikkelson EJ, Rapoport JL, Zavadil AP, Kopin IJ. Effects of imipramine on norepinephrine and blood pressure in enuretic children. Clin Pharmacol Ther 26:647–653, 1979.
63. Lake CR, Pickar D, Ziegler MG, Lipper IS, Slater S, Murphy DL. High plasma norepinephrine levels in patients with major affective disorders. Am J Psychiatry 139:1315–1318, 1982.
64. Lake CR, Sternberg DE, van Kammen DP, Ballenger JC, Ziegler MG, Post RM, Kopin IJ, Bunney WE, Jr. Schizophrenia: Elevated cerebrospinal fluid norepinephrine. Science 207:331–333, 1980.
65. Lake CR, Wood JD, Ziegler MG, Ebert MH, Kopin IJ. Probenecid-induced norepinephrine elevations in plasma and CSF. Arch Gen Psychiatry 35:237–240, 1978.
66. Lake CR, Ziegler MG. Effect of acute volume alterations on norepinephrine and dopamine-beta-hydroxylase in normotensive and hypertensive subjects. Circulation 57:774–778, 1978.
67. Lake CR, Ziegler MG, Coleman MD, Kopin IJ. Fenfluramine potentiation of antihypertensive effects of thiazides. Clin Pharmacol Ther 28:22–27, 1980.
68. Lake CR, Ziegler MG, Coleman MD, Kopin IJ. Sustained sympathetic hyperactivity in hydrochlorothiazide-treated hypertensives. Clin Pharmacol Ther 26:428–432, 1979.
69. Lake CR, Ziegler MG, Kopin IJ. Use of plasma norepinephrine for evaluation of sympathetic neuronal function in man. Life Sci 18:1315–1326, 1976.
70. Landsberg L, Young JB. Fasting, feeding and regulation of the sympathetic nerve cells. N Engl J Med 298:1295–1301, 1978.
71. Langley JN. The difference of behavior of central and peripheral pilomotor nerve cells. J Physiol (Lond) 27:224–236, 1901.
72. Levin BE, Rappaport M, and Natelson BH. Ultradian variations of plasma noradrenaline in humans. Life Sci 25:621–628, 1979.
73. Lund A. Simultaneous fluorimetric determinations of adrenaline and noradrenaline in blood. Acta Pharmacol Toxicol (Copenh) 6:137–146, 1950.
74. Miura Y, Campese V, DeQuattro V, Meyer D. Plasma catecholamines via an improved fluorimetric assay: Comparison with an enzymatic method. J Lab Clin Med 89:421–427, 1977.
75. Murphy DL, Lake CR, Slater S, Lipper S, Shiling D, de la Vega E, and Ziegler MG. Psychoactive Drug Effects on Plasma Norepinephrine and Plasma Dopamine Beta-Hydroxylase in Man. In Catecholamines: Basic and Clinical Frontiers (Vol 1),

E Usdin, IJ Kopin, and J Barchas (eds), 918–920. New York: Pergamon Press, 1979.

76. Nielsen SL, Christensen NJ, Olsen N, Lassen NA. Raynaud's phenomenon: peripheral catecholamine concentration and effect of sympathectomy. Acta Chem Scand 502:57–62, 1980.
77. Ogasawara B, Ogawa K, Sassa H. Effects of nitroglycerin ointment on plasma norepinephrine and cyclic nucleotides in congestive heart failure. J Cardiovasc Pharmacol 3:867–875, 1981.
78. Oliver G, Schafer EA. On the physiologic action of extract of the suprarenal capsules. J Physiol (Lond) 18:230–276, 1895.
79. Passon P, Peuler J. Radioenzymatic assay for plasma norepinephrine and epinephrine. Anal Biochem 51:618–631, 1973.
80. Patten J. Neurological Differential Diagnosis. 259–266. New York: Springer-Verlag, 1977.
81. Perini C, Amann FW, Bolli P, Buhler FR. Personality and adrenergic factors in essential hypertension. Contrib Nephrol 30:64–69, 1982.
82. Perlow M, Ebert M, Gordon EK, Ziegler MG, Lake CR, Chase T. The circadian variation of catecholamine metabolism in the subhuman primate. Brain Res 139:101–113, 1978.
83. Peronnet F, Cleroux J, Perrault H, Cousineau D, de Champlain J, Nadeau R. Plasma norepinephrine response to exercise before and after training in humans. J Appl Physiol 51:812–815, 1981.
84. Petterson J, Hussi E, Janne J. Stability of human plasma catecholamines. Scand J Clin Lab Invest 40:297–303, 1980.
85. Pickar D, Lake CR, Cohen RM, Jimerson DC, Murphy DL. Alterations in noradrenergic function during clorgyline treatment. Commun Psychopharmacol 4:379–386, 1980.
86. Post RM, Lake CR, Jimerson DC, Bunney WE, Jr, Wood JH, Ziegler MG, Goodwin FK. Cerebrospinal fluid norepinephrine in affective illness. Am J Psychiatry 135:907–912, 1978.
87. Redmond DE, Huang VH. Current concepts II. New evidence for a locus coeruleus-norepinephrine connection with anxiety. Life Sci 25:2149–2162, 1979.
88. Renzini P, Brunori CA, Valori C. A sensitive and specific fluorimetric method for the determination of noradrenaline in human plasma. Clin Chim Acta 30:587–594, 1970.
89. Robertson D, Frolich JC, Carr RK, Watson JT, Hollifield JW, Shand DG, Oates JA. Effects of caffeine on plasma renin activity, catecholamines and blood pressure. N Engl J Med 298:181–186, 1978.
90. Rosenblatt JE, Lake CR, van Kammen DP, Ziegler MG, Bunney WE, Jr. Interactions of amphetamine, pimozide and lithium on plasma norepinephrine and dopamine-beta-hydroxylase in schizophrenic patients. Psychiatry Res 1:45–52, 1979.
91. Ross RJ, Zavadil AP, Calil HM, Linnoila M, Kitanaka I, Blombery P, Kopin IJ, and Potter WZ. Effects of desmethylimipramine on plasma norepinephrine, pulse, and blood pressure. Clin Pharmacol Ther 33:429–437, 1983.
92. Roth JA, Rivett AJ. Does sulfate conjugation contribute to the metabolic inactivation of catecholamines in humans? Biochem Pharmacol 31:3017–3021, 1982.
93. Shigeno T. Norepinephrine in cerebrospinal fluid of patients with cerebral vasospasm. J Neurosurg 56:344–349, 1982.
94. Shoulson I, Ziegler MG, Lake CR. Huntington's disease (HD): Determination of

plasma norepinephrine (NE) and dopamine-beta-hydroxylase (DBH). Soc Neurosci Abstracts 2:800, 1976.

95. Smith BH, Sweet WH. Monoaminergic regulation of central nervous system function: I. Noradrenergic Systems. Neurosurgery 3:108–119, 1978.
96. Stolz F. Uber Adrenalin und Alkylaminoacetobienzcatechin. Ber Dtsch Chem Ges 37:4149–4154, 1904.
97. Sundlof G, Wallin GB. The variability of muscle nerve sympathetic activity in resting recumbent man. J Physiol (Lond) 272:383–397, 1977.
98. Swanson LW. The locus coeruleus: A cytoarchitectonic golgi and immunohistochemical study in the albino rat. Brain Res 110:39–56, 1976.
99. Teychenne PF, Lake CR, Ziegler MG. Cerebrospinal Fluid Studies in Parkinson's Disease: Norepinephrine and Gamma-Aminobutyric Acid Concentrations. In Neurobiology of Cerebrospinal Fluid, JH Wood (ed), 197–206. New York: Plenum Press, 1980.
100. Teychenne PF, Lake CR, Ziegler MG, Plotkin C, Wood JH, Calne DB. Central and peripheral deficiency of norepinephrine in Parkinson's disease and the effects of L-DOPA therapy. Soc Neurosci Abstracts 3:417, 1977.
101. Torrey EF, Peterson MR. Schizophrenia and the limbic system. Lancet ii:942–946, 1974.
102. Ungerstedt U. Stereotaxic mapping of the monoamine pathways in the rat brain. Acta Physiol Scand [Suppl] 367:1–48, 1971.
103. Veith RC, Raskind MA, Barnes RF, Gumbrecht G, Ritchie JL, Halter JB. Tricyclic antidepressants and supine, standing, and exercise plasma norepinephrine levels. Clin Pharmacol Ther 33:770–775, 1983.
104. Vulpian CR. Note sur les reactions propres au tissu des capsules surrenales chez les reptiles. Soc Biol 8:223–224, 1856.
105. Wallin BG, Sundlof G, Eriksson B-M, Dominiak P, Grobecker H, Lindblad LE. Plasma noradrenaline correlates to sympathetic muscle nerve activity in normotensive man. Acta Physiol Scand 111:69–73, 1981.
106. Wang P-C, Buu NT, Kuchel O, Genest J. Conjugation patterns of endogenous plasma catecholamines in human and rat. J Lab Clin Med 101:141–151, 1983.
107. Weston PG. Sugar content of the blood and spinal fluid of insane subjects. J Med Res 35:199–208, 1916.
108. Williams AC. Observations on some extrapyramidal diseases. M.D. Thesis, Birmingham U, 1978.
109. Williams AC, Nutt J, Lake CR, Pfeiffer R, Teychenne PE, Ebert M, Calne DB. Actions of Bromocriptine in the Shy-Drager and Steele-Richardson-Olszewski Syndromes. In Dopaminergic Ergot Derivatives and Motor Function, K Fuxe and DB Calne (eds), 271–291. Oxford: Pergamon Press, 1978.
110. Wood JH. Physiology, Pharmacology, and Dynamics of Cerebrospinal Fluid. In Neurobiology of Cerebrospinal Fluid, JH Wood (ed), 1–16. New York: Plenum Press, 1980.
111. Wood JH (ed). Neurobiology of Cerebrospinal Fluid. New York: Plenum Press, 1980.
112. Wood JH. Sites of Origin and Cerebrospinal Fluid Concentration Gradients: Neurotransmitters, Their Precursors and Metabolites, and Cyclic Nucleotides. In Neurobiology of Cerebrospinal Fluid, JH Wood (ed), 53–62. New York: Plenum Press, 1980.
113. Wood JH. Technical Aspects of Clinical and Experimental Cerebrospinal Fluid Investigations. In Neurobiology of Cerebrospinal Fluid, JH Wood (ed), 71–96. New York: Plenum Press, 1980.

114. Yui Y, Kawai C. Comparison of the sensitivity of various post-column methods for catecholamine analysis by high-performance liquid chromatography. J Chromatogr 206:586–588, 1981.
115. Ziegler MG, Brooks BR, Lake CR, Wood JH, Enna SJ. Norepinephrine and gamma-aminobutyric acid in amyotrophic lateral sclerosis. Neurology (NY) 30:98–101, 1980.
116. Ziegler MG, Lake CR, Ebert MH. Norepinephrine elevations in cerebrospinal fluid after D- and L-amphetamine. Eur J Pharmacol 57:127–133, 1979.
117. Ziegler MG, Lake CR, Foppen FH, Shoulson I, Kopin IJ. Norepinephrine in cerebrospinal fluid. Brain Res 108:436–440, 1976.
118. Ziegler MG, Lake CR, Kopin IJ. The sympathetic nervous system defect in primary orthostatic hypotension. N Engl J Med 296:293–297, 1977.
119. Ziegler MG, Lake CR, Kopin IJ. Deficient sympathetic nervous response in familial dysautonomia. N Engl J Med 294:630–633, 1976.
120. Ziegler MG, Lake CR, Kopin IJ. Plasma noradrenaline increases with age. Nature 261:333–335, 1976.
121. Ziegler MG, Lake CR, Williams AC, Teychenne PF, Shoulson I, Steinsland O. Bromocriptine inhibits norepinephrine release. Clin Pharmacol Ther 25:137–142, 1979.
122. Ziegler MG, Lake CR, Wood JH, Brooks BR. Relationship between cerebrospinal fluid norepinephrine and blood pressure in neurologic patients. Clin Exp Hypertens 2:995–1008, 1980.
123. Ziegler MG, Lake CR, Wood JH, Brooks BR, Ebert MH. Relationship between norepinephrine in blood and cerebrospinal fluid in the presence of a blood-cerebrospinal fluid barrier for norepinephrine. J Neurochem 28:677–679, 1977.
124. Ziegler MG, Lake CR, Wood JH, Ebert MH. Norepinephrine in Cerebrospinal Fluid: Basic Studies, Effects of Drugs and Disease. In Neurobiology of Cerebrospinal Fluid, JH Wood (ed), 141–152. New York: Plenum Press, 1980.
125. Ziegler MG, Lake CR, Wood JH, Ebert MH. Circadian rhythm in cerebrospinal fluid noradrenaline of man and monkey. Nature 264:656–658, 1976.
126. Ziegler MG, Wood JH, Lake CR, Kopin IJ. Norepinephrine and 3-methoxy-4-hydroxyphenyl glycol gradients in human cerebrospinal fluid. Am J Psychiatry 134:565–568, 1977.
127. Zivin AJ, Reid JL, Saavedra JM, Kopin IJ. Quantitative localization of biogenic amines in the spinal cord. Brain Res 99:293–301, 1975.

I

Stress

2

The Catecholaminergic Response to Stress and Exercise

Michael G. Ziegler
Ali Jose Milano
Elaine Hull

Human beings respond to most stresses by activation of the sympathetic nervous system (SNS). We are all familiar with the tachycardia, piloerection, and pupillary dilatation that this activation engenders, but we are now able to measure norepinephrine (NE) in blood and quantitate this response. This chapter reviews the human response to stresses, ranging from standing quietly for 5 minutes to exposure to seven times the force of gravity, and from a slow walk to exhaustive exercise.

In 1911, Cannon and de la Paz demonstrated that when a cat is frightened by a barking dog, catecholamines (CA) are released from the adrenal gland into the blood [3]. In 1936, Selye [35] described the sequence of pathologic changes that occurred when an animal was exposed to a variety of stresses, and he named this the "general adaptation syndrome." The stereotyped response to stress leads to adrenocortical and autonomic discharge, and the response may be so violent as to lead to sudden death. When wild rats are subjected in rapid succession to restraint, trimming of the whiskers, and immersion under a jet of water, they may die abruptly [31,32]. Monkeys exposed to a 16-hour stressful avoidance schedule developed electrocardiographic changes characteristic of sympathetic and parasympathetic stimulation and then had ventricular arrest and died [8]. Engel has accumulated 170 examples of sudden death following psychological stress in human beings, including Biblical accounts and current newspaper reports [10]. When there was close medical observation during the stressful event, ventricular fibrillation or myocardial infarction was documented to be the ultimate cause of death.

The studies detailed in this chapter show the impressive magnitude and rapidity of the SNS response to stress. When a person reaches his maximum heart rate through exercise, NE levels are high but only a few minutes more exertion may raise them several-fold higher. It is possible to stress pigs so that sympathetic nervous activity produces gross cardiac lesions. Similar lesions are seen in human beings after fatal head trauma.

AGE AND SYMPATHETIC ACTIVITY

Age increases SNS response and a person's susceptibility to cardiac damage; age has important effects on both the release of NE from the SNS and the response of tissues to NE. A 60-year-old person has plasma NE levels approximately twice those of a 10-year-old child. Electrical activity in sympathetic nerves and the size of the NE response to stress also increase with age [22]. An old person will secrete twice as much NE in response to standing and isometric exercise [22] or to a cold pressor test [28] as will a young person. Both young and old increase their NE 100% in response to standing, but the old person has a higher resting level of NE and a greater absolute increase in NE in response to stress than the young person. The correlation of plasma NE to age is weak and accounts for approximately 20% of the variance of NE levels; thus it is predictably not seen in small studies and is obscured by diseases that alter NE levels.

Several tissue responses to NE decrease with age. The density of β receptors tends to decrease with age [11], which may mediate the decreased sensitivity of the heart to CA seen in older people [38]. A decrease in the number of receptors does not mediate the decrease in maximum heart rate seen in the elderly: one of our subjects demonstrated that he could secrete three times as much NE as needed to achieve his maximum heart rate (see Figure 2.8). The ability to secrete NE increases with physical fitness, but maximum heart rate does not (see Figure 2.9). Even when the β receptor is bypassed by the drug dibutyryl cyclic adenosine 3′,5′ monophosphate (cAMP), the decrease in cardiac response with age remains [12]. Responses to CA decrease with age, especially β-adrenergic–mediated responses such as those found in cardiac [38] and adipose [18] tissues. α-Adrenergic–mediated responses have not been shown to have a similar decline in sensitivity to NE with age, and this might mediate the rise in blood pressure seen with age.

BLOOD SAMPLING

Blood samples for NE assay are obtained by venipuncture, which some people find acutely painful and stressful. We had 15 subjects lie recumbent and inserted a scalp vein needle in an antecubital vein. Blood samples drawn immediately after venipuncture contained 335 pg/ml NE, and samples taken 20 minutes later contained 262 pg/ml NE. Over the same period of time their pulse rate decreased from 80 to 74 beats per minute. The decrease in both NE levels and heart rate was significant and the change in heart rate correlated with the 22% decrease in NE ($r = 0.58$, $p < 0.05$). After lying quietly for 3 hours, NE levels were no different than after 20 minutes. Robertson et al [33] found NE levels of 201 pg/ml in subjects resting for 30 minutes with a heparin lock in place. NE levels were 13% higher when subsequently obtained by venipuncture, but the increase was not significant. Because the decrease in NE level correlates with heart rate, tachycardia is a useful guide to anxiety that may artifactually elevate NE levels.

EFFECT OF ACCELERATION ON SYMPATHETIC ACTIVITY

When we stand, approximately 500 ml of blood pools in our legs [36]. Standing for 10 minutes leads to a further loss of intravascular volume as a 10% hemoconcentration occurs while water moves into interstitial spaces and causes swelling of the feet and legs [43]. The SNS responds to this stress by stimulating the heart and blood vessels to maintain blood pressure. This response has been quantitated by measuring NE levels in reaction to the acceleration produced by as little as a 10-degree tilt and as much as seven times the force of gravity. A 10-degree tilt for 10 minutes produced no detectable change in NE levels, although a 30-degree tilt increased them appreciably. Subsequent tilting to 45 degrees further increased NE levels [34] and a 60-degree tilt increased plasma NE from 70% [22] to 88% [15] above baseline. NE levels increased rapidly after tilting and were nearly maximal at 3 minutes. This increase is largely in response to loss of blood volume to the legs as application of 60 mm Hg pressure to the legs by an antigravity suit diminished the tilting-induced increase in plasma levels of NE from 88% to 37% [15]. Placing subjects on a tilt-table may have psychological as well as gravitational effects. Subjects commonly faint on a tilt-table, particularly if they are young, and Rosenthal et al [34] report one subject who had high NE levels while being tilted and who subsequently fainted. Sitting increases plasma NE by approximately 60% over baseline levels, and standing approximately doubles plasma NE (Figure 2.1) [22]. Although we do not ordinarily think of standing as a stress, the doubling of plasma NE on standing indicates that the body activates potent homeostatic mechanisms to cope with gravity. People who lack these homeostatic mechanisms

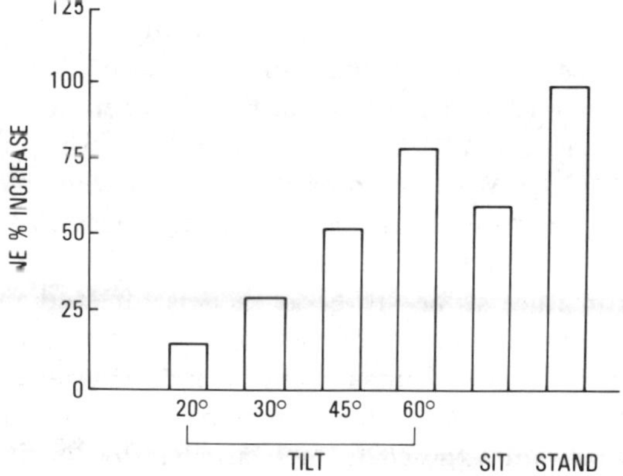

Figure 2.1 The percent increase over baseline norepinephrine (NE) levels while recumbent in subjects who were tilted from 20 to 60 degrees above horizontal or who sat or stood. Data are from Rosenthal et al [34], Hesse et al [15,16], and Lake et al [22].

cannot stand and may die if kept upright for several minutes [44]. As a simple and practical test of the body's ability to respond to stress with a sympathetic response, plasma NE levels may be obtained through an indwelling cannula while the subject is recumbent. People who find venipuncture stressful will have an increase in NE levels of approximately 20%, and those accustomed to venipuncture may have no detectable change in NE. Standing is a more potent stimulus to NE secretion than is a tilt-table and has the practical advantage of requiring no special equipment and of eliciting less frequent fainting in young subjects. When people are to have simultaneous tests requiring instrumentation, however, a tilt-table may be necessary. The usual increases in NE levels found on tilting can be seen in Figure 2.1.

SYMPATHETIC RESPONSE TO ACCELERATION GREATER THAN 1G

Acceleration that is a fraction of 1G can be simulated on a tilt-table and the sympathetic response to these small forces can be seen in Figure 2.1. Modern life routinely exposes human beings to acceleration slightly higher than 1G in elevators and automobiles. In exceptional circumstances, such as commercial roller coaster rides and fighter airplanes, a person may be subjected to acceleration equivalent to 9G. Acceleration greater than 7G lasting more than a few seconds induces syncope in an untrained person and will induce syncope in less than 1 minute in a pilot who is trained to withstand this sort of acceleration force, who is wearing an antigravity suit in a sitting posture, and who is straining to maintain blood pressure. Tolerance to this increased level of acceleration is enhanced if subjects perform a Valsalva maneuver with intermittent straining respirations. Valsalva maneuver increases intrathoracic pressure and thus increases the pressure of arterial blood supply to the brain. The "weight" of the column of blood from the heart to the brain is increased ninefold at 9G and is so "heavy" that ordinary arterial pressure cannot maintain blood flow to the brain. When acceleration force is so high that calculated arterial pressure at eye level is 0, the subject undergoes a blackout and soon faints. We have been unable to obtain blood samples from humans during high acceleration, in part owing to uncertainty about the added risk of an intravascular cannula when the "weight" of the cannula would increase manyfold. Adult miniature swine are good models for studying the response to high acceleration because the height of the column of blood from their hearts to their eyes is similar to that of human beings, and they spontaneously perform straining maneuvers in response to high G as humans are trained to do. Three adult miniature swine were exposed to high acceleration lasting for 100 seconds with acceleration up to 9G and an average acceleration of 7G. The high G exposure was repeated five times, and blood samples from indwelling cannulas were taken from the animals while they were relaxed, while they were placed in a harness prior to their first exposure, and prior to their fifth high G exposure.

While miniature swine are in the relaxed state, they have NE and epinephrine (E) levels that are roughly comparable to human levels (Table 2.1). The stress of

Table 2.1 Effects of Stress of Preparation for High-Gravity Experiments on Plasma Norepinephrine and Epinephrine

State of Animal	*Relaxed*	*Prior to High G (first exposure)*	*Prior to High G (fifth exposure)*
Plasma norepinephrine (pg/ml)	420 ± 88	1500 ± 420	7400 ± 2700
Plasma epinephrine (pg/ml)	100 ± 30	800 ± 300	1000 ± 0

G = gravity.

placing the animals in a harness preparatory to high G exposure led to a large increase in both NE and E. When these animals were exposed to 100 seconds of high G force, plasma NE levels increased to more than 40,000 pg/ml, but 2 minutes later NE levels had decreased to as low as 5000 pg/ml (Figure 2.2). These NE levels are higher than we have ever recorded in humans, but it has not been possible to withdraw blood samples from man during high G. E levels showed a similarly sharp increase in response to the stress of high G (Figure 2.3). Because of this enormous outpouring of CA from the SNS during high G exposure, we wondered if the swine might not deplete their releasable stores of CA. However, both E and NE levels were higher while the animals rested after exposures to high G forces on the same day, and the animals showed greater NE and E responses to the stress of the fifth high G run.

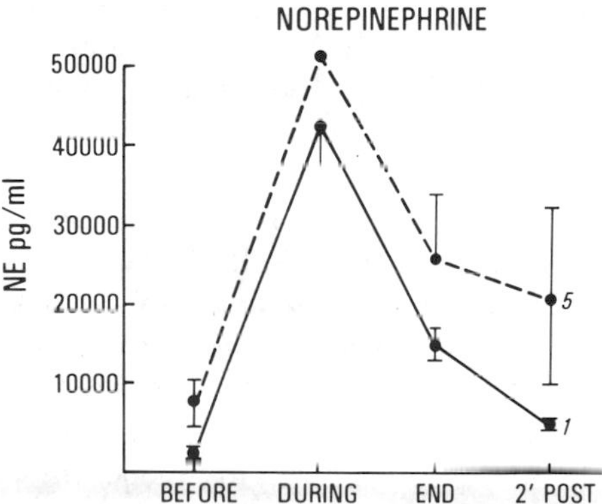

Figure 2.2 Levels of plasma norepinephrine (NE) in adult miniature swine exposed to high-gravity forces for 100 seconds. The solid line shows NE levels in response to the first exposure, and the interrupted line shows the response to the fifth exposure on the same day. Data are expressed as mean ± standard error of the mean (SEM) for five animals.

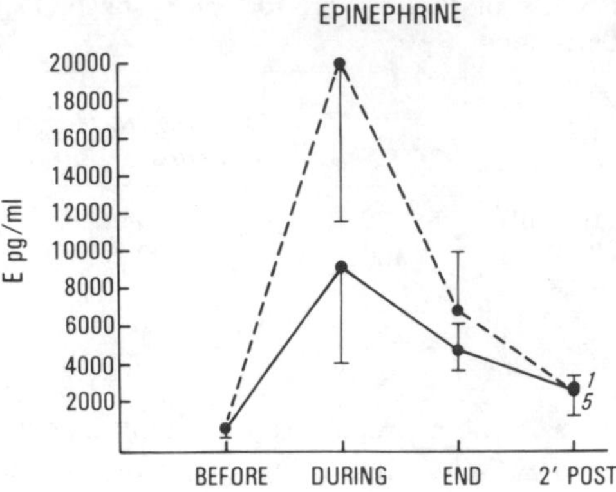

Figure 2.3 Plasma levels of epinephrine (E) in response to a 100-second high-gravity exposure in adult miniature swine. The solid line shows responses to the first and the interrupted line shows responses to the fifth high-gravity experiment of the day. Data are expressed as mean ± standard error of the mean (SEM) for five animals.

The decrease in CA levels immediately following exposure to high G was extremely rapid. For example, plasma NE levels increased to more than 40,000 pg/ml, but by 2 minutes after the high G stress they had decreased to approximately 5,000 pg/ml (see Figure 2.2). This corresponds to a CA half-life of slightly more than one-half minute, although several studies have indicated that the half-life of circulating CA is approximately 2 minutes. The extremely high CA levels attained in these animals might be expected to saturate the high-affinity, low-capacity uptake$_1$, mechanism and thereby prolong half-life rather than shorten it. It may be that a large fraction of the animals' blood supply was sequestered in venous pools in the lower body and was not accessible to the general circulation during high G forces. After high G force stopped, this sequestered blood would be released back into the general circulation and dilute the blood containing high CA levels, which had been sampled during high G. This blood trapping could then help explain the extremely high CA levels attained and short apparent half-life of CA, which would actually be due to an altered volume of distribution. Both the plasma levels of NE and E attained during high G exposure were sufficient to cause marked vasoconstriction. However, the blood NE levels attained in the legs where vasoconstriction is most needed to maintain blood pressure would be lowest.

Dopamine β-hydroxylase (DBH) has a much longer half-life than CA, so any brief period of sympathetic activity should have a relatively small influence on the large circulating pool of DBH [23]. As shown in Figure 2.4, there is a fairly moderate increase in DBH levels during a single high G exposure, but with a more marked accumulation of plasma DBH by the fifth high G exposure.

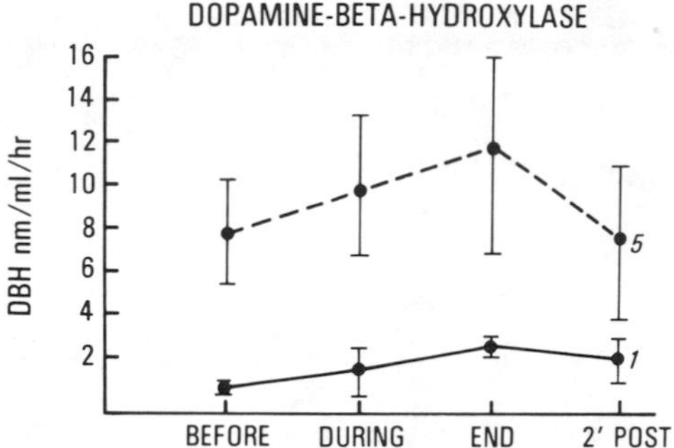

Figure 2.4 Dopamine β-hydroxylase (DBH) levels in response to high-gravity forces in adult miniature swine. The solid line shows a response to the first and the interrupted line shows the response to the fifth high-gravity experiment of the day. Data are expressed as mean ± standard error of the mean (SEM) for five animals.

Although it has not been possible to obtain blood samples from people during exposure to high G, we have obtained samples immediately prior to and 1 minute after high G forces. Two subjects were placed in a sitting posture with an anti-G suit on their legs and exposed to an average force of 4G for 100 seconds. Their plasma NE levels, as shown in Figure 2.5, were markedly increased after exposure to high G, but were still an order of magnitude below the response recorded from the swine. This stress was considerably less than the average 7G force which the swine were exposed to for 100 seconds, so several subjects were tested at a 7G force to their level of voluntary tolerance or for 60 seconds. Their NE levels, shown in Figure 2.6, demonstrate that the shorter exposure to a 7G force was considerably more potent a stimulus than 4G. Their NE levels of 5000 pg/ml in blood samples obtained 1 minute after the cessation of high G exposure were comparable to those seen in swine 2 minutes after their high G exposure. It appears that the human sympathetic nervous response to high G force is similar to that seen in swine, with the exception that the human beings were not as frightened by the procedure and had only mildly elevated CA levels prior to the initiation of high G.

When adult miniature swine are exposed to high G forces, they can develop

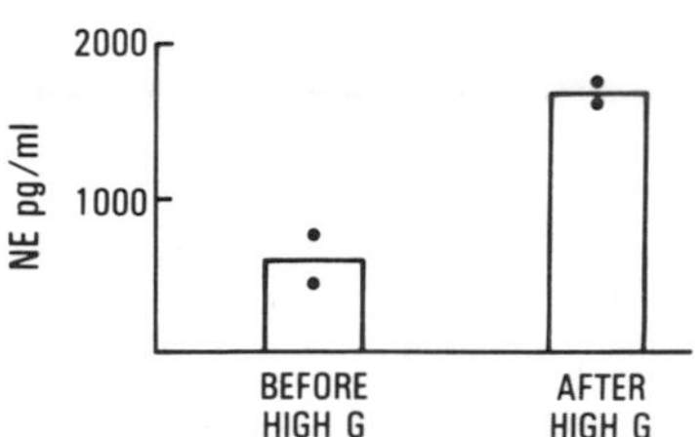

Figure 2.5 Plasma norepinephrine (NE) levels obtained from two pilots prior to and approximately 1 minute after exposure to 4 G for 100 seconds.

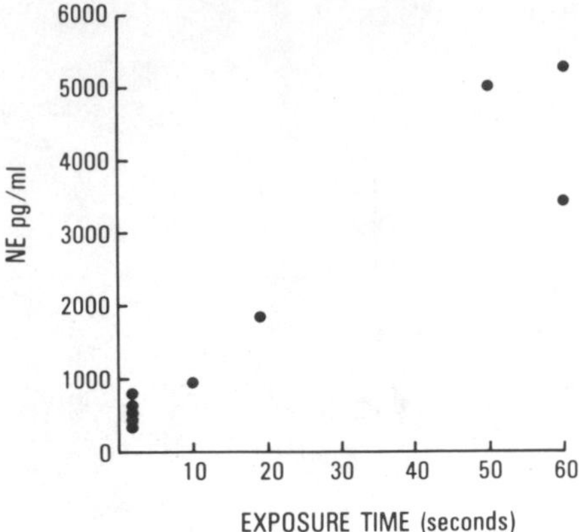

Figure 2.6 Norepinephrine (NE) levels in five subjects prior to (0) and approximately 1 minute after exposure to + 7 G from 10 to 60 seconds.

subendocardial hemorrhages and stress cardiomyopathy [2,25]. Connor [7] has noted subendocardial hemorrhage and focal areas of myocardial necrosis in human beings, which are quite similar to those found by Burton and MacKenzie [2] in swine. These cardiac lesions can be reproduced in animals by the administration of CA [30]. Stimulation of the cervicothoracic ganglion to release NE from cardiac nerve endings can also cause these myocardial lesions [19]. Sympathetic stress can lead to myocardial lesions in animals, and human beings appear capable of a level of sympathetic response to stress similar to that seen in adult miniature swine.

We have found markedly elevated NE levels in patients following severe accidental head injury. In reviewing the clinical and autopsy records of 28 fatally head-injured patients treated at the University of Texas Medical Branch in Galveston, nine of the ten patients who had electrocardiograms (ECGs) performed during the course of their hospitalization had abnormal ECGs. Eight of the 28 patients had cardiac lesions demonstrable at autopsy. The anatomically demonstrated lesions uniformly consisted of superficial areas of subendocardial hemorrhage and necrosis. Adjacent myocardial fibrosis was noted in one patient. The lesions were clustered on the left side of the intraventricular septum and occasionally involved the papillary musculature. This type of lesion is similar to that previously described in the adult miniature swine by Burton and MacKenzie in 1969 [2]. We suspect that severe stress can lead to a level of sympathetic nervous activation in human beings sufficient to cause myocardial damage.

THE NORADRENERGIC RESPONSE TO ISOMETRIC EXERCISE

Isometric exercise leads to rapid stimulation of the SNS with an increase in heart rate and blood pressure shortly after initiation of exercise. Although isometric exercise is not as simple a test of sympathetic function as standing, it has several advantages. The response to isometric exercise should not depend on blood volume as alterations in posture do. The test can be as simple as having a patient grip a partially inflated cuff of a sphygmomanometer and can be quickly standardized between subjects by having all subjects maintain a constant fraction of their maximum exertion for a specified length of time. However, different groups have obtained widely varying results with similar isometric exercise protocols. These variations may be due to differences in muscle mass of exercising subjects and differences in the level of voluntary exertion subjects are willing to produce.

Kozlowski et al [20] designed an exercise protocol in which subjects first gripped a dynamometer with one hand to determine the maximum force they were able to exert. They were then asked to continue squeezing the dynamometer to 30% of their maximum force until exhaustion. They found that maximum NE levels were attained at 4 to 5 minutes and that NE levels increased dramatically from 80 pg/ml to 2000 pg/ml in 4 minutes. However, because they measured plasma NE with a fluorometric assay, it is unlikely that their technique was sufficiently sensitive to measure levels as low as 80 pg/ml of NE. Nazar et al [27] used the same isometric exercise protocol and the same assay and found that isometric exercise increased plasma NE from 860 to 1600 pg/ml in hypertensive subjects and to 2400 pg/ml in normotensive subjects. The baseline plasma NE levels they measured were 10 times as high as those Kozlowski measured, and this discrepancy is probably due to the insensitivity of the fluorometric assay technique that both groups used. This change in baseline would, of course, have a dramatic effect on the reported percentage increase of plasma NE over baseline and so this type of data can be more reliably inferred from studies which use radioenzymatic techniques.

Lake et al [22] measured plasma NE levels with a phenylethanolamine-N-methyltransferase (PNMT)-based radioenzymatic technique and had subjects perform isometric exercise by maintaining 30% of their maximum gripping force for 5 minutes while they were standing. NE levels increased from 538 pg/ml to 778 pg/ml, an increase considerably smaller than that reported by Kozlowski. Watson et al [40] used a similar protocol except that subjects were sitting and performed isometric gripping exercise for only 3 minutes. They studied both normotensive and hypertensive subjects but found no difference in NE levels between the groups. They reported that, in the exercising arm, NE levels increased from 398 to 438 pg/ml, and in the nonexercising arm NE levels went from 498 to 585 pg/ml. They also measured E and found a greater increase in the exercising arm, even though NE levels had increased less in the exercising arm. They attributed this change to an increased blood flow in the exercising arm, which diluted released NE but allowed less opportunity for clearance of E owing to its more rapid blood flow. Vlachakis [39] had subjects exert two-thirds of their maximum gripping effort for 3 minutes while standing and found that subjects with labile hypertension increased their plasma NE by 315 pg/ml in response to isometric exercise. This increase was appreciably greater than that seen in normotensive subjects. Isometric exercise increased plasma NE markedly in all groups of subjects and also induced a notable increase in plasma E. Robertson et al [33] reported that isometric exercise at 30% of maximum handgrip capacity for 3 minutes increased NE levels only 27%.

There appears to be a wide disparity between the amount of NE increase found after isometric exercise, but the greatest discrepancies are attributable to differences in assay techniques. All of these studies found that NE increased markedly after handgrip, while isometric exercise increased plasma NE in hypertensive subjects more [39], the same [40], or less [27] than in normotensive subjects. Handgrip at 30% maximum effort for 3 minutes is not a potent stimulus to NE release [33,40], but handgrip for two-thirds of maximum effort for 3 minutes [39] or one-third or 30% of maximum effort for 5 minutes [22] leads to an appreciable increase in plasma NE levels over those obtained by standing alone.

Vlachakis [39] measured a large increase in plasma NE from handgrip at two-thirds of maximum effort for 3 minutes. It thus appears that a more intense isometric exercise will lead to a more rapid rise in plasma NE, but there is a limit to the intensity of effort obtainable with one arm. Because there is a much larger muscle mass in the legs and abdomen, we studied NE levels in eight subjects who maintained fixed, static leg efforts at 35%, 55%, and 75% of maximum effort against a force plate while performing repetitive Valsalva maneuvers until fatigued. This effort led to heart rates of 101, 124, and 120 respectively at these percentages of maximum effort. The peak levels of plasma NE attained at the termination of exercise were higher for the more intense exercise, even though subjects were able to continue the more intense exercise for a shorter length of time (Figure 2.7). Because higher NE levels were attained over a shorter period

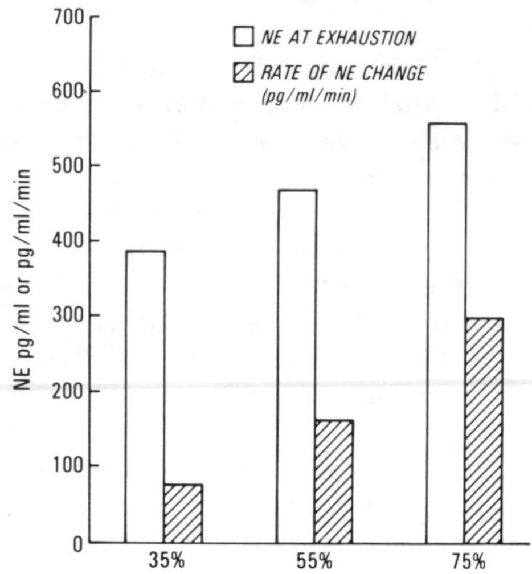

Figure 2.7 Norepinephrine (NE) levels and the rate of increase in NE levels per minute in subjects performing isometric exercise with both legs against a pressure plate at 35%, 55%, and 75% of their maximal effort.

of time, we calculate that the increase in NE levels per minute of exercise is more than three times as great at 75% maximum effort as at 35% of maximum effort (Figure 2.7).

Isometric exercise leads to a sympathetic nervous response characterized by an increase in heart rate, blood pressure, and plasma NE levels. Isometrics can increase NE levels over those obtained by upright posture alone and can be done by procedures as simple as handgripping. It appears that intense isometric exercise over a brief period of time produces both a higher final level of circulating plasma NE and a more rapid rise in NE levels. The degree of sympathetic nervous activation elicited by isometric exercise can be quite large, and this is probably adequate to explain the tachycardia and the increase in blood pressure that occurs with this type of exertion.

ISOTONIC EXERCISE

Running and bicycling are isotonic exercises in which a constant force is applied to move an object and accomplish work. When exercise begins, heart rate increases markedly, initially by withdrawal of parasympathetic tone [5] and then by sympathetic stimulation. The maximum heart rate attained with exercise varies with age and can be predicted fairly accurately in the absence of heart disease [9,37]. After any increase in the level of work, 3 to 4 minutes are needed for the heart rate to reach a new plateau level [29]. During isotonic exercise, cardiac output increases rapidly owing to tachycardia and increased filling pressure from venoconstriction. Deep inspiration causes negative intrathoracic pressure, which helps maintain the increased cardiac filling. In young, healthy adults, cardiac output may increase fivefold over resting levels [9,37].

During isotonic exercise, systolic blood pressure increases in proportion to the workload and mean blood pressure remains unchanged [37] or increases moderately [17]. There is a marked increase in coronary and skeletal blood flow at the expense of the renal and mesenteric vascular beds. At the beginning of exercise, blood flow to the skin increases to facilitate heat loss, but at heavy workloads, the skin may vasoconstrict and redistribute blood to the exercising muscles. Cerebral blood flow remains unchanged at all levels of exercise [9,17].

The maximal rate of exercise can be monitored by the rate of oxygen consumption. Heart rate, cardiac output, and oxygen consumption increase linearly as work load increases [1]. The maximum heart rate is attained at the maximum rate of oxygen consumption and, in the absence of intrinsic cardiac disease, reliably reflects oxygen consumption [29].

Although there are an endless variety of isotonic exercises, two are especially suited to laboratory investigation. Exercise on a bicycle ergometer is easily quantitated and allows the subject to place his arms in a fixed and resting position so that blood pressure and blood samples can be easily obtained. However, bicycle exercise uses only a fraction of the body's total musculature so fatigue usually occurs before maximum rates of oxygen consumption or maximum heart rate are attained. As bicycle testing allows subjects to easily attain 85% of their maximal rate of exertion, it is ideally suited to submaximal exercise protocols. As discussed later in the chapter, the last 15% of a subject's exercise potential may be considerably more stressful than the previous 85%, and testing the last fraction of a subject's capacity for exercise usually requires treadmill testing.

Bicycle Exercise

Claus Weideking (personal communication) measured plasma norepinephrine NE in eight healthy subjects while at rest and after bicycle exercise for 5 minutes at 100, 150, and 200 watts (W). He found no major change in NE levels at the lower exercise level, but a progressive increase in NE levels was observed as exercise increased. The NE levels attained at 150 W were remarkably similar to those recorded in a separate experiment performed by Henquet et al [13] (Figure 2.8). Manhem et al [26] measured NE levels after 6 minutes of exercise at 50 W and 150 W in supine subjects. They sampled blood from numerous sites, including artery, coronary sinus, and renal vein, and calculated that the heart produced NE at the rate of 389 pg/min and the kidney produced NE at the rate of 62 pg/min during exercise at 150 W. At the same time, coronary blood flow increased fourfold and renal blood flow decreased to one fourth of resting levels [24]. NE levels at 150 W exercise recorded in these three studies using healthy, young subjects were quite similar (see Figure 2.8).

Treadmill Exercise

It is more difficult to study people exercising on a treadmill than on a bicycle ergometer, but the treadmill has the advantage of allowing most normal subjects to reach their maximal level of voluntary exertion. Robertson et al [33] found

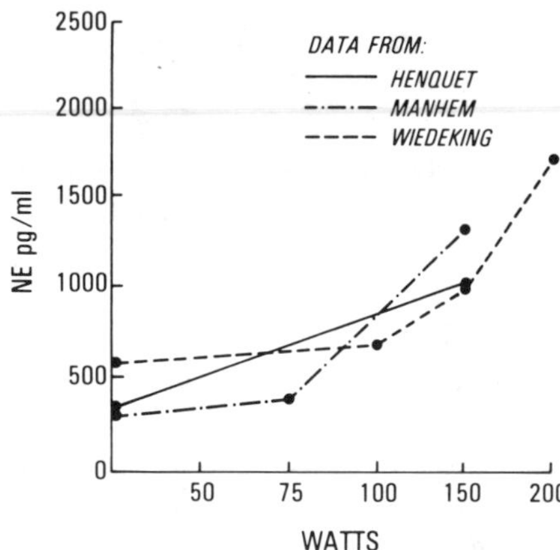

Figure 2.8 Plasma norepinephrine (NE) levels at rest and after various work loads (watts) on a bicycle ergometer. (*Data from Henquet [13], Manhem [26], and Claus Weideking.*)

that treadmill exercise at only 4 mph for 3 minutes was the most effective of six stimuli tested for increasing plasma NE levels. We exercised nine normal subjects on a treadmill and sampled their blood every 3 minutes. We found that the logarithm of plasma NE correlated linearly with the percent maximum heart rate over a wide range (Figure 2.9). Over the range of 40 to 80% of maximum heart rate, NE levels increased exponentially with increasing heart rate, but from 80 to 100% of maximum heart rate, NE levels increased even more rapidly. This was dramatically illustrated by one subject who decided that he wanted to set a new record for endurance running on the treadmill. He attained 100% of his predicted maximum heart rate and at that time had a plasma NE level of 5000 pg/ml. He continued to run for another 3 minutes and increased his plasma NE to 14,500 pg/ml with, of course, no further change in heart rate.

Using percent maximum of heart rate as an index of the rate of exercise has several advantages. It corrects for the slowing of maximum heart rate with age and is closely proportional to rate of oxygen consumption. Heart rate can be displayed continuously by electrocardiographic monitoring for the subject to view while exercising and serves as an immediate stimulus for the subject to meet his exercise goals. Although rate of oxygen consumption might be a better guide to the level of exercise, it needs to be monitored through a face mask, which prevents many subjects from reaching their maximum level of exertion because of discomfort, increased dead space (which raises CO_2 levels), and increased resistance to the work of respiration, which is perceived by many subjects as a limiting factor to exercise.

Physically trained subjects have smaller physical responses to a given amount of work than untrained subjects. It is a common observation that a physically fit person may walk up several flights of stairs without feeling stressed and an untrained person becomes dyspneic, diaphoretic, and tachycardic. Training alters the noradrenergic response to exercise quite rapidly [42]. Subjects on an exercise program of bicycling and running decreased their NE response to a given level of work after 3 weeks and had no further decrease during 6 more weeks of training.

We studied subjects with a wide range of physical fitness and classified them by how long they were able to run on a standard treadmill test before exhaustion.

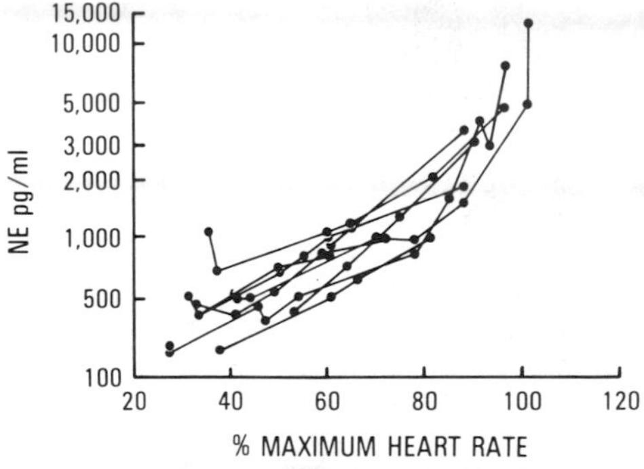

Figure 2.9 Plasma norepinephrine (NE) levels (note logarithmic scale) versus percent maximum heart rate in nine subjects who exercised on a treadmill. Blood samples were drawn every 3 minutes during exercise.

When divided into four groups by the level of treadmill exercise that they were able to attain, groups 1 to 4 reached mean maximum heart rates of 182, 184, 183, and 189 respectively. All groups reached 98% of their predicted maximum heart rate, but group 4 had a higher heart rate because the subjects were slightly younger. They attained their maximum level of exertion because they were told what their predicted maximum heart rate was and their heart rate during exercise was continuously displayed before them.

After 9 minutes of exercise, the most fit group had plasma NE levels of less than half those of their less fit counterparts (Figure 2.10). Although this result was expected, it was surprising that at the greatest level of exercise, fit subjects attained NE levels twice as great as those of the least fit group. Thus, physically fit subjects are able to attain a much greater degree of SNS activation during maximum exercise than are sedentary individuals. This observation is in accord with that of Carr et al [4]; following 4 months of exercise training, women secreted higher levels of β-endorphin and β-lipotropin in response to the same fraction of their maximum exercise level. These substances are secreted from CA neurons along with NE, so physical training increases the secretory capacity of the SNS in response to exercise. Stress can increase the level of CA and their synthetic enzymes in sympathetic tissues [21]. Exercise training also decreases vascular sensitivity to NE [41], so repeated stress can increase the capacity of the SNS to synthesize NE and decrease tissue response to NE. Training also increases the subjective

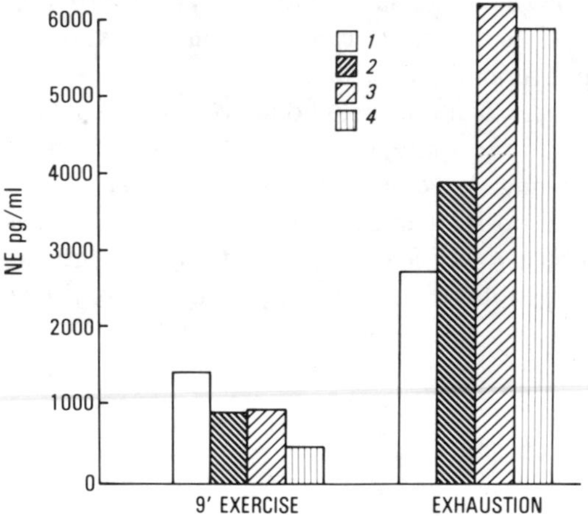

Figure 2.10 Plasma norepinephrine (NE) levels following 9 minutes of exercise and at the point of exhaustion in subjects running on a treadmill. Group 1 was able to exercise for less than 12 minutes on the treadmill, group 2 for 12 to 15 minutes, group 3 for 15 to 18 minutes, and group 4 for longer than 18 minutes.

tolerance of a subject for exertion, and all of these factors may help produce the enhanced NE levels seen in trained subjects during maximal exertion.

When subjects approach their maximum heart rate they are near the limits of cardiac reserve and the ability of the heart to deliver oxygen to exercising muscle. Tissue hypoxia then provides a potent stimulus to NE release. Subjects with chronic hypoxia from obstructive lung disease have elevated plasma NE levels [14], and NE levels in normal subjects during exercise increase more while breathing 14% oxygen than while breathing air [6]. Breathing 100% oxygen decreases the normal NE response to exercise [16]. Under normal circumstances, sympathetic stimulation in response to tissue hypoxia is beneficial as it stimulates cardiac output, increasing oxygen delivery. In some pathologic circumstances, such as lung disease, the sympathetic stimulation may be harmful as it increases metabolic rate and oxygen consumption.

CONCLUSIONS

Most, and perhaps all, stress increases NE release. The rate of NE release is greater with increasing age, but some tissues in older subjects respond less well to NE. Undergoing venipuncture or a change in posture can increase NE release, so the circumstances of blood sampling are important. Standing doubles the NE levels found in recumbent subjects. Acceleration greater than 1 G can increase plasma NE levels 100-fold in 1 minute in experimental animals and probably has a similar effect in human beings. This increase in animals leads to heart damage of a type seen in humans after fatal head trauma.

Exercise is a potent stimulus to NE release, even isometric exercise with one arm. Isometric exercise near the limits of a subject's strength is more potent than prolonged moderate exercise in raising NE levels. Isotonic exercise on a bicycle ergometer gives a fairly uniform sympathetic response in normal subjects at submaximal exertion, but exercise to maximal exertion requires running. Predictably, physically fit subjects release less NE in response to a given workload than poorly trained subjects. Surprisingly, fit subjects are not only capable of more work, but can attain much higher NE levels than sedentary subjects during maximal exercise.

REFERENCES

1. Bates DV. Cardiorespiratory determinants of cardiovascular fitness. Can Med Assoc J 96:697–702, 1967.
2. Burton RR, MacKenzie WF. Cardiac pathology associated with high sustained + Gz. Aviat Space Environ Med 47:711–717, 1976.
3. Cannon WB, de la Paz D. Emotional stimulation of adrenal secretion. Am J Physiol 28:64, 1911.
4. Carr DB, Bullen BA, Skrinar GS, Arnold MA, Rosenblatt M, Beitins IA, Martin

JB, McArthur JW. Physical conditioning facilitates the exercise-induced secretion of beta-endorphin and beta-lipotropin in women. N Engl J Med 305:560–562, 1981.

5. Christensen NJ, Galbo H, Hansen J, Hesse B, Richter EA, Trap-Jensen J. Catecholamines and exercise. Diabetes 28:58–62, 1979.
6. Clancy LJ, Critchley JA, Leitch AG, Kirby BJ, Ungar A, Glenley DC. Arterial catecholamines in hypoxic exercise in man. Clin Sci Mol Med 49:503–506, 1975.
7. Connor RCR. Myocardiac damage secondary to brain lesions. Am Heart J 78:145–148, 1969.
8. Corley KC, Greenhoot J, Mauck HP, Hoff EC. Abnormalities of cardiac rhythm associated with environmental stress. Fed Proc 29:517 (abstract 1520), 1970.
9. Ellestad MH (ed). In Stress Testing: Principles, and Practice Second Edition, Philadelphia: FA Davis, 1980.
10. Engel GL. Sudden and rapid death during psychological stress. Ann Intern Med 74:771–782, 1971.
11. Greenberg LH, Wiess B. Beta-adrenergic receptors in aged rat brain: Reduced number and capacity of pineal gland to develop supersensitivity. Science 201:61–63, 1978.
12. Guarnieri T, Filburn CR, Zitnik G, Roth GS, Lakatta EG. Contractile and biochemical correlates of beta-adrenergic stimulation in the aged heart. Am J Physiol 239:H501–508, 1980.
13. Henquet JW, Kho T, Schols M, Thijssen M, Rahn KH. The sympathetic nervous system and the renin-angiotensin system in borderline hypertension. Clin Sci 60:25–31, 1981.
14. Henriksen JH, Christensen NJ, Kok-Jensen A, Christiansen IB. Increased plasma noradrenaline concentration in patients with chronic obstructive lung disease: Relation to haemodynamics and blood gases. Scand J Clin Lab Invest 40:419–427, 1980.
15. Hesse B, Ring-Larsen H, Nielsen I, Christensen NH. Renin stimulation by passive tilting: The influence of an anti-gravity suit on postural changes in plasma renin activity, plasma noradrenaline concentration and kidney function in normal man. Scand J Clin Lab Invest 38:163–169, 1978.
16. Hesse B, Kanstrup IL, Christensen NJ, Insemann-Hansen T, Hensen JF, Halkjaer-Dristensen J, Petersen FB. Reduced norepinephrine response to dynamic exercise in human subjects during O_2 breathing. J Appl Physiol 51:176–178, 1981.
17. James FW. Exercise Testing in Normal Individuals and Patients with Cardiovascular Disease. In Pediatric Cardiovascular Clinics, MA Engle (ed), 227–246. Philadelphia: FA Davis, 1981.
18. Jelinkova-Tenova M, Hruza Z. The effect of epinephrine on fat metabolism in old rats. Gerontologia 7:168–180, 1963.
19. Klouda MA, Brynjolfsson G. Cardiotoxic effects of electrical stimulation of the stellate ganglia. Ann NY Acad Sci 156:271–280, 1969.
20. Kozlowski S, Brzezinska S, Nazar K, Kowalski W, Franczyk M. Plasma catecholamines during sustained isometric exercise. Clin Sci Mol Med 45:723–731, 1973.
21. Kvetnansky R, Gewirtz GP, Weise VK, Kopin IJ. Enhanced synthesis of adrenal dopamine-beta-hydroxylase induced by repeated immobilization in rats. Mol Pharmacol 7:81–86, 1971.
22. Lake CR, Ziegler MG, Kopin IJ. Use of plasma norepinephrine for evaluation of sympathetic neuronal function in man. Life Sci 18:1315–1326, 1976.
23. Lake CR, Ziegler MG, Coleman MD, Kopin IJ. Lack of correlation of plasma norepinephrine and dopamine-beta-hydroxylase in hypertensive and normotensive subjects. Circ Res 41:865–869, 1977.

24. Lange-Andersen K. The Cardiovascular System in Exercise. In Exercise Physiology, HB Falls (ed), Academic Press: New York & London, 1968.
25. MacKenzie WF, Burton RR, Butcher WI. Cardiac pathology associated with high sustained + Gz to stress cardiomyopathy. Aviat Space Environ Med 47:718–725, 1976.
26. Manhem P, Lecerof H, Hökfelt B. Plasma catecholamine levels in the coronary sinus, the left renal vein and peripheral vessels in healthy males at rest and during exercise. Acta Physiol Scand 104:364–369, 1978.
27. Nazar K, C-Moneta J, Z-Grojec Z. Plasma noradrenaline response to sustained handgrip in patients with essential hypertension. Eur J Appl Physiol 41:181–185, 1979.
28. Palmer CJ, Ziegler MG, Lake CR. Response of norepinephrine and blood pressure to stress increases with age. J Gerontol 33:482–487, 1978.
29. Phillips RE. The Biochemistry and Physiology of Exercise. In Medical Aspects of Exercise Testing and Training: Progress in Cardiac Rehabilitation. LR Frohman and RE Phillips (eds), 1–27. New York: Intercontinental Book, 1981.
30. Reichenbach DD, Benditt EP. Catecholamines and cardiomyopathies: the pathogenesis and potential importance of myofibrillar degeneration. Hum Pathol 1:125–150, 1970.
31. Richter CP. On the phenomenon of sudden death in animals and man. Psychosom Med 19:191–198, 1957.
32. Richter CP. The Phenomenon of Unexplained Sudden Death in Animals and Man. In Physiological Basis of Psychiatry, WH Gant (ed), 148–171. Springfield: Charles C Thomas, 1958.
33. Robertson D, Johnson GA, Robertson RM, Nies AS, Shand DG, Oates JA. Comparative assessment of stimuli that release neuronal and adrenomedullary catecholamines in man. Circulation 59:637–643, 1979.
34. Rosenthal T, Bircy M, Osikowska B, Sever PS. Changes in plasma noradrenaline concentration following sympathetic stimulation by gradual tilting. Cardiovasc Res 12:144–147, 1978.
35. Selye H. A syndrome produced by diverse nocuous agents. Nature 138:32, 1936.
36. Sjostrand T. Regulation of the blood distribution in man. Acta Physiol Scand 26:312, 1952.
37. Starke H, Eliot RS. Assessment of Available Stress Testing Techniques (Treadmill, Bicycle Ergometer, etc). In Stress and the Heart, RS Eliot (ed), 335–367. New York: Futura Publ. Co. Inc., 1974.
38. Vestal RE, Wood AJJ, Shand DB. Reduced beta-adrenoceptor sensitivity in the elderly. Clin Pharmacol Ther 26:181–186, 1979.
39. Vlachakis N. Blood pressure and catecholamine responses to sympathetic stimulation in normotensive and hypertensive subjects. J Clin Pharmacol 19:458–466, 1979.
40. Watson RDS, Littler WA, Eriksson B-M. Changes in plasma noradrenaline and adrenaline during isometric exercise. Clin Exp Pharmacol Physiol 7:399–402, 1980.
41. Wiesman DL, Harris PD, Joshua IG, Miller FN. Decreased vascular sensitivity to norepinephrine following exercise training. J Appl Physiol 51:282–287, 1981.
42. Winder WW, Hickson RC, Hagberg JM, Ehsani AA, McLane JA. Training-induced changes in hormonal and metabolic responses to submaximal exercise. J Appl Physiol 46:766–771, 1979.
43. Ziegler MG, Lake CR, Kopin IJ. Deficient sympathetic nervous response in familial dysautonomia. N Engl J Med 294:630–633, 1976.
44. Ziegler MG, Lake CR, Kopin IJ. The sympathetic nervous system defect in primary orthostatic hypotension. N Engl J Med 296:293–297, 1977.

3

Urinary Catecholamines in Behavioral Research on Stress

Andrew S. Baum
Ulf Lundberg
Neil E. Grunberg
Jerome E. Singer
Robert J. Gatchel

The central role of the endocrine system in arousal and stress is well documented. The involvement of the pituitary and adrenal cortex is established, and some research uses corticosteroids (17-OHCS) to index physiologic responses to stress [66,79]. Patterning of endocrine activities other than those of the adrenal cortex has also been demonstrated [66]. A parallel research tradition focuses on the role of sympathetic arousal in stress as enhanced and extended by adrenal medullary activity. This research shows that increased catecholamine (CA) secretion is associated with exposure to a wide variety of psychological and physical stressors [29]. This chapter considers the links between stress and the adrenal medulla and the methodologic problems associated with measuring this activity. We review research documenting the effects of a number of stress-relevant variables on CA secretion and close with a discussion of the implications of this research.

Cannon [10,11] was one of the first to demonstrate the "emergency function" of the adrenal medullary system in experiments with cats. When confronted with danger, the organism's ability to fight or flee is quickly readied through increased release of epinephrine (E) and overall sympathetic arousal. E, which is secreted by the adrenal medulla, and norepinephrine (NE), a sympathetic neurotransmitter and adrenal medullary hormone, stimulate heart rate, increase blood pressure (BP), selectively constrict blood vessels in order to channel blood to the appropriate organs, and otherwise support sympathetic arousal. This arousal, in turn, prepares

---

The opinions or assertions contained herein are the private ones of the authors and are not to be construed as official or as reflecting the views of the Department of Defense or the Uniformed Services University of the Health Sciences.

the organism for "fight or flight" confrontations with stressors [59]. As a result, the organism can meet the stressor at full strength or retreat quickly. This notion of "preparation for coping" has been supported by a number of studies. Research has linked increased secretion of CA to stimulus conditions characterized by cold, pain, anoxia, exercise, and heat, as well as to psychologic stimuli such as failure, loss, challenge, uncertainty, and threat [21,31].

In general, the adrenal medullary response is induced by events or situations that deviate from one's habitual environment [25]. Among the more potent of these events are anticipation of threat, mental effort, and emotional challenge. The magnitude of CA response to these events is usually related to the subjective intensity of the change and forms part of an ongoing person-environment interaction. According to Lazarus [57], these events are central to the appraised process underlying psychologic stress. The degree to which one experiences stress is determined by the perception of threat as related to one's assessment of one's ability to meet the demands of the situation. Therefore, both subjective and endocrinologic changes closely follow increasing threat, uncertainty, and so on.

Elevations in CA levels suggested by this analysis have been observed in many studies. Figure 3.1 illustrates the relative changes in E excretion during different levels of stress. On the average, the magnitude of the CA response varies from about three times the night-resting urinary level during mild stress to eight

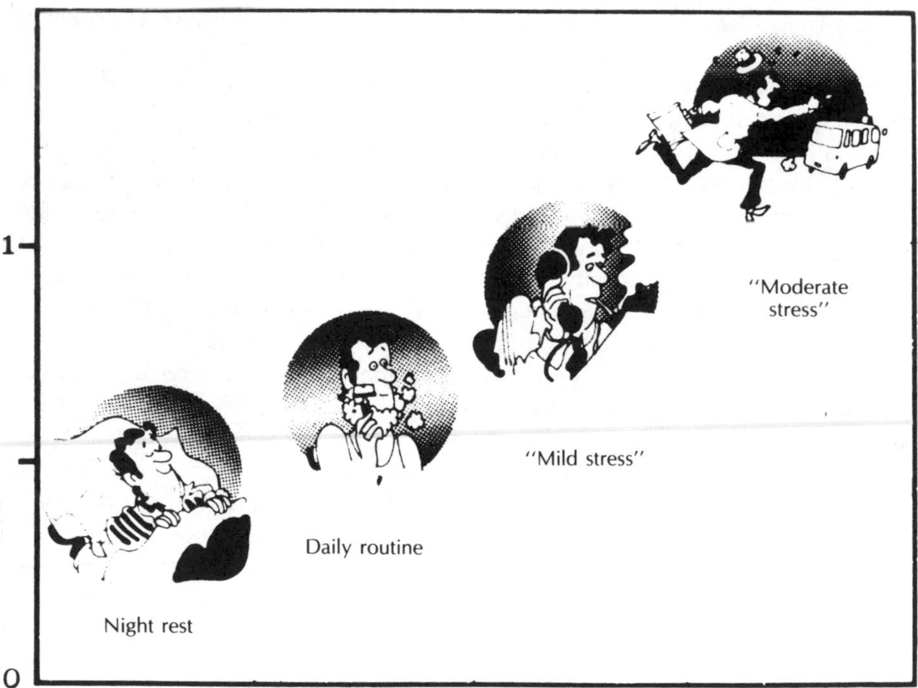

Figure 3.1 Relative changes in epinephrine excretion during different levels of stress. (*Reprinted by permission of M. Frankenhaeuser.*)

to ten times the resting level during intense stress [31]. However, individual urinary excretion levels may vary considerably [48].

Several studies [31,84] show that high CA output is associated with successful coping mechanisms and with the ability to maintain a high performance level during stressful conditions. However, frequently elevated and/or long-term elevated CA levels are assumed to damage various bodily organs and the cardiovascular system [13,46,72,77]. Therefore, chronic elevation in CA levels or frequently repeated instances of arousal may not be associated with positive outcomes or effective coping.

RELATIONSHIP BETWEEN EPINEPHRINE AND NOREPINEPHRINE

Under normal, nonstress conditions, NE excretion is approximately four to five times greater than E excretion. NE responses are generally more sensitive to exercise, physical effort, and physical stress than are E responses. Dimsdale and Moss [19] compared E and NE in plasma during a baseline condition, during public speaking (mental stress), and during physical exercise (physical stress). E excretion increased to more than twice the baseline level during speaking but NE increased only approximately 50%. In contrast, during physical exercise, NE levels reached approximately three times the baseline level, and E increased only approximately 50%. Frankenhaeuser et al [41] examined CA responses during successive exposure to gravitational stress and found that E levels decreased systematically with habituation to the experimental situation, whereas NE levels remained relatively constant. These changes suggest a greater sensitivity of E secretion to the psychologic aspects of the situation and demonstrate the important role played by NE in BP homeostasis during physical stress.

The possible psychologic importance of different E/NE ratios in individual subjects and in various situations is not clear. A hypothesis relating E to fear or anxiety and NE to anger or aggression has gained only weak support [4,44,83]. However, there are data suggesting that abnormal E or NE responses have some psychologic importance. For instance, an abnormal E/NE balance has been reported in maximum security hospital patients [88,89], and a remarkably low NE excretion in men with severe psychopathy awaiting trial was noted by Lidberg et al [60].

Alternative interpretations of varying levels of CA have also been offered. Mason [66] noted that coincident increases in E and NE were most likely when stressors were characterized by uncertainty or ambiguity. When stressors were focused and fear- or anger-producing, NE spikes were observed without associated elevations of E. Support for this notion has also been weak, although true, long-term tests of Mason's hypothesis remain to be done.

To understand why levels of NE and E may differ in response to physical versus psychologic stressors, it is important to consider the sources for production of these CA and what happens to them after they are produced and released. E is a product of the adrenal medulla, and NE is both an adrenal medullary product and a neurotransmitter. This difference may be involved in the resulting disparity in circulating and excreted levels of these two CA in response to physical and psychologic stressors. In addition, there are important differences in the fate of both CA. NE, unlike E, is subject to reuptake—it is taken up at sympathetic nerve endings.

METHODOLOGIC ASPECTS OF CATECHOLAMINE ASSESSMENT

Typically, CA levels are estimated directly from measurement of plasma or urine. Several methods for assaying CA in plasma have been reported, but the use of plasma samples in psychologic experiments, particularly field studies, is somewhat more problematic than the use of urine samples because fluctuations in plasma CA levels are rapid and are extremely sensitive to the subjects' physical movement. Because the half-life of CA in blood is less than 3 minutes, it is often difficult to obtain appropriate blood samples with which to assess the effects of stress. In addition, taking blood is an invasive and potentially reactive process which may itself produce stress. In fact, there is evidence that simple venipuncture is an effective stressor [17,33]. Glass et al [45] have solved some of these problems and, for situations involving *short-term* stress, their methodology for the examination of plasma may be preferable.

Studies of *long-term* stress have typically relied on examination of urinary CA levels. These samples show a slower rate of change than do plasma samples, and they can be used to determine long-term (e.g., 24 hours) changes in levels of CA. The collection of urine samples is easy, noninvasive, and particularly suitable for real-life studies during which the subjects' normal habits and activities should not be changed [34]. A physician's supervision is not required for urine sampling, and samples can be collected over a long period of time without pain, fear, or great inconvenience.

The CA in urine constitute a small but relatively constant fraction of liberated amines in the body [30]. Therefore, the *direction* of change or the relative levels are meaningful, but absolute numbers have limited value. Several assays using spectrophotofluorometric, radioenzymatic, and high-pressure (high-performance) liquid chromatography (HPLC) methods have been devised for measurement of CA [5,6,22]. Of these methods, radioenzymatic assays are particularly cost effective because they are sufficiently sensitive and hundreds of samples can be analyzed in a week or so by one or two trained personnel. The E found in urine can be considered a reliable estimate of adrenal medullary activity because the adrenal medulla is the sole source of circulating E [29,30]. NE levels are somewhat difficult to interpret because NE is secreted by both nerves and the adrenal medulla and is also subject to rapid neuronal reuptake. Despite these complexities, it appears that estimates of CA derived from these assays provide useful indices of stress. As Frankenhaeuser [29] noted:

> Urinary catecholamines represent estimates of sympathetic-adrenal medullary activity integrated over extended time periods, usually one to three hours. Such measurements,

> although not reflecting momentary changes, are particularly well-suited for studying psychosocial influences of every-day life. The fact that measurements can be obtained from human beings carrying out their ordinary daily activities adds to the usefulness of the method in behavioral research. [p. 211]

It is important to note that biochemical markers of stress should not be used alone because they access only one aspect of stress. Because CA levels are sensitive to many things besides stress, additional data must be collected in evaluating stress. Activity can affect levels of E and NE, as can coffee, alcoholic beverages, and cigarette smoking. Gender, age, body weight, and other personal characteristics also affect CA production [30]. It is therefore necessary to gather information about personal habits, daily activities, and the like. The relationship between many of these variables and CA levels is discussed in the section, "Factors Affecting Catecholamine Excretion."

The use of urinary CA levels for long- and short-term stress measurement requires different strategies of sample collection. Urinary CA measurements reflect all CA-stimulating activities that have occurred since the subject last voided. Even in resting, nonstressed subjects, urinary secretions will be sensitive to circadian variations in CA secretion. There are methodologic procedures available for minimizing these potential ambiguities and for increasing the usefulness of the measurements.

1. If the stress to be measured is long-term or repeated, 15- to 24-hour urine samples can be taken. These samples suppress the effects of variation between subjects with different circadian rhythms although they do not eliminate them. It remains possible to obtain an interaction between the occurrence of an acute stressor and a crest or trough in a person's secretory cycle. Long-term samples, however, minimize the biasing effects of idiosyncratic events. For example, a person who experiences a delay on the way to a meeting and runs in an effort to be on time will probably show elevated CA levels at the next voiding, but such one-time elevations should be diluted in a 24-hour collection.

2. Urinary CA can be used to measure the effects of short-term episodes by use of a double-voiding technique. Subjects are asked to void both before and after the event in question. If these measures are taken before and after the completion of an experimental task, the stress induced by the task can be inferred without contamination by preexperimental stress and activity. The limitations of this method include people's ability to void when requested, although this is generally not a great problem [61,81]. Forsman [26] has shown that urine samples obtained at 75-minute intervals following successive periods of stress and inactivity reflect changes in CA levels induced by the different situations. At least for young subjects, residual amounts of urine in the bladder are not large enough to have any noticeable effects on the CA levels obtained in a subsequent condition.

If subjects bring samples from home, particularly of their first morning voiding, further refinements are possible. The overnight CA excretions can be regarded as baseline levels and can be used as covariants to adjust stress-response levels.

3. A previously mentioned consideration in collecting urine samples for CA assay is the circadian pattern of E and NE excretion. Highest levels of CA output appear to occur around noon; the lowest levels occur at night. It is therefore important to ensure that all subjects provide samples during the same time periods and that all samplings are at a constant time across testings. This is particularly crucial for experimental versus control group comparisons. If, in a particular experiment, both experimental and control subjects are scheduled for several times of day, it is advisable to balance conditions by time. It is possible to collect single samplings from experimental subjects and compare these values to similarly collected samples from an appropriate control group. However, this cross-sectional approach is not preferred because of great interindividual variation in urinary output and CA excretion. Large within-subject variability in CA production, however, renders single sample absolute values relatively uninformative. Therefore, it is necessary to use rather large groups for such a single void study. The increased cost of a large number of subjects is offset by the need for only one specimen per subject to be assayed.

CONSISTENCY IN CATECHOLAMINE EXCRETION

As previously noted, CA levels are affected by time of day. Both E and NE levels are low during night rest, increase gradually during morning hours, and reach a peak between 12 noon and 2:00 PM [2]. E has a somewhat more pronounced diurnal pattern than does NE, partly because it is relatively independent of sleep-wakefulness patterns [1,43]. NE levels reflect variations in both posture and activity that are associated with the normal diurnal behavioral pattern and therefore are more affected by alteration in the pattern (e.g., sleep deprivation). Reversal of a sleep-wakefulness pattern (e.g., in shift workers) induces a reversal of CA levels which is not completed until after approximately 1 week [16].

Although early studies failed to find any changes in CA levels during the female menstrual cycle [71], recent studies [23,52,85] using more frequent urine sampling, have shown a small increase in CA levels during the premenstrual period. Intraindividual differences at points in the menstrual cycle are typically smaller than differences between individuals at the same stage.

Despite these kinds of influences, studies of individual CA levels show that both the intraindividual and interindividual consistency is relatively high under controlled conditions [28,46,63,69].

FACTORS AFFECTING CATECHOLAMINE EXCRETION

Age

The absolute amount of CA excreted in 24-hour urine samples is less in children than in adults, and the amount excreted in relation to body weight is higher in children [18,56,61,68]. Different ways to express CA levels in urine have been used in different studies (e.g., 24-hour levels, per kilogram of body weight, per square meter of body surface, and per gram of urinary creatinine). Because considerable variations do occur in creatinine excretion, its use as a reference substance for CA excretion has not been recommended [18,68]. De Schaepdryver et al [18] and Parra et al [68] suggested that body surface be used as a basis for expressing CA. These investigators found that, in age groups varying from 13 to 37.5 years, levels are of approximately the same magnitude. NE levels of old men (60–70 years) are higher than those of young men [3,58,87]. Responses in NE excretion owing to stress seem to be higher in old men. No systematic data on young versus old women are available, but Aslan et al [3] have reported greater CA responses to stress in a small group of postmenopausal women than in young women.

Physical Work

The relationship between CA levels and physical activity has been considered in a number of studies. Elmadjian et al [20] compared the CA levels of hockey players who participated in a game with those of players who watched the game. Active participation in the contest was associated with increased levels of NE and E. Players who merely watched the game had moderate increases in E and no changes in NE levels. As previously mentioned, Dimsdale and Moss [19] found that physical work induced a pronounced increase in NE secretion and only a moderate change in E.

Frankenhaeuser et al [38] studied the effects of increasing amounts of exercise on CA levels. When the amount of exercise was small, CA levels changed very little. At high work loads, however, CA levels increased substantially. Increasing exercise load was also associated with higher rating of effort, more rapid heart rate, and elevated systolic BP, showing that physical work must exceed a "threshold" before CA levels are affected. β blockade, which prevents tachycardia in response to mental and physical stress, was used by Sjoberg et al [82] in a series of experiments with different physical loads. They showed that heart rate was effectively suppressed by the blockade (propranolol), but CA levels were markedly elevated compared to the nonblockade condition.

Mental Work

Frankenhaeuser et al [37] and Lundberg and Forsman [62] showed that both monotonous vigilance tasks and rapid, complex cognitive conflict tasks induced an increase of E excretion (Figure 3.2). Increased output of E also occurred during a matriculation examination [39] and during the defense of a doctoral dissertation [48]. In the latter two cases, the excretion levels were extremely high, indicating that mental effort is a very potent stimulator of E production. However, because in many situations in which mental effort is high there is a concomitant emotional reaction (e.g., during an important examination), it is difficult to separate the

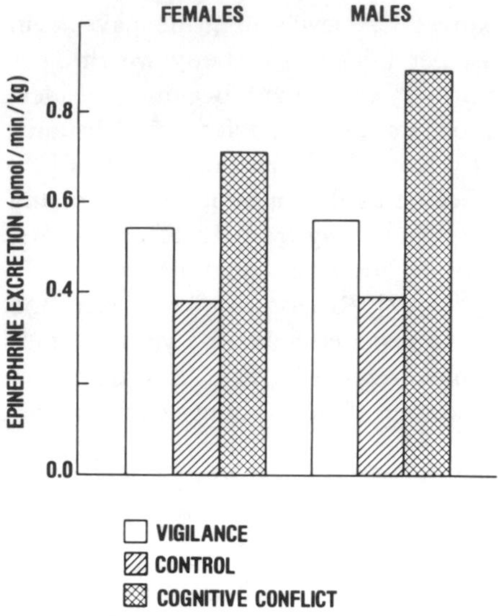

Figure 3.2 Epinephrine excretion levels in males and females during a monotonous vigilance task and a complex cognitive task. (*Based on U Lundberg and L Forsman [62]; reprinted by permission of North-Holland.*)

effects of emotional reaction and mental effort on E output. However, in the same achievement situation, subjects with high E excretion rates performed better than subjects with low excretion rates [37,67]. It is thus likely that better performance in these situations was the result of greater effort and that this variable was reflected in the higher E output of the subjects.

Emotions

The urinary excretion of CA seems to reflect the intensity rather than the subjective quality of an emotional condition. This was demonstrated in an experiment by Patkai [70], in which subjects were exposed to a pleasant situation involving a "bingo" game (with monetary rewards) and an unpleasant situation (watching medicosurgical films). Both situations were associated with elevated E levels as compared with a neutral control condition. Similarly, Levi [59] found that increased E output in both pleasant and unpleasant situations was induced by films. These data follow from a general activation theory of emotion, which defines emotion as an arousal-based physiologic and psychologic experience [11]. These results are also in accord with the infusion experiments by Schachter and Singer [76]. In experimental social settings they showed that the bodily symptoms induced by E infusions were associated with different emotions, depending on how the cognitive interpretations of the situations were manipulated.

Personal Control

In many cases, changes in CA levels are related to psychosocial stressors such as uncertainty, loss of control, crowding, and overload. For example, Frankenhaeuser and Rissler [40] found that having control over aversive events reduced the CA response to them. Research also indicates that a subject who perceives himself to have control over noise has lower CA levels than a subject who does not feel in control [64,65]. Perceptions of control are also related to CA response to crowding on commuter trains [81].

Research in occupational settings has provided further evidence of control-related changes in CA response to stressors and has identified other psychosocial events that may increase CA output. A lack of control over the pace of one's work and extreme workloads (both high and low) appear to be associated with high levels of arousal [34,35,37]. In one study, for example, CA levels of a group of sawmill workers whose work was largely repetitious and machine controlled was compared with levels of a group of workers whose work was varied and self-determined [49]. During work hours, the machine-paced group had higher CA levels than did workers in the self-paced group.

Short-term and Long-term

CA levels may not only reflect short-term changes in arousal, but may also be used as indicators of the "physiologic costs" associated with a particular situation, environment, or life-style.

In a study of female employees at an insurance company in Sweden, levels of CA were measured before, during, and after a period of "overtime" [74,75]. The extra hours (as many as 15 hours per week) were usually worked on Saturdays. During this period of overtime, the E excretion was markedly elevated, not only during working hours, but also in the evening at home. When the women resumed their usual work schedules, E excretion levels returned to normal.

Measurements of CA levels have also been used to track differential responses to acute stressors of many kinds. Glass et al [45] have shown that when exposed to challenge, harassment, and overload, individuals characterized by the type-A behavior pattern exhibit higher CA levels than do people classified as type-B. Higher CA levels in type-A subjects during high challenge have also been reported by Simpson et al [80] and by Friedman et al [42].

Research at Three Mile Island near the site of the 1979 nuclear power plant accident has suggested that continuing uncertainty and perceived threat are associated with chronic elevations in both E and NE [7]. General levels of CA were higher among subjects living near the damaged plant than in control subjects living in other areas more than a year after the accident, and these levels fluctuated with the advent and completion of decontamination procedures (venting of radioactive gas), short-term stressors that were superimposed on long-term concerns (Figure 3.3).

Sex Differences

Although most studies of CA excretion as a human response to stress have been performed on men, studies of women consistently show that they are less likely

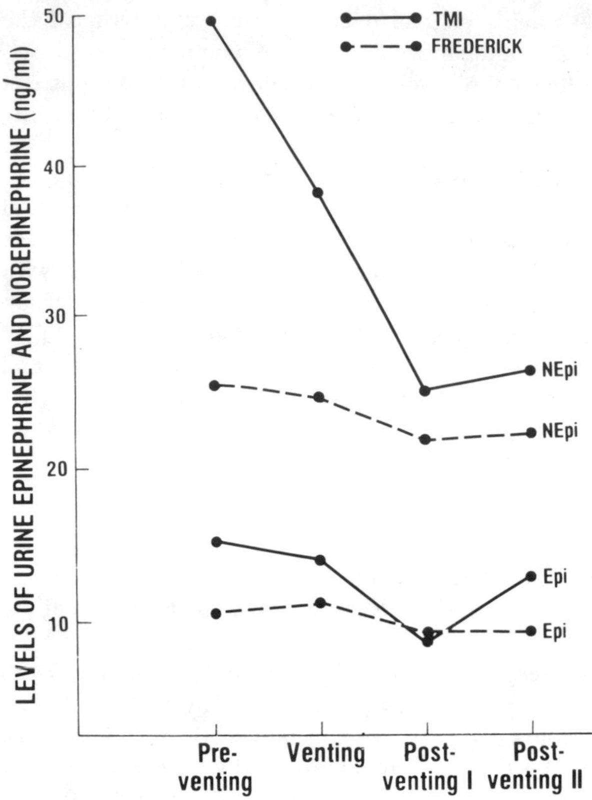

Figure 3.3 Levels of urinary epinephrine (Epi) and norepinephrine (NEpi) over four time periods at Three Mile Island (●——●) and at a control area (●- - -●). (*From Baum et al* [7].)

than men to respond to achievement stress with increased CA secretion [32]. During rest and relaxation, there are generally no differences between men and women, after adjusting for body weight. Sex differences have been found, however, during intelligence testing [51], color-word conflict testing [33,36], and matriculation examinations [39]. In no case were these sex differences in CA responses associated with inferior performance. However, on a subjective level, men generally reported more confidence in their performance than did women, who reported greater distress.

Data suggest that performance efficiency in men is more closely associated with E excretion than it is in women [8,73], but more pronounced E responses have been reported for women in nontraditional occupational roles. For example, in one study, female engineering students were found to excrete as much CA during stress as did their male colleagues [14]. Similarly, very high CA levels were reported in a woman during public defense of her Ph.D. thesis [48]. These data suggest that cognitive factors may, to a certain extent, account for the different CA responses in men and women.

Higher CA levels in boys than in girls have been found in 3- to 6-year-old children at day-care centers [12,61] and in 12-year-old school children [47]. How-

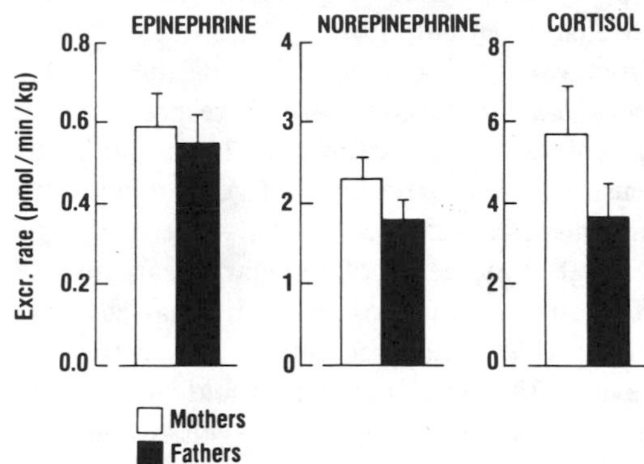

Figure 3.4 Catecholamine and cortisol excretion levels in parents accompanying their 3-year-old children to a hospital for a routine check-up. (Excr. = excretion.) (*Based on data from U Lundberg et al* [*61*].)

ever, during more standardized conditions, no appreciable sex differences were found [61]. It is likely that sex differences found at the day-care centers were induced primarily by differences in activity patterns during the day.

Although it is not yet clear to what extent sex differences in CA excretion during stress are psychologically and/or biologically determined, some support has been obtained for the assumption that psychologic factors are more important than biologic ones. In the study of 3-year-old children visiting a hospital for a routine check-up, it was found that, of the accompanying parents, on arrival the mothers had slightly higher CA and cortisol levels than did the fathers (Figure 3.4).

Because sex differences in CA excretion have generally been found in performance situations, the data in Figure 3.4 suggest that taking a child to the hospital was a greater challenge to the mothers than to the fathers. In this context, it is interesting to note that recent research investigating the effects of estrogen replacement therapy on CA responses of menopausal women showed no changes in responses to stress that could be attributed to estrogen levels [15].

CATECHOLAMINES AND HEALTH

A weak but positive correlation is usually found between CA secretion and indices of emotional stability and adaptation [50]. The organism's ability to excrete CA in response to acute threat and challenge is positively related to well-being and ability to maintain performance efficiency [31,59,84]. However, it is generally assumed that chronically high levels of circulating CA are related to increased morbidity and mortality [13,46,53].

Animal experiments [86] showed that rats that did not survive the stress of electric shocks had exaggerated elevations of plasma CA during stress, which continued to increase after the shocks had ceased. The damaging effects of CA on the myocardium was emphasized by Raab [72], and the important role played by

CA in the pathogenesis of coronary heart disease has been discussed by Krantz et al [54], with special reference to the type-A behavior pattern. Elevated CA levels have also been observed in hypertensive patients [9].

The assumed relationship between elevated CA responses and cardiovascular disease is of interest in light of the observed sex differences in CA responsiveness. Regardless of the nature of the sex differences in CA excretion, boys and adult men experience relatively high concentrations of circulating CA compared to women in the face of stress and during normal self-selected daily activity. This difference may be directly related to the higher incidence of coronary heart disease among men. It is also possible that the current changes in traditional sex role patterns among women may change the morbidity and mortality rates in the two sexes as a result of changes in CA levels [32]. The increased incidence of this disease observed in women after menopause suggests that CA levels, other risk factors, or both change markedly in older women.

CLINICAL APPLICATION

There is currently little direct clinical application of the kinds of CA measures discussed in this chapter. There are, however, a number of potential uses of these measures that may contribute to diagnostic insight and eventually to treatment. For instance, in most of the studies reviewed in this chapter, relative rather than absolute levels of hormones are most important. As an example, concentration or volume of E excreted is less important than changes in these levels over time or across events. Of course, absolute levels are valuable diagnostic tools that may reflect the presence of abnormalities (e.g., adrenal tumors) or excessive intake of particular substances (e.g., caffeine or nicotine). However, normal ranges for CA are wide and levels vary greatly because of their sensitivity to diet, activity, and the like. There is some evidence of relationships between CA levels (particularly NE) and affective disorders (particularly depression). Unfortunately, the validity of such indicators rests on several factors that have not been clearly established. The relationships between central and peripheral levels of NE are not certain, and studies disagree about the relationships between CA and psychiatric distress.

There may be some indirect clinical relevance of these measures that provides new information. For example, there is evidence that suggests a relationship between learned helplessness and depression [78]. Further, the motivational deficits associated with learned helplessness may result in CA response patterns that are different from those exhibited by nonhelpless people [24]. When challenged with a difficult or unsolvable problem, people exhibiting symptoms of helplessness show little or no change in levels of urinary E and NE. In some cases, these individuals exhibit a decrease in excreted CA following challenge. In contrast, people who do not exhibit behavioral or emotional symptoms of helplessness tend to show substantial increases in CA excretion following challenge. Thus, patterns of CA response to challenge may yield information about motivational precursors of depression and helplessness and may contribute to early diagnosis and treatment.

As an additional example, research has shown that some people are more physiologically reactive to psychologic challenge than are others. In some cases this response is related to the type-A behavior pattern, and in others it is viewed as a sensation-seeking phenomenon or as a general tendency to react to stimuli with varying sympathetic vigor [e.g., 55,90]. These patterns are in turn related to coronary heart disease, chronic stress, and posttraumatic stress. Thus, changes in CA levels following challenge may reflect other predisposing conditions that may have clinical importance.

Finally, changes in CA values may indicate individual responses to licit and illicit drugs. For example, examination of changes in CA levels with administration and after cessation of a pharmacologically addictive agent, may reflect physiologic responsivity to that drug, rapidity and tendency to habituate to the drug, and extent of physiologic disequilibrium and withdrawal from the drug. These possibilities are hypothetical but deserve research attention for potential clinical application.

CONCLUSIONS

Researchers have long abandoned a search for a single stress hormone. Current interest focuses on the relationship between stressful events and their role in activation, physiologic processes, and pathogenesis of a variety of diseases. As yet, there is no reasonably complete theory of the mechanisms by which environmental, emotional, or cognitive activities produce similar bodily changes, nor is the role of the affective quality of the event—good or bad—understood. Clearly, no single hormone or group of hormones will be an unequivocal index of stress or coping.

Nevertheless, the involvement of several hormones in the stress process is no longer a matter of conjecture. At the least, the adrenal corticosteroids and the medullary hormones are certainly a part of the stressor-stress-coping-consequences cycle.

This chapter was prepared with assistance from a research grant from the Uniformed Services University of the Health Sciences (CO7216) and support from the Swedish Medical Research Council. We would like to thank T. Kevin Blanc, Martha M. Gisriel, Kathy Moriarty, and Cindy Scher for their editorial assistance.

REFERENCES

1. Akerstedt T. Altered sleep/wake patterns and circadian rhythms. Laboratory and field studies of sympathoadrenomedullary and related variables. Acta Physiol Scand (Suppl. 469), 1979.
2. Akerstedt T, Levi L. Circadian rhythms in the secretion of cortisol, adrenaline and noradrenaline. Eur J Clin Invest 8:57–58, 1978.
3. Aslan S, Nelson L, Carruthers M, Lader M. Stress and age effects on catecholamines in normal subjects. J Psychosom Res 25:33–41, 1981.

4. Ax A. The physiological differentiation between fear and anger in humans. Psychosom Med 15:433–442, 1953.
5. Axelrod J. Catechol-O-methyltransferase from rat liver. Methods Enzymol 5:748–751, 1962.
6. Axelrod J, Tomchick R. Enzymatic O-methylation of catecholamines. J Biol Chem 233:702–705, 1958.
7. Baum A, Gatchel RJ, Fleming R, Lake CR. Chronic and acute stress associated with the Three Mile Island accident and decontamination: Preliminary findings of a longitudinal study. Technical report submitted to the US Nuclear Regulatory Commission, Washington, DC, 1981.
8. Bergman LR, Magnusson D. Overachievement and catecholamine output in an achievement situation. Psychosom Med 41:181–189, 1979.
9. Bertel O, Bühler FR, Kiowski W, Lutold BE. Decreased beta-adrenoreceptor responsiveness as related to age, blood pressure, and plasma catecholamines in patients with essential hypertension. Hypertension 2:130–138, 1980.
10. Cannon WB. The emergency function of the adrenal medulla in pain and the major emotions. Am J Physiol 33:356–372, 1914.
11. Cannon WB. The Wisdom of the Body. Norton, New York, 1932.
12. Cederblad M, Höök B. Beteenderubbningar och katekolaminutsöndring hos treåriga daghemsbarn i Stockholm. (Disturbances in behavior and catecholamine excretion in three year old day-care children in Stockholm.) (In Swedish) Läkartidningen 77:3366–3368, 1980.
13. Christensen NJ. The role of catecholamines in clinical medicine. Acta Med Scand [Suppl.] 624:9–18, 1979.
14. Collins A, Frankenhaeuser M. Stress responses in male and female engineering students. J Human Stress 4:43–48, 1978.
15. Collins A, Hanson U, Eneroth P, Hagenfeldt K, Lundberg U, Frankenhaeuser M. Psychophysiological stress responses in postmenopausal women before and after estrogen replacement therapy. Human Neurobiol, in press, 1984.
16. Dahlgren K. Shiftwork-circadian rhythms and sleep. Field studies of different shift systems. Reports from the Department of Psychology, University of Stockholm, Suppl. 53, 1981.
17. Davis J, Morrill R, Fawcett J, Upton V, Bondy DK, Spiro HM. Apprehension and elevated serum cortisol levels. J Psychosom Res 6:83–86, 1962.
18. De Schaepdryver AF, Hooft C, Delbeke MJ, Van den Noortgaete M. Urinary catecholamines and metabolites in children. J Pediatr 93:266–268, 1978.
19. Dimsdale JE, Moss J. Plasma-catecholamines in stress and exercise. JAMA 243:340–342, 1980.
20. Elmadjian F, Hope JM, Lamson ET. Excretion of epinephrine and norepinephrine in various emotional states. Metabolism 16:608–620, 1967.
21. Euler US von. Twenty years of noradrenaline. Pharmacol Rev 8:29–38, 1966.
22. Euler US von, Lishajko F. Improved technique for the fluorometric estimation of catecholamines. Acta Physiol Scand 51:348–355, 1961.
23. Feichtinger W, Kemeter P, Salzer H, Euller A, Korn A, Fulmek R, Friedrich F. Daily Epinephrine and Norepinephrine Excretion in Urine of Normal Cyclic Women Compared with Prolactin, LH, FSH, Estradiol, Progesterone, Testosterone, and Cortisol. In Psychoneuroendocrinology in Reproduction, L. Zichella and P. Pancheri (eds), 215–223. New York: Elsevier/North Holland Biomedical Press, 1979.

24. Fleming R, Baum A, Reddy DM. Behavioral and biochemical effects of job loss and unemployment stress. Journal of Human Stress 10(1):12–17, 1984.
25. Forsman L. Habitual catecholamine excretion and its relation to habitual distress. Biol Psychol 11:83–97, 1980.
26. Forsman L. Note on estimating catecholamines in urine sampled after 75 minute periods of mental work and inactivity. J Psychosom Res 25:223–225, 1981.
27. Forsman L, Lindblad LE. Effect of mental stress on baroreceptor mediated changes in blood pressure, heart rate, plasma catecholamines and subjective responses in healthy males and females. Psychosom Med, in press, 1984.
28. Forsman L, Lundberg U. Consistency in catecholamine and cortisol excretion in males and females. J Psychosom Res, in press, 1984.
29. Frankenhaeuser M. Experimental Approaches to the Study of Catecholamines and Emotion. In Emotions—Their Parameters and Measurement, L. Levi (ed), 209–234. New York: Raven Press, 1975.
30. Frankenhaeuser M. Sympathetic-Adrenomedullary Activity, Behavior, and the Psychosocial Environment. In Research in Psychophysiology, PH Venables and MJ Christie (eds), 71–94. New York: Wiley, 1975.
31. Frankenhaeuser M. Psychoneuroendocrine Approaches to the Study of Emotion as Related to Stress and Coping. In Nebraska Symposium on Motivation 1978, HE Howe and RA Dienstkier (eds), 123–161. Lincoln: University of Nebraska Press, 1979.
32. Frankenhaeuser M. The Sympathetic-Adrenal and Pituitary-Adrenal Response to Challenge: Comparison Between the Sexes. Proceedings from the German Conference on Coronary Prone Behavior. Altenberg, FRG, June 1981. Basel: Karger, 1984.
33. Frankenhaeuser M, Dunne E, Lundberg U. Sex differences in sympathetic adrenal medullary reactions induced by different stressors. Psychopharmacology (Berlin) 47:1–5, 1976.
34. Frankenhaeuser M, Gardell B. Underload and overload in working life: Outline of a multidisciplinary approach. J Human Stress 2(3):35–46, 1976.
35. Frankenhaeuser M, Johansson G. Task demand as reflected in catecholamine excretion and heart rate. J Human Stress, 2:15–23, 1976.
36. Frankenhaeuser M, Lundberg U, Forsman L. Dissociation between sympathetic-adrenal and pituitary-adrenal responses to an achievement situation characterized by high controllability. Biol Psychol 10:79–91, 1980.
37. Frankenhaeuser M, Nordheden B, Myrsten AL, Post B. Psychophysiological reactions to understimulation and overstimulation. Acta Psychol 35:298–308, 1971.
38. Frankenhaeuser M, Post B, Nordheden B, Sjoberg H. Physiological and subjective reactions to different physical workloads. Percept Mot Skills 28:343–349, 1969.
39. Frankenhaeuser M, Rauste-von Wright M, Collins A, von Wright J, Sedvall G, Swahn CG. Sex differences in psychoneuroendocrine reactions to examination stress. Psychosom Med 40:334–343, 1978.
40. Frankenhaeuser M, Rissler A. Effects of punishment on catecholamine release and efficiency on performance. Psychopharmacology (Berlin) 17:378–390, 1970.
41. Frankenhaeuser M, Sterky K, Jarpe G. Psychophysiological relations in habituation to gravitational stress. Percept Mot Skills 15:63–72, 1962.
42. Friedman M, Byers SO, Diamant J, Rosenman RH. Plasma catecholamine response of coronary prone subjects (Type A) to a specific challenge. Metabolism 24:205–210, 1975.
43. Froberg J. Psychobiological 24-hour Patterns. Theory, Methods, and Summary of

Empirical Studies. Doctoral dissertation, Department of Psychology, University of Stockholm, 1979.

44. Funkenstein DH. Norepinephrine-like and epinephrine-like substances in relation to human behavior. J Ment Dis 124:58–68, 1956.
45. Glass DC, Krakoff LR, Contrada R, Hilton WF, Kehoe K, Mannucci EG, Collins C, Snow B, Elting E. Effect of harassment and competition upon cardiovascular and plasma catecholamine responses in Type A and Type B individuals. Psychophysiology 17:453–463, 1980.
46. Gruchow HW. Catecholamine activity and reported morbidity. J Chronic Dis 29:773–783, 1976.
47. Johansson G. Activation, adjustment and sympathetic-adrenal medullary activity. Field and laboratory studies of adults and children. Reports from the Psychological Laboratories, University of Stockholm [Suppl. 21], 1973.
48. Johansson G. Case report on female catecholamine excretion in response to examination stress. Reports from the Department of Psychology, University of Stockholm, No. 515, 1977.
49. Johansson G, Aronsson G, Lindstrom BO. Social psychological and neuroendocrine stress reactions in highly mechanized work. Ergonomics 21:583–599, 1978.
50. Johansson G, Frankenhaeuser M, Magnusson D. Catecholamine output in school children as related to performance and adjustment. Scand J Psychol 14:20–28, 1973.
51. Johansson G, Post B. Catecholamine output of males and females over a one-year period. Acta Physiol Scand 92:557–565, 1974.
52. Kobus E, Wasilewska E, Bragiel Z. Urinary excretion of catecholamines (CA) and vanillylmandelic acid (VMA) during a normal menstrual cycle. Bull Acad Pol Sci 27:71–74, 1979.
53. Krantz DS, Glass DC, Contrada R, Miller NE. Behavior and Health. National Science Foundation's Second Five Year Outlook on Science and Technology. Washington, DC: US Government Printing Office, 1981.
54. Krantz DS, Glass DC, Schaeffer MA, Davia JE. Behavior Patterns and Coronary Disease: A Critical Evaluation. In Perspectives in Cardiovascular Psychophysiology, JT Cacioppo and RE Petty (eds). New York: Guilford, 1982.
55. Krantz DS, Manuck SB. Measures of Acute Physiologic Reactivity to Behavioral Stimuli. In Proceedings of the National Heart, Lung, & Blood Institute Workshop on Measuring Psychosocial Variables in Epidemiologic Studies of Cardiovascular Disease. A Ostfeld and E Eaker (eds). Bethesda, MD: National Institutes of Health, in press, 1984.
56. Lambert WW, Johansson G, Frankenhaeuser M, Klackenberg-Larsson I. Catecholamine excretion in young children and their parents as related to behavior. Scand J Psychol 10:306–318, 1969.
57. Lazarus RS. Psychological Stress and the Coping Process. New York: McGraw-Hill, 1966.
58. Lehmann M, Keul J. Age-dependent and stress-dependent behavior of plasma-catecholamine. Z Kardiol 69:697, 1980.
59. Levi L. Stress and distress in response to psychosocial stimuli. Acta Med Scand [Suppl.] 528:1–66, 1972.
60. Lidberg L, Levander S, Schalling D, Lidberg Y. Urinary catecholamines, stress, and psychopathy: A study of arrested men awaiting trial. Psychosom Med 40:116–125, 1978.
61. Lundberg U, de Chateau P, Winberg J, Frankenhaeuser M. Catecholamine and cortisol

excretion patterns in three-year-old children and their parents. J Human Stress, 7:3–11, 1981.

62. Lundberg U, Forsman L. Adrenal-medullary and adrenal-cortical responses to understimulation and overstimulation: Comparison between Type A and Type B persons. Biol Psychol 9:79–89, 1979.
63. Lundberg U, Forsman L. Consistency in catecholamine and cortisol excretion patterns over experimental conditions. Pharmacol Biochem Behav 12:449–452, 1980.
64. Lundberg U, Frankenhaeuser M. Adjustment to noise stress. Reports from the Department of Psychology, University of Stockholm, No. 484, 1976.
65. Lundberg U, Frankenhaeuser M. Psychophysiological reactions to noise as modified by personal control over stimulus intensity. Biol Psychol 6:51–59, 1978.
66. Mason JW. A historical view of the stress field. J Human Stress 1:22–36, 1975.
67. O'Hanlon JF, Beatty J. Catecholamine correlates of radar monitoring performance. Biol Psychol 4:293–304, 1976.
68. Parra A, Ramira del Angel A, Cervantes C, Sanchez M. Urinary excretion of catecholamines in healthy subjects in relation to body growth. Acta Endocrinol (Copenh) 94:546–551, 1980.
69. Patkai P. Relations between catecholamine release and psychological functions. Reports from the Psychological Laboratories, University of Stockholm, Suppl. 2, 1970.
70. Patkai P. Catecholamine excretion in pleasant and unpleasant situations. Acta Psychol 35:352–363, 1971.
71. Patkai P, Johansson G, Post B. Mood, alertness, and sympathetic-adrenal medullary activity during the menstrual cycle. Psychosom Med 36:503–512, 1974.
72. Raab W. Preventive Myocardiology: Fundamentals and Targets. Springfield: American Lecture Series, 1970.
73. Rauste-von Wright M, von Wright J, Frankenhaeuser M. Relations between sex-related psychological characteristics during adolescence and catecholamine excretion during achievement stress. Psychophysiology 18:362–370, 1981.
74. Rissler A. Stress reactions at work and after work during a period of quantitative overload. Ergonomics 20:13–16, 1977.
75. Rissler A, Elgerot A. Stress reactions related to overtime at work. Department of Psychology, University of Stockholm, Rapporter, No. 23, 1978.
76. Schachter S, Singer JE. Cognitive, social and physiological determinants of emotional state. Psychol Rev 69:379–398, 1962.
77. Schneiderman N. Animal Behavior Models of Coronary Heart Disease. In Handbook of Psychology and Health, Vol. 3, DS Krantz, A Baum, and JE Singer (eds). Hillsdale, NJ: Erlbaum, 1983.
78. Seligman MEP. Helplessness. San Francisco: WH Freeman Company, 1975.
79. Selye H. The Stress of Life. New York: McGraw-Hill, 1956.
80. Simpson MT, Olewine DE, Jenkins CD, Ramsey FH, Zyzanski SJ, Thomas G, Hames CG. Exercise-induced catecholamines and platelet aggregation in the coronary-prone behavior pattern. Psychosom Med 36:467–487, 1974.
81. Singer JE, Lundberg U, Frankenhaeuser M. Stress on the Train: A Study of Urban Commuting. In Advances in Environmental Psychology, Vol. I, A Baum, JE Singer, and S Valins (eds), 41–56. Hillsdale, NJ: Erlbaum, 1978.
82. Sjoberg H, Frankenhaeuser M, Bjurstedt H. Interactions between heart rate, psychomotor performance and perceived effort during physical work as influenced by beta-adrenergic blockade. Biol Psychol 8:31–43, 1979.

83. Taggart P, Carruthers M, Path MRC, Somerville W. Emotions, catecholamines and the electrocardiogram. Prog Cardiol 7:103–124, 1978.
84. Ursin H, Baade E, Levine S. Psychobiology of Stress. New York: Academic Press, 1978.
85. Wasilweska E, Kobus E, Bargiel Z. Urinary Catecholamine Excretion and Plasma Dopamine-Beta Hydroxylase Activity in Mental Work Performed in Two Periods of Menstrual Cycle in Women. In Catecholamines and Stress: Recent Advances, E Usdin, R Kvetnansky, IJ Kopin (eds), 549–554. New York: Elsevier/North-Holland, 1980.
86. Weick BG, Ritter S, Ritter RC. Plasma catecholamines: Exaggerated elevation is associated with stress susceptibility. Physiol Behav 24:869–874, 1980.
87. Weidmann P, Dechatel R, Schiffman A, Bachmann E, Beretta-Piccoli C, Reubi FC, Ziegler WH, Vetter W. Interrelations between age and plasma renin, aldosterone and cortisol, urinary catecholamines, and the body sodium/volume state in normal man. Klin Wochenschr 55:725–733, 1977.
88. Woodman D, Hinton J. Catecholamine balance during stress anticipation: An abnormality in maximum security hospital patients. J Psychosom Res 22:477–483, 1978.
89. Woodman DD, Hinton JW, O'Neill MT. Plasma catecholamines, stress, and aggression in maximum security patients. Biol Psychol 6:147–154, 1978.
90. Zuckerman M. Biological Basis of Sensation Seeking, Impulsivity, and Anxiety. Hillsdale, NJ: Erlbaum, 1983.

II

Neuropsychiatric Disorders

4

Catecholamines in Anxiety Disorders and Mitral Valve Prolapse

Robert J. Ursano

Understanding anxiety is central to understanding psychopathology and the mind-body interaction. Anxiety has long been considered an indication of a diseased state. In 1869, Beard described neurasthenia, a syndrome which would include the present day anxiety disorders [6]. In 1871, DaCosta [23] reported a syndrome among Civil War soldiers which he called the "irritable heart." In soldiers under substantial battle stress, he described chest pain and recurring palpitations unrelated to any structural lesion. DaCosta's syndrome became a recognized clinical entity, known by various names including "soldier's heart," "neurocirculatory asthenia," and "vasomotor neurosis." Freud introduced the term "anxiety neurosis" in 1895 [32]

As a symptom, anxiety is associated with heightened activation of the autonomic nervous system: palpitations, fatigability, breathlessness, nervousness, chest pain, dizziness, and a host of other physical symptoms [17]. The onset of anxiety may be acute, in which case panic attack occurs. These attacks are described as a sudden onset of terror or apprehension usually accompanied by somatic symptoms and often by feelings of unreality (depersonalization or derealization). Cardiorespiratory symptoms are most common. Patients frequently complain of a more forceful heartbeat, often with a sense of emptiness in the chest. A variety of chest pains may be present, some radiating to the shoulder area. Respiratory symptoms usually include feelings of fullness in the chest and shortness of breath. Patients with panic attacks are frequently so overwhelmingly frightened by their symptoms that they develop anticipatory feelings of helplessness which lead them to stay at home and in other familiar settings, producing the clinical picture of agoraphobia [96].

Patients may also present with symptoms of chronic anxiety related to constant feelings of nervousness, irritability, shakiness, jitteriness, jumpiness, chronic apprehension, and anxious expectation. Some patients may present with symptoms of "irritable colon" [8]. Because depression is a common accompaniment of anxiety disorders, an association between anxiety disorders and primary affective disease

Table 4.1 Clinical Features of Generalized Anxiety Disorder

Age of onset: usually adolescence or young adulthood
Generally anxious, nervous mood lasting at least 6 months and including
  Motor tension (shaky, jittery, trembling, restless, easily fatigued, short of breath)
  Autonomic arousal (sweating, palpitations, light-headedness, high resting pulse)
  Apprehensive expectation and vigilance (worrying, rumination, irritability, insomnia)

remains a possibility. Similarly, the common observation of psychoanalysts that anxiety symptoms become evident following resolution of depressive symptoms suggests a relationship between these two syndromes.

Epidemiologic data indicate that anxiety disorders are a common syndrome which occurs with greater frequency among women and which may cause increased mortality. The usefulness of older epidemiologic data, however, is limited by the use of various definitions of the single syndrome anxiety neurosis. In contrast, the *Diagnostic and Statistical Manual of Mental Disorders* (3rd ed.) (DSM-III) considers generalized anxiety disorder and panic disorder to be separate entities (Tables 4.1 and 4.2). Both panic disorder and generalized anxiety disorder frequently begin in adolescence or early adulthood, usually prior to age 35. Perhaps 5% of the population suffers from either panic disorder or generalized anxiety disorder [18,21,64,78,115]. Generally, investigators agree that anxiety disorders are familial. Twin studies support the increased occurrence of anxiety disorders in monozygotic twins [12,101]. These studies are not, however, totally compatible with family studies, indicating that environmental factors are also highly related to this disease [16]. Panic disorder, in particular, is believed to be familial; estimates of its preva-

Table 4.2 Clinical Features of Panic Disorder

Age of onset: late adolescence or early adult life, but may begin later
Recurrent panic attacks (three within 3 weeks) accompanied by
  Dyspnea
  Palpitations
  Chest pain
  Choking
  Dizziness
  Feelings of unreality
  Parathesias
  Hot and cold flashes
  Sweating
  Faintness
  Trembling
  Fear of dying

lence vary from 1.7 to 8% (Weissman Family Study, New Haven, Connecticut, reported in reference 16).

Women are affected with anxiety disorders two to four times more frequently than men [20,97,119]. Anxiety disorders are reported to affect 10 to 14% of patients in cardiology practices [116,118]. Evidence of increased mortality is conflicting. Wheeler et al [114] found no increased mortality among men with panic disorders, but Coryell et al [20] reported a substantially increased number of deaths in patients with panic disorders from unnatural causes and circulatory system disease. These data, however, include individuals with a history of hypertension at the index evaluation. The frequency of occurrence of secondary depression or obsessional symptoms with panic disorders suggests a connection between these syndromes [16].

Recent clinical advances underscore the development of knowledge about anxiety. The discovery of chlorpromazine provided evidence at the biochemical level that all anxiety was not the same. Chlorpromazine and related pharmacologic agents were useful in psychotic anxiety but not in other types. In contrast, the benzodiazepines were found to be generally useful in treating chronic anticipatory anxiety but not to have an effect on "psychotic anxiety." Klein [55] studied a group of extremely anxious patients who were refractory to all forms of treatment including sedatives and neuroleptics. Their acute anxiety attacks (panic) could be blocked by the use of imipramine, although imipramine had little or no effect on the chronic anxiety symptoms. That each of these three classes of drugs (antipsychotics, benzodiazepines, and tricyclic antidepressants) has its own ability to counter particular "anxiety" symptoms suggests that multiple biologic mechanisms are involved in the production of anxiety.

CATECHOLAMINES IN ANXIETY DISORDERS

The role of the catecholamines (CA) in the unfolding story of the anxiety disorders includes the study of the peripheral effects of the CA and the more recent interest in central nervous system (CNS) noradrenergic mechanisms (see Chapter 1). Cannon and de la Paz in their early study of homeostasis [11] showed activation of the sympathoadrenal system under both physical and emotional stress. In 1919, while studying soldiers with irritable heart, Wearn and Sturgis [112] demonstrated subjective symptoms resembling anxiety following the injection of epinephrine (E). The subjects' experience of symptoms in this and subsequent related studies has been similar but not identical to anxiety; some subjects experienced no emotional changes [30,92].

Whether circulating CA produce symptoms through effects on the CNS or through subjective perception of peripheral effects remains a complicated question. Historically, the most important study into this question has been that of Schachter and Singer in 1962 [92]. The investigators gave E or placebo under various stimulus conditions and concluded that factors determining physiologic arousal and emotional state were independent of each other but each related to situational cues.

The theoretic importance of this study cannot be overlooked for it emphasizes the intimate relationship between cognition and the biologic state of the organism. Mason [67] showed that experimentally induced changes in NE and E in monkeys were related to cognitive factors and coping potential. Animals alerted to the possibility of an unpleasant event showed a different pattern of increase in CA than did those not cued to the upcoming event. Similarly, training alters the E response in humans to parachute jumping: the more trained jumper shows less increase in urinary E than does the beginner [70].

The relationship between anxiety symptoms and increased urinary and plasma CA is well documented [31,61,66,93]. Plasma and cerebrospinal fluid (CSF) CA are elevated in anxious depressed patients [83,121] as well as in patients with generalized anxiety disorder [69] and panic disorder [72]. These levels correlate with ratings of the anxiety symptoms. Most circulating CA, however, are derived from peripheral sources and indicate sympathetic nervous system (SNS) function [59]. Therefore, whether this represents a correlation with a specific psychiatric disorder or rather a generalized indicator of arousal, physical activity, or stress is unclear. Support for the central noradrenergic connection to anxiety derives from studies of 3-methoxy-4-hydroxyphenylethylene glycol (MHPG), a better indicator of central noradrenergic turnover than urinary or plasma NE levels. CSF MHPG is elevated in normal anxiety [3]. Ko et al [58] found elevated plasma MHPG after panic attacks in phobic anxious patients, which correlated with the signs and symptoms of the attack. These MHPG findings support the hypothesis of a central noradrenergic role in anxiety disorders.

The effect of environmental stimuli on changes in CA has been studied both in adults and in developing animals, relating thus to both state and trait anxiety. Thoa et al [107] showed significant changes in CA concentrations in the cingulate cortex, enthorhinal cortex, and the nucleus amygdaloidus centralis in adolescent animals subjected to prolonged isolation. These three areas are part of the limbic system, the major CNS structure mediating emotions. Different stressors produce different alterations in levels of central biogenic amines. Alterations in the central NE in response to different stressors may be particularly important in exposure to severe stress [91] (see Chapters 2 and 3).

The effect of early developmental events on later peripheral and CNS CA activity has been studied in animal models. In mice the combined stress of maternal separation during infancy and isolation after weaning reduces the activity of adrenal tyrosine hydroxylase (TH) and phenylethanolamine N-methyltransferase (PNMT). Animals that are group housed after weaning show increased activity of TH and PNMT. In these studies, the combination of infant manipulation and later isolation produced significant enzyme reductions [2,46]. In a series of experiments, Pfeiffer [79,80,81] showed that rats handled during the first 20 days of life had lower TH activity levels in adulthood than did animals who were not handled. Differences in adaptive changes in TH activity between handled and nonhandled animals were also seen in adult animals following exposure to shock, cold, heat and reserpine. After 3 days of electric shock, handled animals returned more quickly to baseline TH levels than did nonhandled animals. Curiously, confinement to the shock apparatus without shock is sufficient to elevate enzyme activity in the previously handled animals [79,80,81]. Further evidence of the relationship of CA to the history of an animal's conditioning was obtained by Lane et al [60]. Animals originally trained to the same variable interval, 1-minute food schedule but with one group using foot shock and the other a tone, had different levels of CA and serotonin (5-hydroxytryptamine; 5-HT) in various brain regions 5 days or more after the last conditioning. Thus animals exhibiting the same behavior but with different conditioning histories showed different central CA profiles.

Lactate has a well-documented but unclear relationship to anxiety disorders. Pitts and McClure [82] observed that a number of studies reported elevated levels of lactate production on standard exercise in patients with anxiety neurosis. They showed that anxiety symptoms and anxiety attacks could be produced in patients with anxiety neurosis by the infusion of lactate. These symptoms were prevented by the addition of calcium to the lactate. Intravenous administration of disodium-ethylenediaminetetraacetic acid (EDTA), a powerful calcium-binding agent, however, does not produce panic attacks. Liebowitz [62] found a higher plasma NE level prior to lactate infusion in those panic disorder patients who experienced a panic attack with the infusion. Plasma NE did not go up during the panic attack, and acute β-blockade did not affect the panic attacks. He induced a panic attack in 72% of panic disorder patients using Pitts [82] protocol. Imipramine and desipramine blocked the lactate-induced panic [62,88]. Rainey et al [85] found evidence that panic disorder subjects will also develop panic attacks after infusion of isoproterenol, a β-adrenergic agonist.

Propranolol has been shown in several studies to effectively treat the symptoms of anxiety disorders [43,53,106]. The psychological symptoms, unlike the somatic, may only respond at higher dosages (40 mg, four times a day), possibly indicating a central effect at these dosages [53]. Both monoamine oxidase (MAO) inhibitors and imipramine are clinically effective in treating panic disorders and agoraphobia [54–57,90,97,108]. The response of panic and anxiety disorder patients to these noradrenergically active agents, both in clinical practice and under lactate infusion, suggests noradrenergic mechanisms in the production of anxiety disorders.

In the late 1960s and early 1970s, interest focused on CNS noradrenergic pathways. Noradrenergic neurons represent less than 1% of all cells in the brain in contrast to γ-aminobutyric acid (GABA) (55%) and acetylcholine (ACH) (25%) and as such might reasonably be assumed to have a specific function. More than half of all the noradrenergic cell bodies are located in the locus coeruleus (LC). Novel stimuli and noxious stimuli cause firing of these cells. Stimulation of the LC in monkeys creates behavior which looks like fear; ablation leads to a loss of the usual fear response [49,87]. In humans, stimulation induces feelings of fear, and death [71]. Pharmacologic activation of NE cell firing by piperoxane and yohimbine elicits an increase in fear-associated behavior in the restrained monkey [86] and in humans [38,48,102]. However, some reports based on lesion studies using 6-hydroxydopamine question the role of the locus in anxiety [28,68].

Tricyclic antidepressants and benzodiazepines appear to decrease activity of central noradrenergic neurons [1,42,74]. Tricyclic antidepressants and MAO inhibitors may decrease panic symptoms by increasing the NE content at the sites of presynaptic noradrenergic receptors, thereby inhibiting the LC [1]. However, other neurotransmitters are also affected by these drugs. Clinically, clonidine, an alpha-2 agonist which in lower dosages decreases CNS NE, reduces the firing rate of LC cells [13,104] and blocks panic attacks in humans, at least to some extent [47,72]. Both clonidine and imipramine lower plasma MHPG concentrations; failure to show decreased MHPG levels correlates with a lack of clinical response to these drugs [72]. Clonidine is also reported to decrease opiate withdrawal symptoms which are clinically very similar to anxiety symptoms [37,111] and may be mediated by the noradrenergic system. Charney et al [76] found oral yohimbine caused increases in plasma MHPG that correlated with increases in subject-rated anxiety in normal controls, patients with depression, and patients with panic disorder. Pretreatment with clonidine or diazepam prevented the yohimbine-induced anxiety but only clonidine blocked the associated increase in MHPG. The researchers speculated that diazepam may reduce anxiety by a non-noradrenergic mechanism.

MITRAL VALVE PROLAPSE

Beginning in the early nineteenth century, the relationship between anxiety and the heart came under scientific scrutiny. In times of war the link between organic and functional disturbances of the heart was evident. In 1871, DaCosta described "irritable heart" as valvular disease with no murmurs. His description included symptoms of cardiac pain, shortness of breath, rapid pulse, and palpitations. DaCosta felt the causes were most likely to be overactivity and excitement. Throughout the wars of the past century, the name changed but the interest in the relationship between anxiety and cardiac symptoms remained [100]. Gorlin's [39] hyperkinetic heart syndrome and Frohlich et al's [33] hyperdynamic β-adrenergic circulatory state are more recent attempts to focus on this same relationship.

The long history of study into the "head and heart" relationship [100] makes it clear that there are many possible mechanisms of interaction. The intimate relationship between neuropsychologic and cardiac function is well established. Stress [95,113,115], personality style [36,89], and anxiety and depression [9,10,26] all potentially relate to the development or worsening of cardiac conditions. Alterations in peripheral autonomic nervous system output appear to be the major mechanism mediating psychological and cardiac function. Centrally mediated alterations in endocrine function and plasma biochemistry (e.g., fatty acids, cholesterol) may also be important. Cardiac effects are clearly caused by both physiologic and cognitive (symbolic) stressors [117].

Mitral valve prolapse (MVP) is the latest of cardiac conditions to come under scrutiny in terms of its relationship to neuropsychological function (Table 4.3). In MVP, there is a systolic prolapse of one or both of the mitral valve leaflets from their normal position to various points in the left atrial cavity. Many patients with MVP are asymptomatic. The most common complaint is atypical chest pain, but fatigue, dyspnea, palpitations, and light-headedness are often present.

Table 4.3 Clinical Features of Mitral Valve Prolapse

Midsystolic click
Mid-to-late systolic nonejection murmur
Mid-to-late systolic posterior buckling of mitral leaflet on echocardiograph
Chest pain
Palpitations
Arrhythmias
Cerebral ischemic events

The single most characteristic auscultatory abnormality is the presence of a midsystolic nonejection click [27]. A mid-to-late systolic murmur may also be present. Characteristically, the location and intensity of the click and murmur change with the patient's position and with psychological stress [19]. Patients with MVP may have both the click and murmur, one or the other, or neither. The diagnosis of MVP requires either angiography or echocardiography. MVP has a reported prevalance of 4 to 17% of the population and is more common in women than in men [4,24,29,45,51,63]. Individuals with MVP are at increased risk for cardiac arrhythmias, cerebral vascular accidents secondary to microemboli [5], and possibly for sudden death [27,65,84,94,98].

A large number of psychoneurotic symptoms have been reported in patients with MVP [19,45,99,105]. Venkatesh et al [110] reported that 38% of 21 patients with anxiety neurosis also had MVP compared to 10% of controls. Pariser et al [75,76], Gorman et al [41], and Grunhaus et al [44] noted a similarly high prevalence of MVP in panic disorder patients. One report has linked MVP to endogenous depression presenting as gastrointestinal complaints [50]. In 65 patients with MVP, Kane et al [52] did not find an increased frequency of panic disorder, perhaps owing to the relatively small number of subjects for a disease with a prevalence of only 5%. His data do indicate that the majority of individuals with MVP do not have panic or phobic disorders and tend to look like other cardiac referrals on psychiatric symptoms reports. The impaired exercise tolerance demonstrated in anxiety neurosis may be attributable to the subgroup of anxiety disorder patients with MVP [22].

The relationship between MVP and panic or anxiety disorders is not clear. Both panic disorder patients with and without MVP respond to lactate with a panic attack treatable with imipramine [40,41]. Most interestingly, one patient with MVP but not panic disorder experienced panic attacks after lactate infusion [109]. Such single cases, also present in the control groups of other studies, highlight the question of MVP as a predictor of future panic disorder. Because most MVP patients do not have panic attacks, however, it seems unlikely that it is causatively related to panic disorder. Both MVP and panic disorder may be related to an underlying autonomic nervous system dysfunction.

Increased levels of urinary and plasma CA are reported in symptomatic MVP patients [7,77,120]. MVP patients with a prolonged Q-T interval on electrocardiogram (ECG) have the highest plasma CA levels [84]. Propranolol is frequently the treatment of choice for MVP, thought to be effective because of β-adrenergic receptor blockade. An autonomic dysfunction seems the most likely explanation of the altered CA levels in MVP [35,120]. Panic attacks and excessive increases in heart rate have been observed in patients with MVP when isoproterenol was infused [15]. These responses to the infusion of isoproteronol are similar to the findings of Frohlich et al [33,34] and Easton and Sherman [25] in the hyperdynamic β-adrenergic heart syndrome. Frohlich found 9 of 14 patients had a "hysterical outburst," similar to a panic attack, and an increased heart rate response after isoproterenol infusion, which he interpreted as being caused by a heightened β-adrenergic responsiveness. These outbursts could not be replicated with atropine and were blocked by propranolol. The data indicating some form of autonomic dysfunction in MVP are considerable; however, the exact nature and location of this disturbance remains undetermined.

CONCLUSIONS

The anxiety disorders are currently exciting areas of research involving both central and peripheral nervous system mechanisms. Generalized anxiety disorder and panic disorder are the major areas of present interest. The association of MVP with panic disorder has aroused interest in the common origins of these two syndromes. The role of anxiety in its other clinical forms—physical disease (e.g., gastrointestinal) and phobias—warrants further exploration. The clarification of the relationship between anxiety and depression, which both clinically and in the adrenergic theories of anxiety are closely related, holds promise of new theoretic ground.

The epidemiology of the anxiety disorders requires reexamination using present-day nomenclature. Panic disorder, a more discrete syndrome than generalized anxiety disorder, may be more easily explored epidemiologically. The clinical presentation and pharmacologic treatment of panic disorder and generalized anxiety disorder are frequently not as distinct as the diagnostic nomenclature might suggest. In the clinical setting, phobic conditions are frequently intertwined with these syndromes. In most laboratory models of anxiety, physiologic responses rather than cognitive variables are most prominent; as such they more resemble panic disorder. The role of cognitive function as the mediator of anxiety, most clearly seen in phobias, requires further exploration.

Cardiac responses associated with anxiety disorders require accurate definition and diagnosis to explore the interface of the heart and brain. The diagnosis of MVP can be totally accurate only at autopsy; angiography is the definitive clinical diagnostic test. Short of this, the typical echocardiographic findings accompanied with the auscultatory findings provide the best probability of a definite diagnosis. To date, no distinction has been found between panic attacks with or without MVP, either on challenge testing or pharmacologic treatment.

Considerable evidence has been collected in animal models and human subjects linking noradrenergic activity to anxiety. Measures of circulating CA and central CA activity are elevated in subjects exposed to anxiety-producing settings and in anxiety disorder patients. Pharmacologic and electrical stimulation of the major site of noradrenergic neurons in the brain, the LC elicits fear and anxiety symptoms. Lesions of the LC in animals block these responses. More support for the role of CA in these disorders comes from the clinical arena. Further pharmacologic dissection of central brain mechanisms related to the LC will clarify the role of this structure in anxiety. All anxiolytic agents used clinically have noradrenergic activity, but the different and at times conflicting mechanisms of noradrenergic activity of these agents makes a simple model of action difficult. Recent findings of benzodiazepine receptors [103] and primate anxietylike responses to β-carboline [73] require further examination in the light of the data on LC function and the clinical utility of noradrenergically active drugs. Inhibition of central noradrenergic firing through different mechanisms (e.g., GABA receptors, α_2 stimulation) may be the factor linking the pharmacologically useful treatments for anxiety disorders.

The mechanism of lactate-inducted panic attacks is unclear. No animal studies with lactate and LC measures have been done. Measures of MHPG before and after lactate-induced panic attacks would help clarify any effect lactate may have on central noradrenergic activity. The possibility that lactate induces fear behavior in animals conditioned to this behavior can be investigated, as well as the effects of lactate on locus firing. At present, the lactate infusion is not useful as a clinical test because it has not been standardized and verified on appropriate populations. However, it may in the future provide a systematic guide to pharmacologic intervention in complicated cases.

The association of MVP with noradrenergic hyperactivity as measured by plasma CA is clear; however, the nature of this association is not. No animal models of MVP are known. Patients with MVP and panic attacks respond similarly to non MVP panic disorder subjects under both provocation and treatment. Measures of MHPG in MVP patients might help identify central noradrenergic dysfunction. Panic attacks after lactate or isoproterenol infusion in MVP patients without a previous diagnosis of panic disorder have not been systematically studied. If MVP is found to be an indicator of autonomic dysfunction, panic attacks in MVP patients would be expected without a diagnosis of panic disorder. Thus MVP would serve as a predictor of possible future panic attacks. Longitudinal studies of asymptomatic MVP patients, including measures of CA activity, may clarify the temporal relationship between MVP, panic disorder, and noradrenergic dysfunction.

One of the intriguing sidelights of the adrenergic studies of anxiety has been the findings of the relationship of conditioning history to changes in both central and peripheral adrenergic function. Klein's [55] clinical proposal concerning early separations in humans as predisposing the brain to certain modes of functioning and biochemical constitution—and presumably to different drug responses—may bring together clinical and laboratory findings. Similarly, the clinical observation that the presence of a trusted other raises an individual's threshold to panic suggests again that environmental manipulation can alter brain structures and functions related to anxiety. The exploration of the mechanisms mediating this interaction of environment and biology may be furthered by studies in primate laboratories.

REFERENCES

1. Aghajanian GK, Cedarbaum JM, Wang RY. Evidence for norepinephrine-mediated collateral inhibition of LC neurone. Brain Res 136:570–577, 1977.
2. Axelrod J, Mueller RA, Henry JP, Stephens PM. Changes in enzymes involved in biosynthesis and metabolism of noradrenaline and adrenaline after psychosocial stimulation. Nature 225:1059, 1970.
3. Ballenger JC, Post RM, Jimerson D, Lake CR, Lerner P, Bunney W, Goodwin FK. Cerebrospinal fluid and noradrenergic correlations with normal anxiety. Syllabus and Scientific Proceedings of the American Psychiatric Association Annual Meeting, p 235. Washington, DC: American Psychiatric Association, 1981.
4. Barlow JB, Pacock WA. The problem of nonejection systolic clicks and associated mitral systolic murmurs: emphasis on the bellowing mitral leaflet syndrome. Am Heart J 90:636–655, 1975.
5. Barnett M. Mitral valve prolapse and stroke. Presented to the annual meeting of the American Neurological Association, Washington, DC, Sept 22–24, 1978.
6. Beard GM. Neurasthenia or nervous exhaustion. Boston Med Surg J 3:217–221, 1869.
7. Boudoulas H, Reynolds JC, Mazzaferri E, Wooley C. Metabolic studies in mitral valve prolapse syndrome. Circulation 61:1200–1205, 1980.
8. Brown F. Heredity in psychoneuroses. Proc R Soc Med 35:785–799, 1942.
9. Bruhn JG, Chandler B, Wolf S. A psychological study of survivors and non-survivors of myocardial infarction. J Psychosom Med 31:8–19, 1969.
10. Bruhn JG, Parades A, Adsett AC, Wolf S. Psychological predictors of sudden death in myocardial infarction. J Psychosom Res 18:187–191, 1974.
11. Cannon WB, de la Paz B. Emotional stimulation of adrenal secretion. Am J Physiol 28:64–70, 1911.
12. Carey G, Gottesman I. Twin and Family Studies of Anxiety, Phobic and Obsessive Disorders. In Anxiety: New Research and Changing Concepts, DE Klein and JG Rabkin (eds), 117–136. New York: Raven Press, 1981.
13. Cedarbaum JM, Aghajanian GK. Noradrenergic neurons of the locus coeruleus: Inhibition by epinephrine and activation by the alpha antagonist piperoxane. Brain Res 112:413–419, 1976.
14. Charney DS, Heninger GR, Redmond DE. Noradrenergic function in human anxiety states. New Research Abstracts, No. 96. Washington, DC: American Psychiatric Association Press, 1983.
15. Clark R, Boudoulas H, Schaal S, Schmidt H. Adrenergic hyperactivity and cardiac abnormality in primary disorders of sleep. Neurology (NY) 30:113–119, 1980.
16. Cloninger CR, Martin PL, Clayton P, Guze S. A Blind Follow-up and Family Study of Anxiety Neurosis: Preliminary Analysis of the St. Louis 500. In Anxiety: New Research and Changing Concepts, DE Klein and JG Rabkin (eds), 137–154. New York: Raven Press, 1981.
17. Cohen M, White P. Life situations, emotions and neurocirculatory asthenia (anxiety neurosis, neurasthenia effort syndrome). Res Proc Assoc Res Nerv Ment Dis 29:832–869, 1950.
18. Cohen ME, Badal DW, Kilpatrick A, Reed EW, White D. The high familial prevalence of neurocirculatory asthenia. Am J Hum Genet 3:126–158, 1951.
19. Coombs R, Shah P, Shulman R, Klorman R, Sylvester L. Effects of psychological

stress on click and rhythms in mitral valve prolapse. American Heart Association, Monograph No. 56, (No. 57, Part II):III:111, 1977.

20. Coryell W, Noyes R, Clancy J. Excess mortality in panic disorders. Arch Gen Psychiatry 37:701–703, 1982.
21. Crowe RR, Pauls DL, Slymen DJ, Noyes R. A family study of anxiety neurosis. Arch Gen Psychiatry 37:77–79, 1980.
22. Crowe RR, Pauls DL, Venkatesh A, Van Valkenburg C, Noyes R, Martins JB, Kerber RE. Exercise and anxiety neurosis: Comparison of patients with and without mitral valve prolapse. Arch Gen Psychiatry 36:652–653, 1979.
23. DaCosta JM. On irritable heart, a clinical form of functional cardiac disorder and its consequences. Am J Med Sci 61:17, 1871.
24. Darsee JR, Mikolich JR, Nicholoff NB, Lesser LE. Prevalence of mitral valve prolapse in presumably healthy young men. Circulation 59:619–622, 1979.
25. Easton DJ, Sherman DG. Somatic anxiety attacks and propranolol. Arch Neurol 33:689–691, 1976.
26. Engel G. Psychologic stress, vasodepressor (vasovagal) syncope and sudden death. Ann Intern Med 89:403–412, 1978.
27. Engel P, Hickman J. Mitral valve prolapse—a review. Aviat Space Environ Med 51:273–286, 1980.
28. File SE, Deakin JF, Longden A, Crow TJ. An investigation of the role of the LC in anxiety and agonistic behavior. Brain Res 169:411–420, 1979.
29. Fontana M, Pence H, Leighton R, Wooley C. The varying clinical spectrum of the systolic click-late systolic murmur syndrome. Circulation 41:807–816, 1970.
30. Frankenhaeuser M. Experimental Approaches to the Study of Catecholamines and Emotion. In Emotions: Their Parameters and Measurement, L Levi (ed), 209–234. New York: Raven Press, 1975.
31. Frankenhaeuser M. Behavior and circulating catecholamines. Brain Res 31:241–262, 1971.
32. Freud S. On the Reasons for Detaching a Particular Syndrome from Neurasthenia Under the Description of "Anxiety Neurosis." In Standard Edition of the Complete Psychological Works of Sigmund Freud, Vol. 3, J Strachey (ed), p. 90. London: Hogarth Press, 1962.
33. Frohlich ED, Dustan HP, Page DH. Hyperdynamic beta-adrenergic circulatory state. Arch Intern Med 117:614–619, 1966.
34. Frohlich ED, Tarazi RC, Dustan HP. Hyperadrenergic circulatory state. Arch Intern Med 126:1–7, 1969.
35. Gaffney FA, Karlsson ES, Campbell W, Schutte JE, Nixon JV, Willerson JT, Blomquist CG. Autonomic dysfunction in women with mitral valve prolapse syndrome. Circulation 59:894–901, 1979.
36. Garrity TF, Somes GW, Marx M. Personality factors in resistance to illness after recent life changes. J Psychosom Res 21:23–32, 1977.
37. Gold MS, Redmond DE, Jr, Kleber HD. Noradrenergic hyperactivity in opiate withdrawal supported by clonidine reversal of opiate withdrawal. Am J Psychiatry 136:100–102, 1979.
38. Goldenberg M, Snyder CH, Aranow H, Jr. New test for hypertension due to circulating epinephrine. JAMA 135:971–976, 1947.
39. Gorlin R. The hyperkinetic heart syndrome. JAMA 182:823–829, 1962.

40. Gorman JM, Fyer AD, Glicklich J, King D, Klein D. Effect of sodium lactate on patients with panic disorder and mitral valve prolapse. Am J Psychiatry 138:247–249, 1981.
41. Gorman JM, Fyer AF, Glicklich J, King D, Klein D. Mitral valve prolapse and panic disorders: Effect of imipramine. In Anxiety: New Research and Changing Concepts, DF Klein and J Rabkin (eds), 317–326. New York: Raven Press, 1981.
42. Grant SJ, Huang YH, Redmund DE Jr. Benzodiazepines attenuate single unit activity in LC. Life Sci 27:2231–2236, 1980.
43. Granville-Grossman KL, Turner P. The effect of propranolol on anxiety. Lancet ii:788–790, 1960.
44. Grunhaus L, Golger S, Rein A, Lewis B. Mitral valve prolapse and panic attacks. Israel J Med Sci 18:221–223, 1982.
45. Hancock EW, Cohn K. The syndrome associated with mid-systolic click and late systolic murmur. Am J Med 41:183–196, 1966.
46. Henry JP, Stephens PM, Axelrod J, Mueller RA. Effect of psychosocial stimulation on the enzymes involved in the biosynthesis and metabolism of noradrenaline and adrenaline. Psychosom Med 33:227, 1971.
47. Hoehn-Saric R, Merchant A, Keyser M, Smith V. Effects of clonidine on anxiety disorders. Arch Gen Psychiatry 38:1278–1282, 1981.
48. Holmberg G, Gershon S. Autonomic and psychic effects of yohimbine hydrochloride. Psychopharmacology (Berlin) 2:93–116, 1961.
49. Huang YH, Redmond DE, Snyder DR, Mass JW. In vivo location and destruction of the LC in the stumptail macaque (*Macaca arctoides*). Brain Res 100:157–162, 1975.
50. Jean-Louis P. Click syndrome and late midsystolic murmur (idiopathic mitral valve prolapse) and endogenous (unipolar) depression: probable genetic association. Lyon Med 238:543–544, 1977.
51. Jeresaty R. Mitral valve prolapse–click syndrome. Prog Cardiovasc Dis 15:623–652, 1973.
52. Kane JM, Woerner M, Zeldie S, Kramer R, Saraway S. Panic and Phobic Disorders in Patients with Mitral Valve Prolapse. In Anxiety: New Research and Changing Concepts, DF Klein and J Rabkin (eds), 327–340. New York: Raven Press, 1981.
53. Kathol RG, Noyes R Jr, Slymen DJ, Crowe RR, Clancy J, Kerber R. Propranolol in chronic anxiety disorder. Arch Gen Psychiatry 37:1361–1365, 1980.
54. Kelly D, Guirgois W, Frommer E, Mitchell-Heggs N, Sargant W. Treatment of phobic states with antidepressants. Br J Psychiatry 116:387–398, 1970.
55. Klein D. Anxiety Reconceptualized. In Anxiety: New Research and Changing Concepts, DE Klein and JG Rabkin (eds), 235–263. New York: Raven Press, 1981.
56. Klein DF, Fink M. Psychiatric reaction patterns to imipramine. Am J Psychiatry 119:432–438, 1962.
57. Kline NS. Drug treatment of phobic disorders. Am J Psychiatry 123:1447–1450, 1967.
58. Ko G, Elsworth J, Roth R, Rifkin BG, Leigh H, Redmond DE, Jr. Panic induced elevation of plasma MHPG levels in phobic-anxious patients: Effects of clonidine and imipramine. Arch Gen Psychiatry 40:425–430, 1983.
59. Kopin I, Lake CR, Ziegler MG. Plasma levels of norepinephrine. Ann Intern Med 88:671–680, 1978.
60. Lane J, Sands M, Co C, Cherek DD, Smith JR. Biogenic amine turnover in discrete

rat brain regions as correlated with conditioned emotional response and its conditioning history. Brain Res 240:95–108, 1982.

61. Levi L. Stress and distress in response to psychosocial stimuli. Acta Psychiatr Scand [Suppl] 528:1–157, 1972.
62. Liebowitz M. Biochemical precipitation of panic attacks: Cardiovascular aspects of vulnerability provocation and blockade. Presented at Psychiatry-Cardiology Interface: a Clinical Challenge. Columbia University Symposium, American Psychiatric Association Annual Meeting, New York, April 30–May 6, 1983.
63. Markiewicz W, Stoner J, London E, Hunt S, Popp R. Mitral valve prolapse in one hundred presumably healthy young females. Circulation 53:464–473, 1976.
64. Marks I, Lader M. Anxiety states (anxiety neurosis): a review. J Nerv Ment Dis 156:3–18, 1973.
65. Marshall CE, Shoppell SD. Sudden death and the ballooning posterior leaflet syndrome. Arch Pathol 98:134–138, 1974.
66. Mason JW. A review of psychoendocrine research on the sympathetic adrenal medullary system. Psychosom Med 30:613–653, 1968.
67. Mason JW. Emotion as Reflected in Patterns of Endocrine Integration. In Emotions: Their Parameters and Measurements, L Levi (ed), pp. 143–181. New York: Raven Press, 1975.
68. Mason ST, Roberts DCS, Fibiger HC. Noradrenaline and neophobia. Physiol Behav 21:353–361, 1978.
69. Mathew RJ, Ho BT, Kralik P, Taylor DL, Clayhorn JL. Catecholamines and monoamine oxidase activity in anxiety. Acta Psychiatr Scand 63:245–252, 1981.
70. Mikulaj L, Kvetnansky R, Murgas K, Parizkova J, Vencel P. Catecholamines and Corticosteroids in Acute and Repeated Stress. In Catecholamines and Stress, E Usdin, R Kvetnansky, and I Kopin (eds), 445–459. New York: Pergamon Press, 1976.
71. Nashold BS, Wilson WP, Slaughter P. The Midbrain and Pain. In Advances in Neurology, John J Bonica (ed), vol. 4, 191–196. New York: Raven Press, 1974.
72. Nesse R, Cameron O, Curtis G, McCann D. Adrenergic function in panic disorder. New Research Abstracts, No. 56, Washington, DC: American Psychiatric Association Press, 1983.
73. Ninan P, Insel TR, Cohen RM, Skolnick P, Paul SM. A benzodiazepine receptor mediated model of anxiety. Science 218:1332, 1982.
74. Nybeck H, Walters JR, Aghajanian GK, Roth RH. Tricyclic antidepressants: Effects on firing rate of brain noradrenergic neurons. Eur J Pharmacol 32:302–312, 1975.
75. Pariser SF, Jones BA, Pinta E, Young EA, Fontana ME. Panic attack: Diagnostic evaluations of 17 patients. Am J Psychiatry 136:105–106, 1979.
76. Pariser SF, Pinta E, Jones B. Mitral valve prolapse syndrome and anxiety neurosis/panic disorder. Am J Psychiatry 135:246–247, 1978.
77. Pasternac A, Tubau JF, Puddu P, Krol RB, Champlain J. Increased plasma catecholamine levels in patients with symptomatic mitral valve prolapse. Am J Med 73:783–790, 1982.
78. Pauls DL, Bucher KD, Crowe RR, Noyes R. A genetic study of panic disorder pedigrees. Am J Hum Genet 32:639–644, 1980.
79. Pfeiffer WD. Modification of Adrenal Tyrosine Activity in Rats Following Manipulation in Infancy. In Catecholamines and Stress, E Usdin, R Kvetnansky, and I Kopin (eds), 265–270. New York: Pergamon Press, 1976.

80. Pfeiffer WD, Davis LC. Effects of handling in infancy on responsiveness of adrenal tyrosine hydroxylase in maturity. Behav Biol 10:239–245, 1974.
81. Pfeiffer WD, Denenberg VH, Zarrow NX. Decreased tyrosine hydroxylase activity in the adrenal gland of adult rats that were handled in infancy. Physiol Behav 10:411–413, 1973.
82. Pitts FN, Jr, McClure JN, Jr. Lactate metabolism in anxiety neurosis. N Engl J Med 227:1329–1336, 1967.
83. Post RM, Lake CR, Jimerson D, Bunney WE, Wood JH, Ziegler MG, Goodwin FK. Cerebrospinal fluid norepinephrine in affective illness. Am J Psychiatry 135:907–912, 1978.
84. Puddu PE, Tubau JF, Krol R, deChamplain J, Pasternac A. Prolonged QT interval and autonomic inbalance: A clue for the prevention of sudden death in mitral valve prolapse. Am J Cardiol 47:480, 1981.
85. Rainey JM, Pohl RB, Williams M, Kniiter E, Freedman R, Ettedgui E. A Comparison of Lactate and Isoproterenol Anxiety States. Presented at Seventh World Congress of Psychiatry. Vienna, Austria, 1983.
86. Redmond DE, Huang YH. New evidence for a locus coeruleus–norepinephrine connection with anxiety. Life Sci 25:2149–2162, 1979.
87. Redmond DE, Huang YH, Snyder DR, Maas JW. The behavioral effects of stimulation of the LC in the stumptail monkey (*Macaca arctoides*). Brain Res 116:502–510, 1975.
88. Rifkin A, Klein D, Dillon D, Levitt M. Blockade by imipramine or desipramine of panic induced by sodium lactate. Am J Psychiatry 138:676–677, 1981.
89. Rosenman RH, Brand RG, Jenkins CD, Freidman M, Straus R, Wurm M. Coronary heart disease in the Western Collaborative Group Study: A final follow-up experience of 8½ years. JAMA 233:872–877, 1975.
90. Roth M, Meyers DH. Anxiety neurosis and phobic states. II. Diagnosis and management. Br Med J 1:559–562, 1969.
91. Saito H, Morita A, Miyazaki I, Takagi K. Comparison of the Effects of Various Stresses on Biogenic Amines of the Central Nervous System and Animal Symptoms. In Catecholamines and Stress, E Usdin, R Kvetnansky, and I Kopin (eds), 95–103. New York: Pergamon Press, 1976.
92. Schachter S, Singer JE. Cognitive, social, and physiological determinants of emotional state. Psychol Rev 69:379–399, 1962.
93. Schildkraut JJ, Kety SS. Biogenic amines and emotion. Science 156:21–30, 1967.
94. Schwartz MH, Teichholz, LE, and Donoso E. Mitral valve prolapse: A review of associated arrhythmias. Am J Med 62:377–389, 1977.
95. Schwartz PJ, Stone HL. The role of the autonomic nervous system in sudden coronary death. Ann NY Acad Sci 382:162–181, 1971.
96. Sheehan DV. Panic attacks and phobias. N Engl J Med 307:156–158, 1982.
97. Sheehan DV, Ballenger J, Jacobsen G. Treatment of endogenous anxiety with phobic hysterical and hypochondriacal symptoms. Arch Gen Psychiatry 37:51–58, 1980.
98. Shoppell S, Marshall C, Brown R, Bruce T. Sudden death and the familial occurrence of mid-systolic click, late systolic murmur syndrome. Circulation 48:1128–1134, 1973.
99. Shoppell S, Orr W, Gwynn C. The ballooning posterior leaflet syndrome: MMPI profiles in symptomatic and asymptomatic groups. Chest 66:690–692, 1974.
100. Skerritt PW. Anxiety and the heart—a historical review. Psychol Med 13:17–25, 1983.
101. Slater B, Shields J. Genetic aspects of anxiety. Br J Psychiatry Special Publication No. 3, Studies of Anxiety, 62–71. Ashford, Kent, Engl: Headley Bros, 1969.

102. Soffer A. Regitine and benodaine in the diagnosis of pheochromocytoma. Med Clin North Am 387:375–385, 1954.
103. Squires RF, Braestrup C. Benzodiazepine receptors in rat brain. Nature 266:732–734, 1977.
104. Svensson TH, Bunney BS, Aghajanian GK. Inhibition of both noradrenergic and serotonergic neurons in brain by the alpha-adrenergic agonist clonidine. Brain Res 92:291–306, 1975.
105. Szmiulowicz J, Flanney J. Mitral valve prolapse syndrome and psychological disturbance. Psychosomatics 21:419–421, 1980.
106. Tanna VT, Penningroth RP, Woolson RF. Propranolol in the treatment of anxiety neurosis. Compr Psychiatry 18:319–326, 1977.
107. Thoa NB, Tizabiy Y, Jacobowitz DM. The Effect of Prolonged Isolation on the Catecholamine and Serotonin Concentration of Discrete Areas of Rat Brain. In Catecholamines and Stress, E Usdin, R Kvetnansky, and I Kopin (eds), 61–67. New York: Pergamon Press, 1976.
108. Tyrer P, Candy J, Kelly DA. A study of the clinical effects of phenelzine and placebo in the treatment of phobic anxiety. Psychopharmacologia (Berlin) 32:237–254, 1973.
109. Ursano R, Lake CR, Chernow B, Zaloga G, Becker B. Unpublished data, 1983.
110. Venkatesh A, Pauls DF, Crowe R, Noyes R, Van Valkemburg C, Martins JF, Kerber RR. Mitral valve prolapse in anxiety neurosis. Clin Res 26:656A, 1978.
111. Washton AM, Resnick BB. Clonidine for opiate detoxification: Outpatient clinical trials. Am J Psychiatry 137:1121–1122, 1980.
112. Wearn JT, Sturgis CC. Studies on epinephrine. I. Effects of the injection of epinephrine in soldiers with "irritable heart." Arch Intern Med 24:247–268, 1919.
113. Weinblatt E, Ruberman W, Goldbers I, Frank CW, Shapiro S, Chaudhary BS. Relation of education to sudden death after myocardial infarction. N Engl J Med 229:60–65, 1978.
114. Wheeler EO, White PD, Reed EW, Cohen ME. Neurocirculatory asthenia. JAMA 142:878–889, 1950.
115. Wheeler EO, White PD, Reed EW, Cohen ME. Familial incidence of neurocirculatory asthenia. J Clin Invest 27:562, 1948.
116. White PD, Jones TD. Heart disease and disorders in New England. Am Heart J 3:302–318, 1928.
117. Wolf S. Cardiovascular reactions to symbolic stimuli. Circulation 18:287–292, 1938.
118. Wood P. DaCosta's Syndrome (or effort syndrome). Br Med J I: 767–772, 805–811, 845–851, 1941.
119. Woodruff RA, Jr, Guze SB, Clayton PJ. Anxiety neurosis among psychiatric outpatients. Compr Psychiatry 13:165–170, 1972.
120. Wooley CF, Reynolds J, Mazzafeiri E. Mitral valve prolapse syndrome—evidence for a hyperadrenergic state. Am J Cardiol 43:368, 1979.
121. Wyatt R, Portnoy B, Kupfer D, Snyder F, Engelman K. Resting plasma catecholamine concentrations in patients with depression and anxiety. Arch Gen Psychiatry 24:65–70, 1971.

5

Central Catecholamine Systems: Interaction with Neurotransmitters in Normal Subjects and in Patients with Selected Neurologic Diseases

Paul F. Teychenne
Giora Feuerstein
C. Raymond Lake
Michael G. Ziegler

The function of cerebral cortex, cerebellar cortex, midbrain and basal ganglia depends on an interplay between many neurotransmitter systems. In Parkinson's disease, Huntington's chorea, migraine and seizure disorders, multiple neurotransmitter systems must be considered, although the clinical expression of each is due to a disorder in predominantly one neurotransmitter system (e.g., Parkinson's disease is mainly due to decreased nigrostriatal dopamine [DA] activity).

NEUROTRANSMITTERS RELATED TO NOREPINEPHRINE IN THE BASAL GANGLIA

Noradrenergic Systems

Noradrenergic projections are divergent, originating from a few thousand cells in the pons and medulla oblongata and innervating the diencephalon, cerebral cortex, cerebellar cortex, and spinal cord. The system mediates general function (e.g., attention, mood, and vigilance) rather than specific sensory information [35,67].

The locus coeruleus (LC) (A6 in Figures 5.1 and 5.2A) (central pontine gray matter, ventral to the fourth ventricle) contains 1500 neurons on each side.

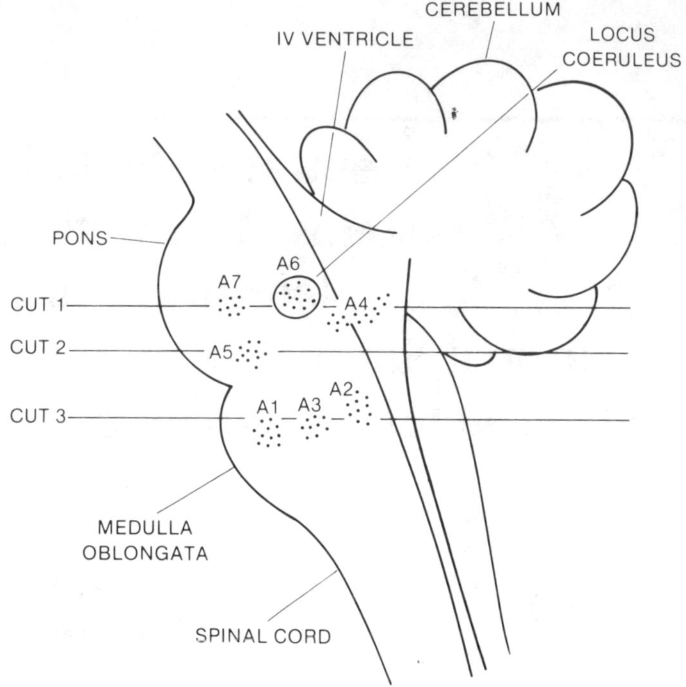

Figure 5.1. Location of noradrenergic neuron cell bodies. Sagittal section of brainstem, pons, and medulla oblongata showing location of the seven groups of noradrenergic cells. Cuts 1, 2, and 3 represent horizontal sections through the noradrenergic cell clusters.

The LC is the major nidus of noradrenergic cells supplying the brain and spinal cord but input arises from these other noradrenergic cells:

1. A4 cells (caudal from LC to floor of fourth ventricle)
2. A7 subcoeruleus neurons (ventral from LC along the medial surface of the fifth motor nucleus to pontine reticular formation in front of superior cerebellar peduncle)
3. A5 cells (lateral tegmentum pons)
4. A1, A2, and A3 cells (lateral tegmentum medulla oblongata)

The A1, A2, A3, A5, and A7 cells (lateral tegmental noradrenergic neurons) are loosely scattered in pons and medulla oblongata and lie outside the LC, but their fibers intermingle with LC axons. Posterior tegmental cells descend to the spinal cord, and anterior tegmental cells ascend to the cerebrum and diencephalon. Most noradrenergic cells project ipsilaterally, though 25% project contralaterally [35].

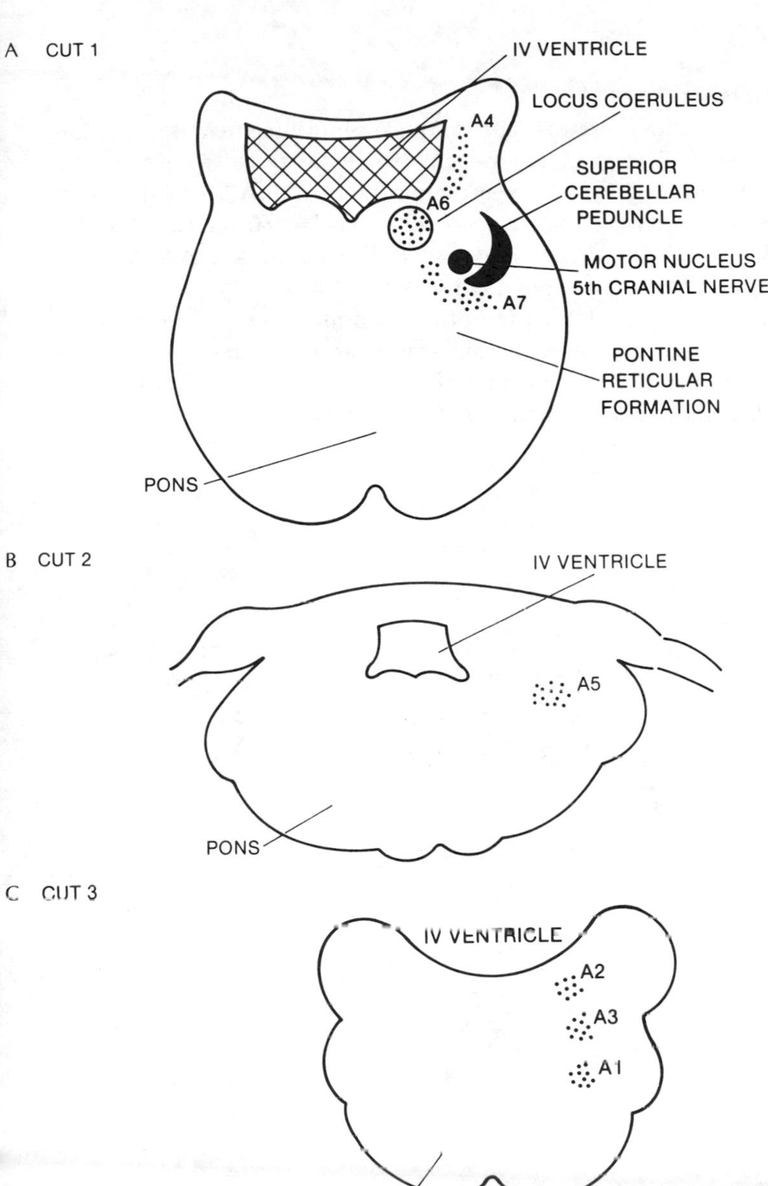

Figure 5.2(A) Noradrenergic neurons are represented on both sides of the brainstem but are shown here only on one side. A4 extends to roof of fourth ventricle, A7 extends into lateral tegmentum of pons. (B) A5 noradrenergic neurons in the lateral tegmentum of the pons. These neurons are present on both sides of the pons but are here represented on one side. (C) Distribution of A1, A2, and A3 noradrenergic neurons in the lateral tegmentum of the medulla oblongata. They are represented here on one side but are present on both sides.

Noradrenergic Tracts

Three ascending pathways exist (Figure 5.3): (1) central tegmental tract (dorsal noradrenergic bundle) from LC; (2) ventral tegmental tract (from A1, A2, A3, A5, A7, and LC); and (3) dorsal periventricular tract (from A2, LC, subcoeruleus). There is also one posterior tract, the coerulocerebellar (from LC, A4, A5, and A7 to cerebellum) and one descending spinal tract (from A1, A2, A5, LC, and subcoeruleus) to brainstem and spinal cord [47].

The dorsal noradrenergic tract supplies the cerebral cortex and branches to the diencephalon. The ventral noradrenergic tract passes to the diencephalon via the medial forebrain bundle. The dorsal periventricular tract supplies the periventricular region, the diencephalon, and the cerebral cortex.

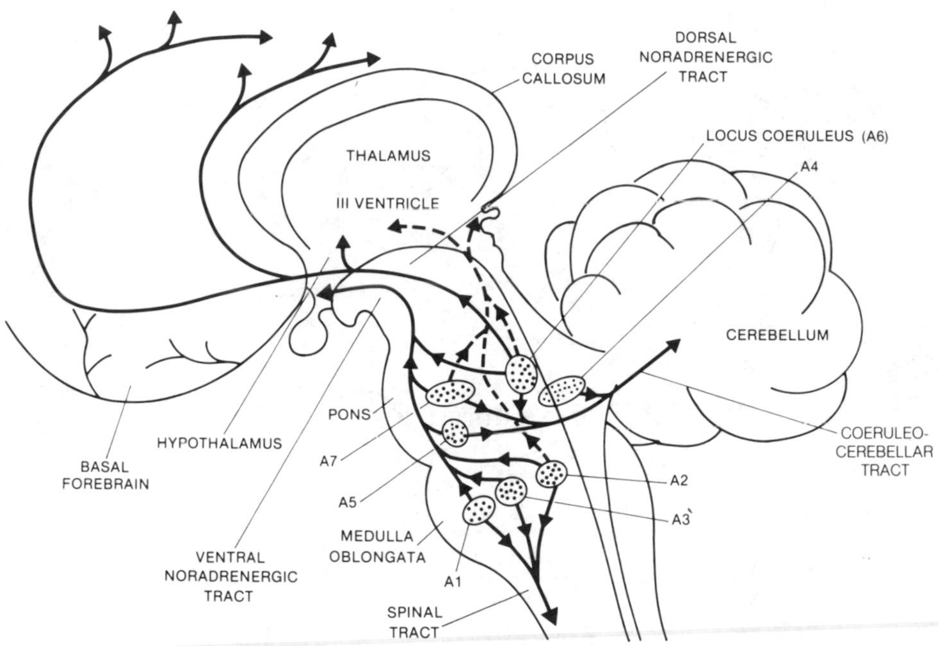

Figure 5.3 The ventral noradrenergic tract (from A1, A2, A3, A5, A6, and A7 noradrenergic neurons) innervates the hypothalamus, basal forebrain, and limbic system. The dorsal noradrenergic tract (from A6 [LC] noradrenergic neurons) branches to the diencephalon and then innervates the cerebral cortex curving over the genu of the corpus callosum to supply the medial cortex and through the frontal lobe to supply the lateral cortex. The spinal tract (from A1, A2, and A3 noradrenergic neurons) passes down to the intermediolateral columns and central gray matter of the spinal cord. The coerulocerebellar tract (from A6, A4, A5, and A7 noradrenergic neurons) passes to the cerebellum. The dorsal periventricular tract (from A2, A6, and A7 noradrenergic neurons) passes to the periventricular area. The LC (A6), subcoeruleus (A7), and A5 also project to the descending spinal tract (not represented in this diagram).

Investigators disagree somewhat on the path of the noradrenergic axons to the cerebral cortex [35,67]. The dorsal noradrenergic tract passes up the ventrolateral reticular formation and curves over the genu of the corpus callosum to the medial cortex, and other noradrenergic neurons pass through the frontal pole and turn back as longitudinal fibers giving off radial terminals to each layer of the lateral cortex.

The diencephalon, amygdaloid cortex, entorhinal cortex, and basal forebrain are supplied by the dorsal and ventral noradrenergic tracts through the medial forebrain bundle [30,35]. The amygdala and basal forebrain are innervated by the LC with collateral branches to the thalamus [35].

A1 cells supply the hypothalamus via the ventral tegmental tract and overlap without topographic organization, in origin or termination, of noradrenergic neurons [75]. A1 fibers connect the autonomic nuclei (tractus solitarius and visceral motor nucleus of the vagus) with the periventricular and supraoptic nuclei of the hypothalamus, thus integrating hypothalamic responses to visceral stimuli and coordinating autonomic and endocrine responses [88]. The solitary tract receives information from atrial stretch receptors, aortic baroreceptors, and carotid body chemoreceptors and helps regulate blood pressure (BP). The A1 and A2 noradrenergic cell clusters also project to the intermediolateral cell column of the spinal cord [56]. The coeruleocerebellar tract passes through the superior and middle cerebellar peduncle (near the fourth ventricle) to the cerebellum carrying mainly ipsilateral but also contralateral input[35,76]. The descending noradrenergic fibers pass by the anterior and lateral columns of the spinal cord to the spinal gray matter. A1, A2, and A5 neurons supply the intermediolateral columns and central gray matter; the LC projects ipsilaterally and contralaterally to the ventral horns [35,40,55]. Noradrenergic fibers synapse beside motoneurons and autonomic preganglionic neurons and influence their action [35]. Subcoeruleus descending fibers innervate reticular formation and cranial nerve nuclei [35].

Function of Noradrenergic Cells

Microiontophoretically applied norepinephrine (NE) and repetitive stimulation of the LC inhibit the spontaneous activity of cerebral cortex, cerebellar cortex, and hippocampus through β-adrenergic receptors [24,74]. NE activates the synthesis of receptor cyclic 3′, 5′ adenosine-monophosphate (cAMP) by activation of β-receptors. The LC inhibits itself through collaterals from its axons acting on α_2-adrenergic autoreceptors [1]. NE, even at doses which do not depress spontaneous activity and LC stimulation, enhances cerebellar γ-aminobutyric acid (GABA) inhibition. NE alters postsynaptic response to other transmitters which directly transfer information [106].

On the left side of the brain, NE concentrations are highest in the motor pulvinar and ventrolateral regions of the left (dominant) thalamus. Cryogenic surgery here relieves dyskinesia and the tremor of parkinsonism. By contrast, ventral posterior lateral and medial nuclei of the right (nondominant) thalamus have the highest concentration of NE, receive the entire somatosensory input, and project to the right parietal cortex, which monitors body image and geographic orientation [73].

Cholinergic drugs (oxotremorine) or acetylcholinesterase inhibitors (physostigmine) increase NE turnover via muscarinic receptors, and oxotremorine stimulates NE synthesis [66]. The LC is inhibited by iontophoretically applied NE and the α_2-adrenergic agonist clonidine, but is excited by acetylcholine [38]. Conversely, decreased forebrain NE blocks the cataleptic effect of muscarinic cholinergic agonists and potentiates the locomotor activity induced by muscarinic cholinergic blockers [60]. Cholinergic receptors may be located on noradrenergic terminals or LC cells [62,95].

EPINEPHRINE SYSTEMS

Nerve cells containing epinephrine (E) as their neurotransmitter have been localized in the rostral part of the reticular formation and are termed the C1 cell cluster. A second group of E cells are located in the dorsolateral part of the medulla oblongata (the C2 cell cluster) [40]. The pathways of these neurons have been mapped by an immunohistofluorescence technique with antibodies raised to adrenal phenylethanolamine-N-methyltransferase (PNMT), which synthesizes E from NE. However, the distribution and morphology of PNMT-containing neurons coincide with some of the CA nerve terminals and cell bodies shown by the Falck-Hillarp technique. Thus, the C1 group shares some of the A1 area of CA cells and the C2 group appears to be identical with the rostral part of the A2 area [50]. The axons of the C1 and C2 cell groups project rostrally to the hypothalamus and caudally to the spinal cord. Some of the C2 group nerve cells are located in the rostral half of the nucleus tractus solitarii (NTS), and E projections are found in the nuclei involved in the baroreceptor reflex arc, NTS, and the dorsal motor nucleus of the vagus. The E-containing cells of both C1 and C2 clusters also project to the intermediolateral cell column of the spinal cord [40]. The distribution of PNMT in the rat brain corresponds to that of E [49]. An E-sensitive adenyl cyclase is present in brain regions surrounding cell bodies containing PNMT [57,104]. SKF 64139, an inhibitor of PNMT, markedly lowers E levels in rat brainstem nuclei [84,87]. These data support the idea that the PNMT-containing cells, though closely related to the NE cell cluster, function as a separate adrenergic neuronal system in the brainstem, using E as their major neurotransmitter.

Epinephrine-related Functions

Although information regarding the function of E-producing cells is scarce, some central autonomic functions seem to be related to the E system. PNMT activity is markedly elevated in the A1 and A2 regions of spontaneous hypertensive rats [68,85], and E levels are elevated in specific brainstem nuclei of various experimental models of hypertensive rats [32,36,37,83,103]. E cells and pathways seem to be involved in central cardiovascular control.

However, E [31] and PNMT activity [86] are also found in brain areas unrelated to cardiovascular control. The hypothalamus and some limbic system nuclei are relatively densely innervated by E-containing nerve endings originating in the Cl and C2 cells, suggesting a role for E in neuroendocrine and behavioral processes. This possibility is further supported by profound changes in E content in specific hypothalamic nuclei of rats exposed to short- or long-term stress situations [51, 52,103]. Thus, the central E system seems to be involved along with the other catecholaminergic pathways dopamine (DA), (NE) in control of fundamental autonomic and complex behavioral responses.

DOPAMINE SYSTEMS

DA cells (A9) in the pars compacta (substantia nigra) and adjacent ventrolateral mesencephalic reticular formation (A8), which projects to the neostriatum (caudate nucleus and putamen), are shown in Figures 5.4 and 5.5. Lateral and medial substan-

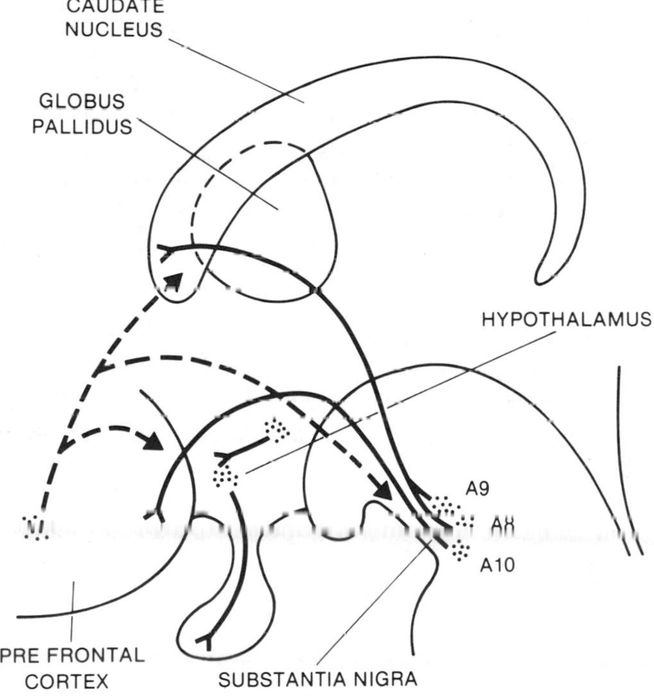

Figure 5.4 Dopamine tracts from the substantia nigra and ventral tegmental area (VTA) terminate in the caudate nucleus and limbic system respectively. Prefrontal cortex catecholamine tracts pass back to the caudate nucleus, nucleus accumbens, substantia nigra, and VTA. Intrahypothalamic tracts and hypothalamic-pituitary tracts are shown.

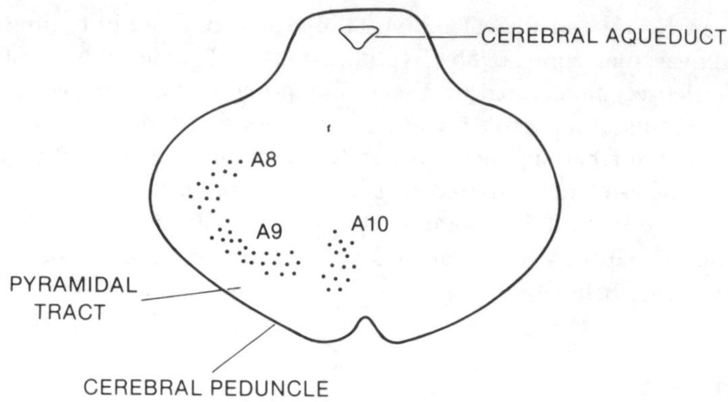

Figure 5.5 The substantia nigra (A8 dopamine neurons in the ventrolateral mesencephalic formation and the A9 dopamine neurons in the pars compacta) and the ventral tegmental area (A10 dopamine neurons).

tia nigra cells project to lateral and medial neostriatum respectively. This nigrostriatal DA tract ascends medially and ventrally through the medial forebrain bundle with collaterals to the globus pallidus [26,35,53]. The A10 DA cells (medial to substantia nigra in ventral tegmental areas [VTA]) pass in the medial and ventral part of the nigrostriatal projection to the limbic system (nucleus accumbens, olfactory tubercle) [26]. The A10 neurons have a restricted projection compared to nigral DA neurons, but do innervate the prefrontal cortex [35,90]. CA neurons pass back from medial prefrontal cortex to striatum, nucleus accumbens, VTA, and the substantia nigra [6,26].

Some of the nucleus accumbens receives DA from A9 cells. In Parkinson's disease, degeneration occurs in striatal (caudate) and limbic (accumbens) DA terminals but not in the olfactory area [77].

Other DA neurons pass from arcuate and periventricular nuclei to the pituitary and median eminence contacting peptide terminals controlling gonadotropin secretion. DA neurons pass from the dorsal posterior hypothalamus to the dorsal anterior hypothalamus and lateral septal nuclei.

Function of Dopamine Cells

Iontophoretically applied DA inhibits neuronal discharge, and this inhibition is potentiated by phosphodiesterase inhibitors. However, electrical stimulation of the VTA and substantia nigra induces both excitation and inhibition.

DA agonists produce low-intensity stereotypy (coordinated locomotion and sniffing) from the nucleus accumbens and olfactory tubercles and high-intensity stereotypy (gnawing and licking) from the striatum. Conversely, DA antagonists produce hypomobility (mesolimbic) and catalepsy (striatal) [22,23].

Lesions in the VTA and medial prefrontal cortex induce hyperactivity in rats and enhance behavioral responses to amphetamine, but lesions of substantia nigra DA pathways produce the opposite effects. The frontal cortical DA system inhibits motor behavior [79]. Lesions of the A10 neurons to the prefrontal cortex produce cognitive deficits [90].

Interaction of Dopamine and Norepinephrine

Bilateral transection of the noradrenergic ventral bundle decreases DA turnover in the nucleus accumbens and increases it in the nucleus tractus diagonalis. Unilateral transection, however, decreases DA concentration in both caudate nuclei, in the olfactory tubercle, and in the nucleus accumbens, but it increases DA in the ipsilateral reticulata and in both VTAs. The noradrenergic ventral bundle has broad projections and interacts with DA cells [72]. Decreased LC activity either increases haloperidol catalepsy or produces no change [42,72,78,102]. Depletion of NE stores produces catalepsy and potentiates haloperidol catalepsy [2].

Some DA/NE interactions are modulated by cholinergic mechanisms. The cholinergic agonist oxotremorine releases DA via muscarinic receptors located on the DA nerve terminals. It also increases striatal DA turnover by stimulating NE neurons, which modulate DA nigrostriatal pathways through β receptors. Clonidine inhibits the oxotremorine increase in DA turnover by stimulating presynaptic α_2 receptors on NE neurons and decreasing the firing of the LC. Destruction of the LC-dorsal noradrenergic bundle decreases DA activity in the striatum [62,66].

DA agonists, through presynaptic DA receptors, decrease stimulated release of NE [46], but increase NE turnover so that presynaptic DA receptors have little physiologic role in noradrenergic neurotransmission [27,65].

NE receptor activation is important in L-dopa–induced hyperkinesia as α-adrenergic blockers and dopamine β-hydroxylase (DBH) inhibitors reduce L-dopa hyperkinesia [4].

STRIATONIGRAL PATHWAYS

Inhibitory (GABA) and excitatory (substance P) neurons of the globus pallidus and caudate nucleus project back to pars reticulata GABAergic neurons, which project out to the thalamus, superior colliculus, and reticular formation (Figure 5.6). These pars reticulata neurons carry striatal output to the mesencephalon and send GABAergic collaterals to inhibit DA cells of the pars compacta. The pars reticulata GABAergic neuron is more sensitive to GABA than the DA cell

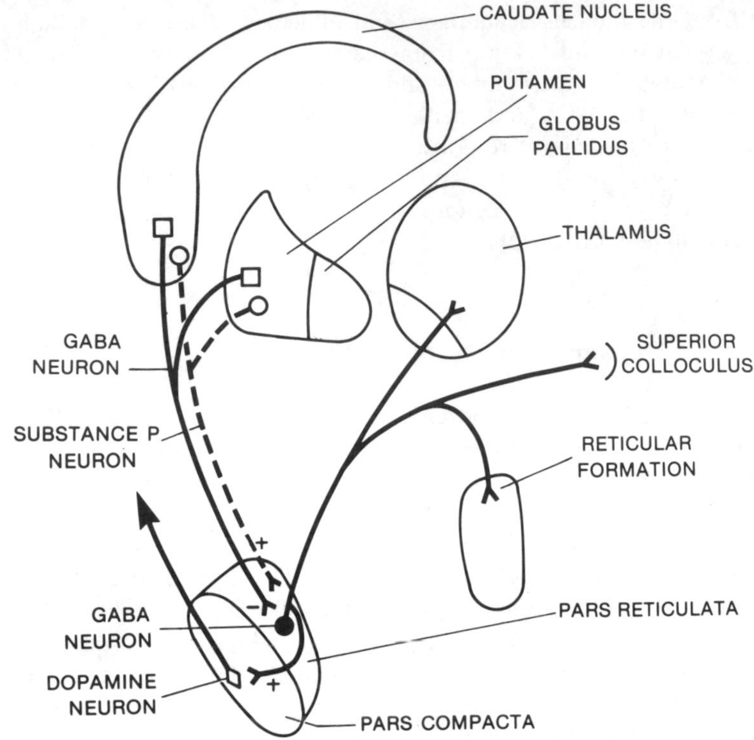

Figure 5.6. The γ-aminobutyric acid (GABA) neurons from the caudate nucleus inhibit the excitatory pars reticulata GABA neuron, thus indirectly decreasing DA activity, which is stimulated by the pars reticulata GABA neuron. The GABA circuit from the pars reticulata to the thalamus, reticular formation, and superior colliculi forms another output pathway for the basal ganglia, in addition to that pathway passing directly from the basal ganglia to the ventrolateral nucleus of the thalamus. Excitatory substance P neurons pass down from the caudate nucleus and globus pallidus to the substantia nigra.

and, when inhibited, stops exciting the DA cell. Thus, GABA agonists injected intravenously or into the substantia nigra increases DA activity [12].

The striatonigral GABAergic pathway is an output for behavior and motor patterns (turning, stereotyped gnawing, and catalepsy) arising in the striatum secondary to nigrostriatal DA activity. Turning stereotypy from asymmetric dopaminergic stimulation of the caudate is reduced and catalepsy increased by striatonigral lesions or blockade of nigral GABA transmission. Stimulation of the nucleus accumbens can inhibit VTA DA cells, and this inhibition is blocked by GABA antagonists, but intravenous GABA agonists excite A10 DA neurons. This may explain why muscimol worsened schizophrenic psychosis [100].

SEROTONIN CELLS

The nine clusters of serotonin (5-hydroxytryptamine; 5-HT) neurons lie near the midline and raphe regions of the pons and upper brainstem. The caudal group (B1–B3) projects to the medulla and spinal cord, and the rostral group (B7–B9) projects to the cortex and brainstem. The dorsal raphe nucleus projects to the substantia nigra and striatum, and the median raphe nucleus projects to the hippocampus [63]. NE cells innervate 5-HT cells in the dorsal raphe [5]. Lesions severing the A1 and A2 parts of the ventral noradrenergic bundle reduce 5-HT in the median raphe nucleus but not in the dorsal raphe nucleus [63].

Function of Serotonergic Neurons

5-HT inhibits DA's action in the nucleus accumbens, striatum, and substantia nigra, whereas decreased 5-HT reduces neuroleptic catalepsy [33]. By contrast, 5-HT agonists increase DA agonist–induced contralateral circling in raphe-lesioned rats [16], and apomorphine stereotypy is attenuated by midbrain raphe lesions and 5-HT receptor antagonists [92].

DA may need 5-HT for postsynaptic action. 5-HT injected into the pars reticulata can induce contralateral circling independent of nigrostriatal DA activity [71]. The anatomic connections between noradrenergic cells and 5-HT cells may have a physiologic function.

PEPTIDE NEURONS

High concentrations of neuropeptides are found in the basal ganglia. Substantia nigra substance P decreases with lesions of the striatum or striatonigral projection [82]. Caudate and putamen enkephalin neurons project radially, concentrically, and topographically to the globus pallidus [20] (Figure 5.7). Enkephalin neurons terminate presynaptically on DA terminals in the striatum [17]. Cholecystokinin (CCK) is present in the same neuron as DA, projecting from the VTA to the nucleus accumbens. Somatostatin, concentrated in substantia nigra and striatum, exists in NE neurons, substance P exists in 5-HT neurons, and both acetylcholine and vasoactive intestinal peptides coexist in the same cells [8,41]. Thyrotropin-releasing hormone (TRH) (in nucleus accumbens) and neurotensin (in substantia nigra, neostriatum, and limbic nuclei) are heterogeneously distributed in the basal ganglia [45].

Function of Peptide Neurons

Substance P increases firing of nigral neurons, increases motor activity, decreases hypokinesia, and reduces haloperidol rigidity but not normal tone. Somatostatin increases haloperidol rigidity. Substance P and somatostatin act postsynaptically

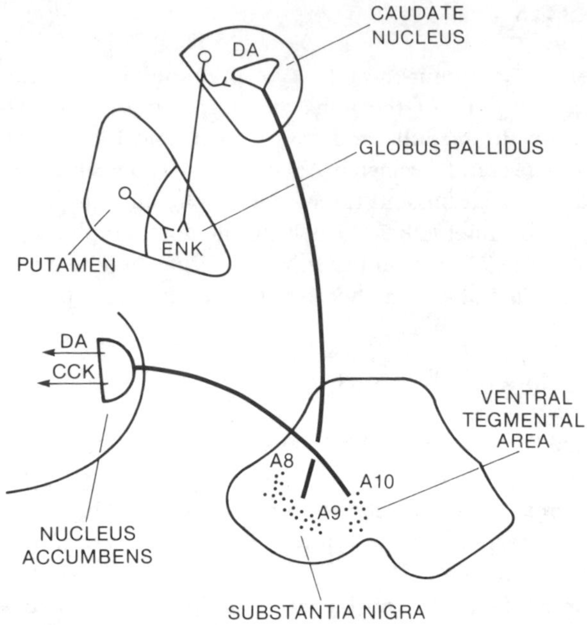

Figure 5.7. The dopamine (DA) neuron from the ventral tegmental area to the nucleus accumbens contains cholecystokinin (CCK). Enkephalin neurons (ENK) pass from caudate nucleus and putamen to the globus pallidus. ENK terminate on presynaptic DA terminals of the nigrostriatal pathway.

and do not alter reserpine-induced rigidity. Neurotensin produces analgesia, muscular relaxation, decreased motor activity, and hypothermia [45,82].

TRH was found to exert behavioral effects in human beings and animals. The stimulatory effects of TRH do not mimic the effects of known antidepressants as regards inhibition of monoamine reuptake [99] or monoamine oxidase (MAO) activity [10]. However, the overall rate of brain CA metabolism is increased. Kellar et al [48] found that TRH increases 3-methoxy-4-hydroxyphenylglycol (MHPG) concentration and tyrosine hydroxylase (TH) activity; Riegle et al [81] found that NE efflux from brain was increased after pharmacologic doses of TRH, and Marek et al [59] showed that TRH increases the turnover of DA and NE in rat brain. Thus the neuropeptide-releasing factors act in central regulation of the CA system in addition to their role in neuroendocrine control.

Morphine and endorphins induce catalepsy, DA turnover in the striatum, firing of pars compacta cells, and prolactin release, as well as antagonize apomorphine and amphetamine-induced stereotypy. However, increase in turnover does not necessarily mean more neurotransmitter in the synapse; on the contrary, it may be accompanied by *less* neurotransmitter in the synapse as in the case of reserpine or MAO treatment. Rats dependent on morphine are cross-tolerant to haloperidol, and opiates inhibit DA stimulation of adenyl cyclase in monkey amygdala and rat striatal membranes [69].

Opiate peptides do not prevent DA from interacting with its binding site but do prevent it from activating adenyl cyclase. They inhibit DA release through putative presynaptic opiate receptors on DA terminals. These actions are reversed by the opiate antagonist naloxone [13,69]. Depletion of brainstem NE potentiates morphine catalepsy and locomotor depression but not morphine stimulation [3,83].

CCK, a potent excitatory agent in discrete areas of the mesencephalon [64], decreases DA turnover in the caudate nucleus and nucleus accumbens but does not affect locomotion [34].

Enkephalins and substance P make target cells less susceptible to other signals; when they stop releasing inhibitory signals they act as excitants [8].

NEUROCHEMICAL CHANGES IN CLINICAL CONDITIONS

Parkinson's Disease

The symptoms of Parkinson's disease include tremor, rigidity, slowness, and an inability to initiate movement. Postural hypotension, atonic bladder, spastic bladder, increased salivation, and increased sweating occur. Many patients have a flexed posture and often fall. Some are demented, confused, anxious, and occasionally psychotic. Most have small, untidy writing and experience difficulty in dressing, washing, eating, or rolling over in bed.

There is a decreased level of DA and L-aromatic amino acid decarboxylase (L-aromatic AAD) in the substantia nigra with degeneration of the nigrostriatal pathway and other DA tracts such as from the frontal cortex and VTA to the limbic system. Degeneration also occurs in noradrenergic cells, LC, dorsal motor nucleus of the vagus, and sympathetic ganglia. Brain 5-HT level is low, and some patients reverse their sleep cycle with nocturnal insomnia.

NE (as well as DA) is related to the disturbed motor activity of Parkinson's disease. Reserpine rigidity is partially reversed with DA agonists and further reversed by the α_2-noradrenergic agonist clonidine [96]. DA reversal of reserpine rigidity is prevented by α_2-adrenergic antagonists [1,96].

Apomorphine stereotypy is prevented by reduced 5-HT activity in the nucleus linearis intermedius, and L-dopa is not effective in patients with low cerebrospinal fluid (CSF) 5-hydroxyindoleacetic acid (5-HIAA) [22]. The following results summarize the values of CSF and plasma NE concentration and DBH activity in patients with parkinsonism and in control subjects.

Collection of Cerebrospinal Fluid Samples

Lumbar punctures were performed while the patients were supine and lying on their left side, after complete rest for 2 hours and no food for 3 hours. A 4-ml sample of CSF for NE and DBH assay was obtained after 16 ml of CSF had been removed for other tests. This sample was placed in a tube containing 5 mg ascorbic acid, chilled, and frozen (−70° C) 30 minutes later for assay within 6 weeks.

Collection of Plasma Samples

The subjects were supine at complete rest. A 19-gauge butterfly cannula, connected to a heparin lock, was inserted into an antecubital vein. After 20 minutes (when BP and pulse were stable), a 12-ml sample of blood was taken through the cannula, transferred into a chilled tube containing acid-citrate-dextrose anticoagulant, and placed on ice. Patients then stood for 5 minutes, and a second blood sample was collected. Plasma was separated by centrifugation at 4° C within 30 minutes of collection. The plasma was stored at −70° C for assay within 6 weeks. BP and pulse were recorded at rest and when erect.

Norepinephrine and Dopamine β-Hydroxylase Assay

CSF and plasma NE were measured by the radioenzymatic method of Ziegler et al [108]. In this reaction, catalyzed by phenylethanolamine-N-methyltransferase (PNMT), NE is converted to ^{3}H-E. The ^{3}H methyl group is enzymatically transferred from ^{3}H methyl-S-adenosylmethionine (SAM) to the primary amine of NE, and ^{3}H-E is measured by liquid scintillation spectrometry. The assay can detect 20 pg/ml of NE.

Williams [105] found that CSF and plasma NE levels in Parkinson's disease were low (Table 5.1). Teychenne et al reported that CSF [96] and plasma NE [97] were significantly lower in patients with untreated Parkinson's disease compared to patients treated with L-dopa where levels were normal (Table 5.2). When untreated parkinsonian patients and L-dopa–treated patients were divided into those who had tremor and those who did not, the mean CSF NE level was significantly higher in those patients with tremor than in those without; no significant difference in the plasma NE level was found, although the L-dopa–treated patients had higher plasma NE levels (Table 5.3).

Table 5.1 Cerebrospinal Fluid and Plasma Norepinephrine Levels for Parkinson's Disease and Controls*

Subjects (N)	*CSF NE (pg/ml)*	*Plasma NE (pg/ml)*
Normal (19)	374 ± 36	351 ± 63
Parkinson's disease (14)	215 ± 34†	233 ± 50

CSF = cerebrospinal fluid; NE = norepinephrine; N = number of patients.
* Data are shown as mean ± standard error of the mean (SEM).
† $p < 0.05$ compared with normal (student t test).
SOURCE: AC Williams [105].

Table 5.2 Cerebrospinal Fluid and Plasma Norepinephrine Concentrations in Treated and Untreated Subjects with Parkinson's Disease and Controls*

Subjects (N)	*Age (years)*	*CSF NE (pg/ml)*	*Plasma NE (pg/ml)*
Untreated Parkinson's disease (7)	57 ± 4	137 ± 25	189 ± 22
Treated Parkinson's disease (14)	60 ± 4	362 ± 145†	320 ± 58†
Control (25)	55 ± 1	209 ± 25†	371 ± 42‡

CSF = cerebrospinal fluid; NE = norepinephrine.
* Data are shown as mean ± standard error of the mean (SEM).
† $p < 0.5$ compared with untreated subjects.
‡ $p < 0.001$ compared with untreated patients.
SOURCE: PF Teychenne [96,97].

Supine parkinsonian subjects had lower levels of plasma NE. In spite of lower basal NE levels, the untreated patients with Parkinson's disease had an adequate increment in plasma NE in response to a standing test (Table 5.4). Thus, normal controls had a 78% increase in plasma NE as compared to 102% increase in plasma NE of the patients with Parkinson's disease.

In an additional study, where untreated parkinsonian patients were compared to L-dopa–treated parkinsonians and normal subjects (Table 5.5), it was found that L-dopa treatment elevates the lower resting plasma NE levels (which is significantly lower in untreated patients with Parkinson's disease; $p < 0.01$) to the normal range of plasma NE. However, standing for 5 minutes (from supine position) increased plasma NE in all the groups studied, but the largest relative increment was observed in the untreated parkinsonian patients: 116% versus 73% in treated parkinsonian patients and 60% in control patients. In all these groups there was a significant increase in diastolic blood pressure, which probably indicates increased peripheral resistance owing to sympathetic activation by standing. Although the sympathetic nervous system has somewhat lower tone in the resting patient with Parkinson's disease, it is still capable of responding adequately to mild stress

In two sets of patients the DA agonists lergotrile and bromocriptine significantly decreased the concentration of CSF NE (Tables 5.6 and 5.7).

The mean plasma DBH activity was the same in parkinsonian patients regardless of treatment (Table 5.8). Plasma and CSF DBH activity was similar in parkinsonian patients and controls (Table 5.9).

Decreased CSF NE in untreated patients with Parkinson's disease suggests low NE in the basal ganglia. L-dopa produces DA and NE, increasing the concentration of both transmitters. Increased plasma NE after L-dopa and a peripheral dopa decarboxylase inhibitor suggests that this dose of carbidopa does not completely inhibit peripheral dopa decarboxylase.

In vitro DA stimulation of presynaptic DA receptors on noradrenergic terminals inhibits NE release [109]. DA, however, does not inhibit noradrenergic neurotransmission, possibly because it is a precursor of NE. Bromocriptine and lergotrile

Table 5.3 Cerebrospinal Fluid and Plasma Norepinephrine in Controls and Patients with and without Significant Tremor*

Group	*Number and Gender of Patients*	*Age (year)*	*Score for Tremor (%)*	*CSF NE (pg/ml)*	*Plasma NE (pg/ml)*	*L-dopa/ Carbidopa Dose (mg/day)*
Parkinsonian: drug-free, tremor	8 (5 M, 3 F)	58 ± 3	40 ± 3	317 ± 48†,‡	205 ± 41‡	—
Parkinsonian: drug-free	8 (5 M, 3 F)	63 ± 3	13 ± 3	122 ± 20§	191 ± 23¶	—
Parkinsonian: tremor	9 (5 M, 4 F)	61 ± 3	40 ± 2	407 ± 82	420 ± 86	922/92 ± 254/25
Parkinsonian	4 (3 M, 1 F)	64 ± 2	8 ± 3	181 ± 98¶	268 ± 78	933/93 ± 377/37
Controls	16 (9 M, 7 F)	53 ± 2	—	489 ± 39	353 ± 45	—

CSF = cerebrospinal fluid; NE = norepinephrine; L-dopa = levodopa; M = male; F = female.
* The two-tailed nonpaired student t test was used in all statistical analyses. Data are shown as mean ± standard error of the mean (SEM).
† $p < 0.01$ compared with parkinsonian, drug-free subjects.
‡ $p < 0.02$ compared with control.
¶ $p < 0.01$ compared with control.
§ $p < 0.001$ compared with control.
SOURCE: PF Teychenne [96,97].

Table 5.4 Supine and Erect (after 5 minutes of standing) Plasma Norepinephrine in Parkinson's Disease and in Controls*

Patients (N)	*Supine Plasma NE (pg/ml)*	*Standing Plasma NE (pg/ml)*
Control (19)	351 ± 63	625 ± 70
Parkinson's disease (14)	233 ± 50†	471 ± 88

NE = norepinephrine.
* Data are shown as mean ± standard error of the mean (SEM).
† $p < 0.05$ compared with control.
SOURCE: AC Williams [105].

Table 5.5 Supine and Erect Plasma Norepinephrine and Blood Pressure in Treated and Untreated Subjects with Parkinson's Disease and in Controls

Group (N)	*Age**	*Mean Supine Plasma NE (pg/ml)*	*Mean Erect Plasma NE (pg/ml)*	*Mean Supine BP (mm Hg)*	*Mean Erect BP (mm Hg)*
Untreated Parkinson's disease (13)	59 ± 2	188 ± 18†	407 ± 38	112 ± 3 / 68 ± 2	116 ± 4 / 78 ± 2
Treated Parkinson's disease (17)	62 ± 2	408 ± 37	704 ± 129	102 ± 3 / 77 ± 2	117 ± 4 / 83 ± 3
Control (10)	40 ± 3	305 ± 37	489 ± 49	121 ± 3 / 76 ± 2	118 ± 3 / 87 ± 4

NE = norepinephrine; BP = blood pressure.
* Data are shown as mean ± standard error of the mean (SEM).
† $p < 0.01$ compared with control.
SOURCE: PF Teychenne [97].

Table 5.6 Mean Concentration of Cerebrospinal Fluid Norepinephrine in Parkinsonian Patients Before and During Lergotrile Administration*

Patients (N)	*Age*	*CSF NE Before Lergotrile Therapy (pg/ml)*	*CSF NE During Lergotrile Therapy (pg/ml)*
10	57 ± 3	238 ± 65	159 ± 56†

CSF = cerebrospinal fluid; NE = norepinephrine.
* Data are shown as mean ± standard error of the mean (SEM).
† $p < 0.03$ compared with before lergotrile therapy (two-tailed paired t test).
SOURCE: PF Teychenne [96].

Table 5.7 Mean Concentration of Cerebrospinal Fluid Norepinephrine in Parkinsonian Patients Before and During Bromocriptine Administration

Patients (N)	*Mean CSF NE Before Bromocriptine Therapy (pg/ml)*	*Mean CSF NE During Bromocriptine Therapy (pg/ml)*
6	201	99*

CSF = cerebrospinal fluid; NE = norepinephrine.
* $p < 0.02$ compared with before bromocriptine therapy.
SOURCE: MG Ziegler et al [109].

Table 5.8 Plasma Dopamine β-Hydroxylase in Treated and Untreated Parkinson's Disease*

Group (N)	*Dose Levodopa (Sinemet) (mg/day)*	*Plasma DBH*
Untreated Parkinson's disease (11)	—	325 ± 64
Treated Parkinson's disease (11)	1219 ± 206	355 ± 99

DBH = dopamine β-hydroxylase.
* Data are shown as mean ± standard error of the mean (SEM).
SOURCE: PF Teychenne et al [97].

displace ^{3}H-clonidine from α_2-adrenergic autoreceptors on noradrenergic cells [80]. Bromocriptine inhibits NE release by stimulating presynaptic receptors but increases NE turnover [65]. Physiologically, bromocriptine inhibits noradrenergic neurotransmission [80]. Bromocriptine and lergotrile, a related cross-tolerant ergoline [98], decrease the concentration of CSF NE [96,109]. In vivo, the presynaptic action of bromocriptine may dominate its postsynaptic adrenergic activity [25].

The concentration of CSF NE in untreated parkinsonism correlates with

Table 5.9 Plasma and Cerebrospinal Fluid Dopamine β-Hydroxylase in Parkinson's Disease and Controls*

Groups	*Plasma DBH*	*CSF DBH*
Parkinson's disease	482 ± 87	1.0 ± 0.19
Control	567 ± 85	0.78 ± 0.09

DBH = dopamine β-hydroxylase; CSF = cerebrospinal fluid.
* Data are shown as mean ± standard error of the mean (SEM).
SOURCE: AC Williams [105].

the severity of tremor ($r = 0.62$), but no correlation exists between tremor and plasma NE. Bromocriptine and lergotrile are more effective against tremor than L-dopa. An imbalance between NE and DA may induce tremor [107], and bromocriptine therapy may depend on dopaminergic and noradrenergic actions. Low plasma NE in untreated parkinsonism correlates with low supine diastolic BP. There may be a peripheral as well as central noradrenergic deficit in Parkinson's disease, but there is no change in DBH activity in parkinsonism. However, DBH is a poor index for sympathetic activity, especially during acute changes in sympathetic activity.

Huntington's Chorea

Huntington's chorea is an inherited autosomal dominant disorder which surfaces in childhood in 10% of those afflicted with epilepsy and chorea, myoclonus, or dystonia. The course is rapid, and rigidity occurs early. In most victims, the disease presents itself in the fourth to fifth decade, progresses slowly, and is accompanied by the development of chorea, dementia, and brain atrophy, particularly atrophy of the caudate nucleus. The concentrations of GABA, glutamic acid decarboxylase, choline acetyltransferase, angiotensin-converting enzyme, and substance P are reduced, and the activities of TH and monoamine oxidase B (MAO-B) in the striatum, substantia nigra, and cerebral cortex are increased. There is a reduction in DBH activity and levels of NE and DA, but, because of tissue atrophy, DA is relatively increased in the striatum, substantia nigra, and nucleus accumbens. Homovanillic acid (HVA) is increased in the cerebral cortex but not in the basal ganglia [21]; plasma DBH activity is slightly higher in Huntington's chorea, and haloperidol induces no change in plasma DBH activity. CSF HVA is lower in patients with increased tone and bradykinesia [7,11,14,58,93].

Plasma for NE and DBH was collected as described in the section on Parkinson's disease from resting supine subjects. Plasma NE and DBH [101] concentra-

Table 5.10 Resting Supine Plasma Norepinephrine and Dopamine β-Hydroxylase in Huntington's Chorea*

Group (N)	*Age*	*Plasma NE (pg/ml)*	*Plasma DBH Activity*	*BP (mm Hg)*
Huntington's chorea (6)	51 ± 2.4	182 ± 15†	396 ± 107	114 ± 4 / 71 ± 3
Control (8)	51 ± 4.2	379 ± 66	747 ± 121	119 ± 4 / 75 ± 4

NE = norepinephrine; DBH = dopamine β-hydroxylase; BP = blood pressure.
* Data shown are mean ± standard error of the mean (SEM).
† $p < 0.05$ compared with control (t test).
SOURCE: I Shoulson et al [89].

tions were significantly lower in Huntington's chorea than in controls. Resting supine systolic and diastolic BP were normal [89] (Table 5.10).

In these patients there is a reduced cholinergic and GABAergic function with relatively increased DA activity producing involuntary movements such as L-dopa dyskinesia. Bromocriptine decreases chorea at low dose and increases it at high dose. Bromocriptine may not stimulate DA presynaptic inhibitory receptors as CSF HVA is increased after bromocriptine. Bromocriptine may act as both a DA agonist and antagonist because postsynaptic antagonism by bromocriptine increases DA turnover and HVA [54]. GABA, GABAergic agonists, or putative cholinergic agonists do not help Huntington's chorea.

Seizure Disorders

Reduction of brain NE and DA increase the susceptibility to, severity and duration of, electroconvulsive shock and pentylenetetrazol-induced seizures. L-dopa reverses this lowered seizure threshold by replenishing both transmitters [43,61].

DA agonists reduce the susceptibility to photically induced convulsions in the baboon. Ventricular infusion of DA reverses convulsions induced by CA-depleting agents; DA antagonists block this reversal [61]. Selective depletion of forebrain NE but not DA increases seizure activity provoked by repeated electrical stimulation of the amygdala (kindling) in rats [18,29]. NE depletion potentiates seizures by disinhibiting the spread of seizure discharge from the stimulated site rather than increasing epileptic activity in the site itself.

5-HT and GABA may be involved in seizures. Mice susceptible to audiogenic seizure have lower levels of brain NE, 5-HT, and GABA than seizure-resistant strains. Lowering of these transmitters increases susceptibility; increased NE, 5-HT, and GABA protect against audiogenic seizures. No correlation exists between DA concentrations and audiogenic susceptibility [44].

To study seizure disorders in human beings, lumbar punctures were performed on hospitalized patients as described in the section on Parkinson's disease (resting, supine, lying on left side) within 48 hours of either idiopathic or alcohol-withdrawal seizures. The subjects with idiopathic seizures, but not the alcoholic patients, had EEGs diagnostic of a seizure disorder. The mean concentration of CSF NE in the idiopathic seizure patients was higher than that in the age-matched normal controls (Table 5.11).

Kainic acid (a selective neurotoxin affecting cell bodies but not axons near the injection site) injected into the dentate gyrus of the hippocampus produces rapid seizures associated with a marked depletion of NE in all cortical areas innervated by the LC. There is a twofold increase in the NE breakdown product 3-methoxy-4-hydroxyphenylglycol sulfate (MHPG-SO_4), consistent with an accelerated release of NE. Acute transection of the dorsal noradrenergic bundle does not prevent cortical NE depletion after hippocampal kainate injection. Kainic acid does not directly deplete NE. Thus, it appears that paroxysmal seizure activity can cause NE release at the injection site independent of stimulation from the

Table 5.11 Cerebrospinal Fluid Norepinephrine Concentration in Alcohol-Withdrawal Seizures, Idiopathic Seizures, and Control*

Group (N)	*Age*	*CSF NE (pg/ml)*
Alcohol-withdrawal seizures (8)	47 ± 6	545 ± 87
Idiopathic seizures (12)	43 ± 4	555 ± 118
Control (18)	44 ± 3	439 ± 40

CSF = cerebrospinal fluid; NE = norepinephrine.
* Data shown are mean ± standard error of the mean (SEM).
SOURCE: PF Teychenne et al [96].

LC [70]. High to normal CSF NE in humans (with idiopathic seizures) soon after seizure activity may mean that (1) patients with idiopathic seizure disorders have low CSF NE which is increased to normal or high levels by the seizure, or (2) NE levels are normal in subjects with idiopathic seizures.

Alcohol-Withdrawal Seizures

Controversy exists regarding NE turnover and levels in alcoholic subjects. A persistent and significant decrease in the concentration of NE in the whole brain and hypothalamus was observed in 1- to 21-day-old rats exposed to ethanol prenatally or postnatally. Some investigators found that ethanol increased the turnover of NE in adult animals, but regional studies showed that NE turnover was decreased in the hypothalamus and increased in the pons and medulla regions with no change in the frontal or parietal cortex, cerebellum, amygdala, hippocampus, or LC. Others noted decreased accumulation of labeled NE metabolites and decreased rate of noradrenergic neuronal firing, suggesting less NE release after acute ethanol administration [94]. These variant results could be due to differences in alcohol concentration and duration of exposure [9,15,39].

Subjects with seizures after alcohol withdrawal have a higher mean concentration of CSF NE than age-matched normal controls, but the difference is not significant (see Table 5.11).

The CSF concentration of the NE metabolite MHPG in alcoholic patients is elevated during intoxication, correlates with blood alcohol levels, and successively declines during subsequent abstinence (1 to 3 weeks). When intoxicated, healthy subjects have a higher concentration of CSF MHPG than after intoxication.

During withdrawal, alcoholics have high CSF NE, which falls during recovery, but is still higher than in subjects with other neurologic disorders [39]. Alcohol administration stimulates NE metabolism in the central nervous system (CNS) of human beings [9].

The high to normal CSF NE that occurs within days of alcohol-withdrawal seizures could be consistent with these findings, although we have no evidence of increased release or turnover of NE in our subjects. In aged patients with senile dementia and in chronic alcoholics, the level of DA, NE, 5-HT, and choline acetyltransferase in the caudate nucleus is lower than normal. The process of neuronal aging is enhanced in alcoholics, with pathologic changes similar to those in senile dementia [15].

Migraine

Migraine, which occurs in 10% of the population, is marked by recurrent headaches and two or more of the following features: unilateral headache, nausea, visual or other neurologic disturbances, family history of migraine, history of bilious attacks and travel sickness.

Migraine symptoms are associated with low levels of 5-HT in the brain, which increase the sensitivity of the vomiting center in the medulla oblongata and lead to irritability. Bright light and stress (which can precipitate migraine) reduce 5-HT levels in the brain. Methysergide, a competitive 5-HT antagonist, however, prevents migraine. Platelets release 5-HT during migraine and, although 5-HT induces arterial constriction (dilation with low 5-HT), an intravenous infusion of 5-HT can relieve migraine. Some fatty acids release platelet 5-HT, and a significant rise in linoleate, palmitate, and oleate occurs in some migraine sufferers during migraine. An increase in plasma 5-HT may lead to a relative deficiency because of catabolism and excretion [19].

Reserpine, a precipitant of migraine, acutely releases but chronically depletes stored 5-HT and NE. The tunica adventitia of migraine temporal arteries have increased binding for NE. Migraine increases the release of NE and DBH, and may be triggered by stress. Clonidine, an α_2-adrenergic agonist, decreases NE release but may or may not alleviate migraine. β-adrenergic blockers may prevent migraine, and biofeedback may relieve migraine while decreasing plasma CA. There is a deficit of platelet MAO-B during migraine, which could lead to defective inactivation of vasoactive amines [19].

Bromocriptine increased NE turnover but inhibited release of NE [80,109]. It increased brain 5-HT and decreased brain 5-HIAA concentration, probably by inhibiting 5-HT release [80]. Nine of 10 migraine patients were unable to tolerate bromocriptine; 30 to 120 minutes after a 2.5-mg dose they developed headache with nausea, vomiting, flittering scotomas, and feebleness. One patient had syncope, and, in many, systolic BP dropped by 10 to 30 mm Hg with a less distinct fall in diastolic BP. This did not occur in normal subjects [28] and is evidence of the complex chemical interactions in migraine.

Glutamate, an excitatory neurotransmitter and precursor of GABA, is elevated in blood and CSF from migraine subjects. High concentrations of monosodium L-glutamate cause a migraine-like picture (burning sensation in the face with headache known as chinese restaurant syndrome) [19].

CSF endorphin and enkephalin levels are low in patients with migraine compared to controls. There may be impairment in the antinociceptive system, increasing the pain of migraine [19].

CONCLUSIONS

Several neurologic diseases are associated with alteration in central and peripheral noradrenergic systems. The interaction of central noradrenergic neurons with DA, 5-HT, GABA, and peptide neurons can alter NE activity in neurological diseases associated with changes in neurotransmitter concentrations. For example, Parkinson's disease primarily affects DA, but CSF NE levels are low in parkinsonian patients and correlate with specific aspects of the disease. Many of the drugs used to treat neurologic disorders act on noradrenergic systems. We are just beginning to understand the alterations in NE activity that help make these drugs useful.

We thank Miss Frances Shaw, Ms. Betsy Ann Youngholm, and Ms. Mary Holzsweig for their indispensable secretarial and administrative services.

REFERENCES

1. Aghajanian GK, Cedarbaum JM, Wang RY. Evidence for norepinephrine-mediated collateral inhibition of locus coeruleus neurons. Brain Res 136:570–577, 1977.
2. Al-Shabibi MH, Doggett NS. On the central noradrenergic mechanism involved in haloperidol induced catalepsy in the rat. J Pharm Pharmacol 30:529–530, 1978.
3. Anden NE, Strombom U, Svensson TH. Locomotor stimulation by L-dopa: Relative importance of noradrenaline receptor activation. Psychopharmacology (Berlin) 54:243–248, 1977.
4. Arbilla S, Langer SZ. Morphine and β endorphin inhibit release of noradrenaline from cerebral cortex but not dopamine from rat striatum. Nature 271:559–560, 1978.
5. Baraban JM, Aghajanian GK. Noradrenergic innervation of serotonergic neurons in the dorsal raphe: Demonstration by electron microscopic autoradiography. Brain Res 204:1–11, 1981.
6. Beckstead RM. An autoradiographic examination of cortico-cortical and subcortical projections of the mediodorsal-projection (prefrontal) cortex in the rat. J Comp Neurol 184:43–62, 1979.
7. Bird ED. Chemical pathology of Huntington's disease. Annu Rev Pharmacol Toxicol 20:533–551, 1980.
8. Bloom FE. Neuropeptides. Sci Am 245:148–168, 1981.
9. Borg S, Kvande H, Sedvall G. Central norepinephrine metabolism during alcohol intoxication in addicts and healthy volunteers. Science 213:1135–1137, 1981.
10. Breese GC, Cooper BR, Prange AJ, Cott JM, Lipton MA. Pharmacological Studies of Thyroid-Imipramine Interactions in Animals. In The Thyroid Axis, Drugs, and Behavior, AJ Prange (ed), 115–127. New York: Raven Press, 1974.
11. Buck SH, Burks TF, Brown MR, Yamamura HI. Reduction in basal ganglia and substantia nigra substance P levels in Huntington's disease. Brain Res 209:464–469, 1981.

12. Bunney BS, Grace AA, Hommer DW. Changing concepts of nigral dopamine system function within the basal ganglia: Relevance to extrapyramidal disorders. J Neural Transm 16[Suppl]:17–23, 1980.
13. Calderini G, Consolazione A, Garattini S, Algeri S. Different effects of methionine-enkephalin and (D-Ala^2) methionine-enkephalin amide on the metabolism of dopamine and norepinephrine in rat brain: Fact or artifact. Brain Res 146:392–399, 1978.
14. Caraceni T, Calderini G, Consolazione A, Riva E, Algeri S, Girotti F, Spreafico R, Branciforti A, Dall'Olio A, Morselli PL. Biochemical aspects of Huntington's chorea. J Neurol Neurosurg Psychiatry 40:581–587, 1977.
15. Carlsson A, Adolfsson R, Aquilonius S, Gottfries C, Oreland L, Svennerholm L, Winblad B. Biogenic Amines in Human Brain in Normal Aging, Senile Dementia, and Chronic Alcoholism. In Ergot Compounds and Brain Function: Neuroendocrine and Neuropsychiatric Aspects, M Goldstein (ed), 295–304. New York: Raven Press, 1980.
16. Carter CJ, Pycock CJ. The role of 5-hydroxytryptamine in dopamine-dependent stereotyped behavior. Neuropharmacology 20:261–265, 1981.
17. Chesselet MF, Cheramy A, Reisine TD, Glowinski J. Effects of Opiates on Dopamine Release in the Cat Caudate Nucleus In Vivo. In Apomorphine and Other Dopaminomimetics, Basic Pharmacology, GL Gessa and GU Corsini (eds), vol. 1, 79–84. New York: Raven Press,1981.
18. Corcoran ME, Mason ST. Role of forebrain catecholamines in amygdaloid kindling. Brain Res 190:473–484, 1980.
19. Crook M. Migraine: A biochemical headache. Biochem Rev 9:351–357, 1981.
20. Cuello AC, Del Fiacco M, Paxinos G, Somogyi P, Priestley JV. Neuropeptides in striato nigral pathways. J Neural Transm 51:83–96, 1981.
21. Cunha L, Oliveira CR, Diniz M, Amaral R, Concalves AF, Pio-Abreu J. Homovanillic acid in Huntington's disease and Sydenham's chorea. J Neurol Neurosurg Psychiatry 44:258–261, 1981.
22. Curzon G. The biochemistry of the basal ganglia and Parkinson's disease. Postgrad Med J 53:719–725, 1977.
23. Di Chiara G, Morelli M, Imperato A, Porceddu ML. Substantia Nigra as an Efferent Station for Dopaminergic Behavioral Syndromes Arising in the Striatum. In Apomorphine and Other Dopaminomimetics. Basic Pharmacology, GL Gessa and GU Corsini (eds), vol. 1, 41–64. New York: Raven Press, 1981.
24. Dillier N, Laszlo J, Muller B, Koella WP, Olpe HR. Activation of an inhibitory noradrenergic pathway projecting from the locus coeruleus to the cingulate cortex of the rat. Brain Res 154:61–68, 1978.
25. Dolphin AC, Jenner P, Sawaya MCB, Marsden CD, Testa B. The effects of bromocriptine on locomotor activity and cerebral catecholamines in rodents. J Pharm Pharmacol 29:727–734, 1977.
26. Domesick VB. The Anatomical Basis for Feedback and Feedforward in the Striatonigral System. In Apomorphine and Other Dopaminomimetics. Basic Pharmacology, GL Gessa and GU Corsini (eds), vol. 1, 27–39. New York: Raven Press, 1981.
27. Dubocovich ML, Galzin A, Langer SZ. Presynaptic inhibition by dopamine receptor agonists of noradrenergic neurotransmission in the rabbit hypothalamus. J Pharmacol Exp Ther 221:461–471, 1982.
28. Durko A. Hyperresponsiveness of migraine patients to bromocriptine. Headache 21:166, 1980.

29. Ehlers CL, Clifton DK, Sawyer CH. Facilitation of amygdala kindling in the rat by transecting ascending noradrenergic pathways. Brain Res 189:274–278, 1980.
30. Fallon JH, Koziell DA, Moore RY. Catecholamine innervation of the basal forebrain. Comp Neurol 180:509–532, 1978.
31. Feuerstein G, Zerbe RL, Ben-Ishay D, Kopin IJ, Jacobowitz DM. Catecholamines and vasopressin in forebrain nuclei of hypertension prone and resistant rats. Brain Res Bull 7:671–676, 1981.
32. Feuerstein G, Zerbe RL, Ben-Ishay D, Kopin IJ, Jacobowitz DM. Catecholamines and vasopressin in forebrain nuclei of hypertension prone and resistant rats. Brain Res 251:169–173, 1982.
33. Fuenmayor T. Effect of a reduction in brain 5-hydroxytryptamine on the concentration of homovanillic acid in the rat caudate nucleus. Proceedings of the Behav Pharmacol Soc 391, 1978.
34. Fuxe K, Andersson K, Locatelli V, Agnatic LF, Hökfelt T, Skirboll L, Mutt V. Cholecystokinin peptides produce marked reduction of dopamine turnover in discrete areas of the brain following intraventricular injection. Eur J Pharmacol 67:329–331, 1980.
35. Fuxe K, Hökfelt T, Olson L, Ungerstedt U. Central monoaminergic pathways with emphasis on their relation to the so-called "extrapyramidal motor system." Pharamcol Ther [B] 3:169–210, 1977.
36. Fuxe K, Vincent M, Andersson K, Harfstrand A, Agnati LF, Sassard J, Benferati F, Hökfelt T. Selective reduction of adrenaline turnover in the dorsal midline area of the caudal medulla oblongata and increase of hypothalamic adrenaline levels in the Lyon strain of genetically hypertensive rats. Eur J Pharmacol 77:187–191, 1982.
37. Goldstein M, Sauter AM, Baba Y, Lew JY. The effect of PNMT inhibition on epinephrine levels in the central nervous system of control and spontaneous hypertensive rats. International Congress of Neuroscience Abstracts, 425, Kopenhagen, 1977.
38. Guyenet PG. The coeruleospinal noradrenergic neurons: Anatomical and electrophysiological studies in the rat. Brain Res 189:121–133, 1980.
39. Hawley RJ, Major LF, Schulman EA, Lake CR. CSF levels of norepinephrine during alcohol withdrawal. Arch Neurol 38:289–292, 1981.
40. Hökfelt T, Fuxe K, Goldstein M, Johansson O. Immunohistochemical evidence for the existence of adrenaline neurons in the rat brain. Brain Res 66:235–251, 1974.
41. Hökfelt T, Rehfeld JF, Skirboll L, Ivemark B, Goldstein M, Markey K. Evidence for coexistence of dopamine and CCK in mesolimbic neurons. Nature 285:476–477, 1980.
42. Honma T, Fukushima H. Role of brain norepinephrine in neuroleptic induced catalepsy in rats. Pharmacol Biochem Behav 7:501–506, 1977.
43. Horton R, Anlezark G, Meldrum B. Noradrenergic influences on sound induced seizures. J Pharmacol Exp Ther 214:437–442, 1980.
44. Johnson DD, Jaju AT, Ness L, Richardson JS, Crawford RD. Brain norepinephrine, dopamine and 5-hydroxytryptamine concentration abnormalities and their role in the high seizure susceptibility of epileptic chickens. Can J Physiol Pharmacol 59:144–149, 1981.
45. Jolicoeur F, Rondeau D, St.-Pierre S, Rioux F, Barbeau A. Peptides and the Basal Ganglia. In Apomorphine and Other Dopaminomimetics. Basic Pharmacology, GL Gessa and GU Corsini (eds), vol. 1, 19–25. New York: Raven Press, 1981.
46. Kalsner S, Chan C-C. Inhibition by dopamine of the stimulation induced efflux of

[^{3}H] noradrenaline in renal arteries: Limitations of the unitary hypothesis of presynaptic regulation of transmitter release. Can J Physiol Pharmacol 58:504–512, 1980.
47. Karoum F, Commissiong JW, Neff NH, Wyatt RJ. Biochemical evidence for uncrossed and crossed locus coeruleus projections to the spinal cord. Brain Res 196:237–241, 1980.
48. Keller H, Bartholini G, Pletscher A. Enhancement of cerebral noradrenaline turnover by thyrotropin releasing hormone. Nature 248:528–529, 1974.
49. Koslow SH, Schlumpf M. Quantitation of adrenaline in rat brain areas by mass fragmentography. Nature 251:530–531, 1974.
50. Kuhar MJ, Atweh SF. Distribution of some suspected neurotransmitters in the central nervous system. Rev Neurosci 3:35–76, 1978.
51. Kvetnansky R, Kopin IJ, Saavedra JM. Changes in epinephrine in individual hypothalamic nuclei after immobilization stress. Brain Res 155:387–390, 1978.
52. Kvetnansky R, Mitro A, Palkovits M, Brownstein MJ, Torda T, Vigas M, Mikulaj L. Catecholamines in individual hypothalamic nuclei of acutely and repeatedly stressed rats. Neuroendocrinology 23:257–267, 1977.
53. Lindvall O, Bjorklund A. Dopaminergic innervation of the globus pallidus by collaterals from the nigrostriatal pathway. Brain Res 172:169–173, 1979.
54. Loeb C, Roccatagliata G, Albano C, Besio G. Bromocriptine and dopaminergic function in Huntington's disease. Neurology (NY) 29:730–734, 1979.
55. Loewy AD, McKellar S, Safer CB. Direct projections from the A5 catecholamine cell group to the intermedio-lateral cell column. Brain Res 174:309–314, 1979.
56. McKellar S, Lowey AD. Efferent projections of the A1 catecholamine cell group in the rat: An autoradiographic study. Brain Res Bull 241:11–29, 1982.
57. Makman MH, Matsumoto Y, Drorkin B, Lew JY, Goldstein M. Localization of adenylate cyclase stimulated by epinephrine in specific regions of medulla oblongata of rat brain. Neuroscience 1:317, 1975.
58. Mann JJ, Stanley M, Gershon S, Rosser M. Mental symptoms in Huntington's disease and a possible primary aminergic neuron lesion. Science 210:1369–1371, 1980.
59. Marek K, Hanbrich DR. Thyrotropin-releasing hormone–increased catabolism of catecholamines in brains of thyroidectomized rats. Biochem Pharmacol 26:1817–1818, 1977.
60. Mason ST. Central noradrenergic-cholinergic interaction and locomotor behavior. Eur J Pharmacol 56:131–137, 1979.
61. Mason ST, Corcoran ME. Seizure susceptibility after depletion of spinal or cerebellar noradrenaline with 6-OHDA. Brain Res 170:479–507, 1979.
62. Mason ST, Roberts DCS, Fibiger HC. Noradrenergic influences on catalepsy. Psychopharmacology (Berlin) 60:53–57, 1978.
63. Massari VJ, Tizabi Y, Jacobwitz DM. Potential noradrenergic regulation of serotonergic neurons in the median raphe nucleus. Eur Brain Res 34:177–182, 1979.
64. Meyer DK, Beinfeld MC, Oertel WH, Brownstein MJ. Origin of cholecystokinin containing fibers in the rat caudatoputamen. Science 215:187–188, 1982.
65. Mogilnicka E, Klimek VL. Dopaminergic stimulation enhances the utilization of noradrenaline in the central nervous system. J Pharm Pharmacol 29:569–570, 1977.
66. Morgan WW, Pfeil KA. Evidence for a cholinergic influence on catecholaminergic pathways terminating in the anterior and medial basal hypothalamus. Brain Res 173:47–56, 1979.
67. Morrison JH, Mollivin ME, Grzanna R. Noradrenergic innervation of cerebral cortex: Widespread effects of local cortical lesions. Science 205:313–316, 1979.

68. Nakamura K, Nakamura K. Role of brainstem and spinal noradrenergic and adrenergic neurons in the development and maintenance of hypertension in spontaneously hypertensive rats. Naunyn Schmiedebergs Arch Pharmacol 305:127–133, 1978.
69. Neff NH, Parenti M, Gentleman S, Olianas MC. Modulation of Dopamine Receptors by Opiates. In Apomorphine and Other Dopaminomimetics. Basic Pharmacology, GL Gessa and GU Corsini (eds), vol. 1, 193–200. New York: Raven Press, 1981.
70. Nelson MF, Zaczek R, Coyle JT. Effects of sustained seizures produced by intrahippocampal injection of kainic acid on noradrenergic neurons: Evidence for local control of norepinephrine release. J Pharmacol Exp Ther 214:694–702, 1980.
71. Oberlander C, Hunt PF, Dumont C, Boissier JR. Dopamine-independent rotational responses to unilateral intranigral injection of serotonin. Life Sci 28:2595–2601, 1981.
72. O'Donohue TL, Crowley WR, Jacobowitz DM. Biochemical mapping of the noradrenergic ventral bundle projection sites: Evidence for a noradrenergic-dopaminergic interaction. Brain Res 172:87–100, 1979.
73. Oke A, Keller R, Mefford I, Adams RN. Lateralization of norepinephrine in the human thalamus. Science 200:1411–1413, 1978.
74. Olpe HR, Glatt A, Laszlo J, Schellenberg A. Some electrophysiological and pharmacological properties of the cortical noradrenergic projection of the locus coeruleus in the rat. Brain Res 186:9–19, 1980.
75. Palkovits M, Zabonszky L, Feminger A, Mezey E, Fekete MIK, Herman JP, Kanyieska B, Szabo D. Noradrenergic innervation of the rat hypothalamus: Experimental biochemical and electron microscopic studies. Brain Res 191:161–171, 1980.
76. Pasquier DA, Gold MA, Jacobowitz DM. Noradrenergic perikarya (A5–A7), subcoeruleus projections to the cat cerebellum. Brain Res 196:270–275, 1980.
77. Price KS, Farley IJ, Hornykiewicz O. Neurochemistry of Parkinson's Disease: Relation Between Striatal and Limbic Dopamine. In Advances in Biochemical Psychopharmacology, PJ Roberts (ed), vol. 19, 293–300. New York: Raven Press, 1978.
78. Pycock CJ. Noradrenergic involvement in dopamine-dependent stereotyped and cataleptic responses in the rat. Arch Pharm (Weinheim) 298:15–22, 1977.
79. Pycock CJ, Kerwin RW, Carter CJ. Effect of lesion of cortical dopamine terminals on subcortical dopamine receptors in rats. Nature 286:74–77, 1980.
80. Reavill C, Jenner P, Marsden CD. Puzzles of the Mechanism of Action of Bromocriptine. In Apomorphine and Other Dopaminomimetics. Basic Pharmacology, GL Gessa and GU Corsini (eds), vol. 1, 229–239. New York: Raven Press, 1981.
81. Reigle TG, Arni J, Platz PA, Schildkraut JJ, Plotnikoff NP. Norepinephrine metabolism in the rat brain following acute and chronic administration of thyrotropin-releasing hormone. Psychopharmacologia (Berlin) 37:1–6, 1974.
82. Rinne UK. Recent advances in research on Parkinsonism. Acta Neurol Scan 57[Suppl 67]:77–113, 1978.
83. Roberts DCS, Mason ST, Fibiger HC. 6-OHDA lesion to the dorsal noradrenergic bundle alters morphine-induced locomotor activity and catalepsy. Eur J Pharmacol 52:209–214, 1978.
84. Saavedra JM, Grobecker H, Axelrod J. Adrenaline-forming enzyme in brain stem: Elevation in genetic and experimental hypertension. Science 191:483–484, 1975.
85. Saavedra JM, Grobecker H, Axelrod J. Changes in central catecholaminergic neurons in spontaneously (genetic) hypertensive rats. Circ Res 42:529–534, 1978.
86. Saavedra JM, Palkovits M, Brownstein MJ, Axelrod J. Localization of phenylethanolamine N-methyltransferase in rat brain nuclei. Nature 248:694–696, 1974.
87. Sauter AA, Lew JY, Baba Y, Goldstein M. Effect of phenylethanolamine N-methyl-

transferase and dopamine-β-hydroxylase inhibition on epinephrine levels in the brain. Life Sci 21:261–266, 1977.

88. Sawchenko PE, Swanson LW. Central noradrenergic pathways for the integration of hypothalamic neuroendocrine and autonomic responses. Science 214:685–687, 1981.
89. Shoulson I, Ziegler MG, Lake CR. Huntington's disease (HD): Determination of plasma norepinephrine (NE) and dopamine-β-hydroxylase (DBH). Neuroscience Abstracts 2:800, 1976.
90. Simon H, Scatton B, LeMoal M. Dopaminergic A10 neurons are involved in cognitive functions. Nature 286:150–151, 1980.
91. Skirboll LR, Hökfelt T, Grace AA, Hammer DW, Rehfeld JF, Maskey K, Goldstein M, Bunney BS. The Coexistence of Dopamine and a CCK-like Peptide in a Subpopulation of Midbrain Neurons: Immunocytochemical and Electrophysiological Studies. In Apomorphine and Other Dopaminomimetics. Basic Pharmacology, GL Gessa and GU Corsini (eds), vol. 1, 65–78. New York: Raven Press, 1981.
92. Slater P. Circling produced by serotonin and dopamine agonists in raphe-lesioned rats: A serotonin model. Pharmacol Biochem Behav 13:817–821, 1980.
93. Spokes EGS. Neurochemical alterations in Huntington's chorea. A study of post-mortem brain tissue. Brain 103:179–210, 1980.
94. Tabakoff B, Yanai J, Ritzmann RF. Noradrenaline and seizures. Science 203:1265–1266, 1979.
95. Taube MD, Starke K, Bosowski E. Presynaptic receptor systems on noradrenergic neurons of rat brain. Naunyn Schmiedebergs Arch Pharmacol 299:123–141, 1977.
96. Teychenne PF, Lake CR, Ziegler MG. Cerebrospinal Fluid Studies in Parkinson's Disease. In Neurobiology of Cerebrospinal Fluid, JH Wood (ed), vol. 1, 197–206. New York: Plenum Press, 1980.
97. Teychenne PF, Lake CR, Ziegler MG, Plotkin C, Wood JH, Calne DB. Central and peripheral deficiency of norepinephrine in Parkinson's disease and the effects of L-dopa therapy. Neuroscience Abstracts 3:47, 1977.
98. Teychenne PF, Rosin AJ, Plotkin CN, Calne DB. Cross tolerance between two dopaminergic ergot derivatives—bromocriptine and lergotrile. Br J Clin Pharmacol 9:47–50, 1980.
99. Tuomisto J, Mannisto P. Amine uptake and TRH. Lancet 1:836–837, 1973.
100. Waszczak BL, Walters JR. Intravenous GABA agonist administration stimulates firing of A10 dopaminergic neurons. Eur J Pharmacol 66:141–144, 1980.
101. Weinshilboum R, Axelrod J. Serum dopamine-β-hydroxylase activity. Circ Res 28:307–315, 1971.
102. Weinstock M, Zavadil AP, Muth EA, Crowley WR, O'Donohue TL, Jacobowitz DM, Kopin IJ. Evidence that noradrenaline modulates the increase in striatal dopamine metabolism induced by muscarinic receptor stimulation. Eur J Pharmacol 68:427–435, 1980.
103. Wijnen HJLM, Versteeg DHG, Palkovits M, DeJong W. Increased adrenaline content of individual nuclei of the hypothalamus and the medulla oblongata of genetically hypertensive rats. Brain Res 135:180–185, 1977.
104. Wikening D, Dvorkin B, Makman MH, Lew JY, Matsumoto J, Baba Y, Goldstein M, Fuxe K. Catecholamine-stimulated cyclic AMP formation in phenylethanolamine N-methyltransferase–containing brain stem nuclei of normal rats and of rats with spontaneous genetic hypertension. Brain Res 186:133–143, 1980.
105. Williams AC. Observations on some extrapyramidal diseases. M.D. Thesis, Birmingham University, 1978.

106. Woodward DJ, Moises HC, Waterhouse BD, Hoffer BJ, Freedman R. Modulatory actions of norepinephrine in the central nervous system. Fed Proc 38:2109–2116, 1979.
107. Yamazaki M, Tanka C, Takaori S. Significance of central noradrenergic system of harmaline-induced tremor. Pharmacol Biochem Behav 10:421–427, 1979.
108. Ziegler MG, Lake CR, Kopin IJ. Norepinephrine in cerebrospinal fluid. Brain Res 108:436–440, 1976.
109. Ziegler MG, Lake CR, Williams AC, Teychenne PF, Shoulson I, Steinsland O. Bromocriptine inhibits norepinephrine release. Clin Pharmacol Ther 25:137–142, 1979.

6

Noradrenergic Responses in Postural Hypotension: Implications for Therapy

Michael G. Ziegler
C. Raymond Lake

Debate concerning the role of the sympathetic nervous system (SNS) in hypertension has caused more heat than light. In disorders of postural hypotension, however, the sympathetic nervous response to standing often illuminates the cause of the disorder. Even in hypotensive disorders such as volume depletion, where the SNS functions normally, indices of sympathetic activity can help make the diagnosis and guide therapy. Heart rate has long served as a simple clinical guide to sympathetic tone. Plasma norepinephrine (NE) levels now provide a quantitative biochemical index of sympathetic nervous activity. Because hypotensive disorders inevitably involve diseases of the SNS or compensatory response of SNS to a disease, these disorders can be conveniently divided according to patients' NE levels.

Sympathetic tone normally doubles on standing (see Chapters 1 and 2) in response to an effective decrease in blood volume. Fluids flow downhill so that when we stand, 300 to 600 ml of blood pools in our legs [42]. If we continue to stand for 10 minutes, water swells into our feet and legs from blood and causes a 10% hemoconcentration [48]. We compensate for this "self-phlebotomy" with an increase in heart rate, peripheral resistance, and venous tone. If these compensatory mechanisms are inadequate, blood pressure falls, the brain is inadequately perfused, and symptoms of lightheadedness and fatigue ensue. Standing causes an average 5 mm Hg rise in diastolic blood pressure. Postural hypotension occurs when there is a significant drop in diastolic blood pressure accompanied by symptoms attributable to inadequate perfusion of the brain. A drop in systolic blood pressure is a less reliable marker of postural hypotension because in people more than 50 years of age, systolic pressure normally decreases on standing. Postural hypotension may occur intermittently in response to cardiac arrhythmias, heat, exercise, drugs, or voiding a full bladder. Since lightheadedness and fatigue can be produced by so many causes, the diagnosis of intermittent postural hypotension can only be made if the symptoms are reproduced and blood pressure is measured.

It is sometimes difficult to diagnose the disease that causes postural hypotension, but the mechanism responsible for the lowered blood pressure should be known before treatment is initiated. The unclear etiology of hypotensive disorders has resulted in labeling people with "syndromes" and the diagnosis of "idiopathic orthostatic hypotension" [49]. However, it should always be determined which organ system is responsible for the postural hypotension because appropriate therapy depends on this determination. For example, the hypotension caused by the reduced cardiac output of congestive heart failure is treated by salt restriction, but the hypotension of sodium depletion is treated with increased dietary salt. Although there are dozens of diverse entities that decrease standing blood pressure, they all act by impairing one of the major mechanisms necessary for blood pressure maintenance [47]; therapy is directed toward repairing or compensating for their failure.

MECHANISMS OF POSTURAL BLOOD PRESSURE MAINTENANCE

Blood pressure can be maintained only in the presence of an adequate blood volume. The extracellular fluid volume, including blood volume, is governed by the amount of sodium retained by the body. Although excess dietary sodium is the norm for modern man, diuretics and renal disease often lead to sodium depletion and a decreased extracellular fluid volume. The volume of the intravascular fraction of extracellular fluid is primarily determined by the oncotic pressure of plasma albumin and the volume of red blood cells. Both hypoalbuminemia and anemia cause tachycardia on standing and, when severe, cause postural hypotension.

In the presence of an adequate blood volume, maintenance of blood pressure on standing requires a redistribution of blood flow in the first few seconds after standing. When a person stands, baroreceptors decrease the neural input into the brainstem vasomotor centers. This information is processed by the vasomotor centers, and sympathetic nervous activity is increased and parasympathetic activity decreased. The sympathetic nerves sharply increase their output of NE; subsequently, the heart responds with increased chronotropic and inotropic activity, arterioles constrict and lead to a sharply increased peripheral vascular resistance, and capacitance vessels contract, increasing the return of blood to the heart. These events lead to prompt maintenance of normal blood pressure as longer-term processes are initiated by the kidney, which secretes renin, ultimately leading to enhanced vasoconstrictor activity and sodium retention. The therapy of postural hypotension depends on diagnosing which component of this system is defective. A diagnosis can be made on the basis of the physical examination and available laboratory tests.

DIAGNOSIS OF THE SYSTEMIC DEFECT CAUSING POSTURAL HYPOTENSION

Diseases that cause postural hypotension act through several mechanisms which give strikingly different NE responses to standing (Figure 6.1).

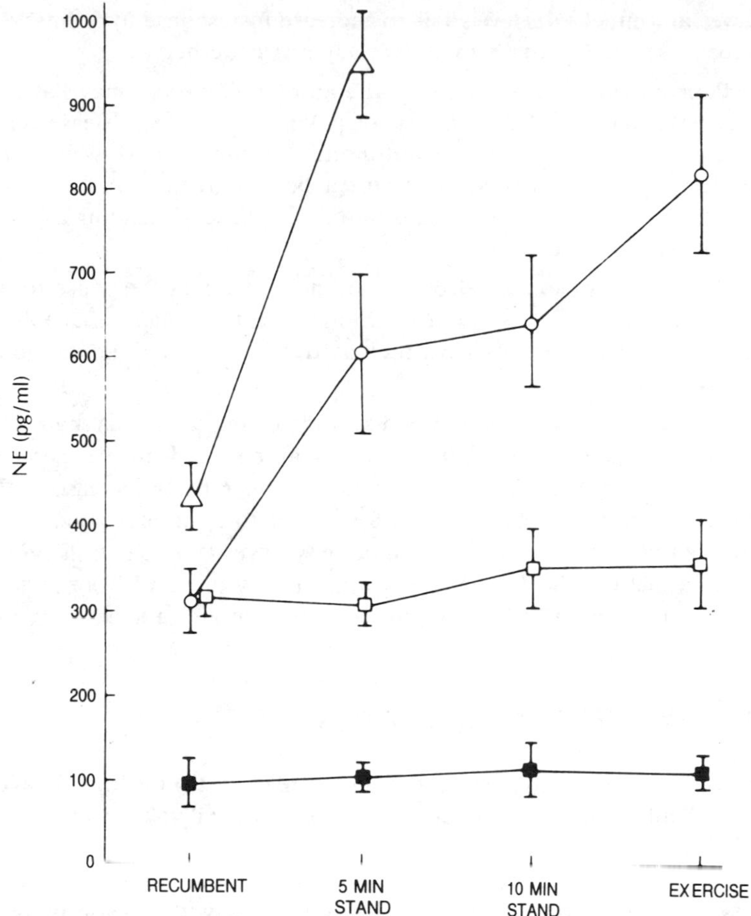

Figure 6.1 Plasma norepinephrine (NE) levels while recumbent, after standing for 5 and 10 minutes, and after 5 minutes of isometric exercise while standing. Solid squares represent idiopathic orthostatic hypotension; open squares represent Shy-Drager syndrome; open circles represent normal subjects, and open triangles represent normal subjects after furosemide diuresis. Values are shown as mean ± standard error of the mean. (*Reproduced with permission from the* Annual Review of Medicine, *Vol. 31. Copyright 1980 by Annual Reviews, Inc.*)

1. Patients with postural hypotension from central nervous system (CNS) lesions have other symptoms of CNS disorders, which may range from paraplegia as the result of a spinal cord lesion to parkinsonism and cerebellar dysfunction as a result of the Shy-Drager syndrome [46,49]. They have a fairly fixed heart rate and other symptoms of autonomic dysfunction, such as impotence and incontinence. Their NE levels while recumbent are normal since their peripheral sympa-

thetic nerves are intact. NE levels fail to increase in response to ordinary stimuli, however, because the CNS fails to activate sympathetic nerves.

2. Patients with a neuropathy of the autonomic nerves may have no CNS lesions, but have many of the symptoms of patients with CNS disease. They have a fixed heart rate and symptoms of autonomic dysfunction. However, their NE levels are very low while they are recumbent because their noradrenergic nerves are damaged. There is, of course, no plasma NE response to standing as the sympathetic nerves are damaged.

3. Patients may have a defective cardiac or vascular response to NE as a result of intrinsic heart disease or from humoral causes, such as anaphylaxis or carcinoid tumor. These patients have increased NE levels and an exaggerated response of NE to standing.

4. Patients with a decreased blood volume owing to anemia, hypoalbuminemia, or sodium depletion have a tachycardia at rest and an exaggerated heart rate response to standing. The increased heart rate reflects increased NE levels which further increase on standing in an attempt to maintain blood pressure in the face of volume depletion. These patients may have signs of peripheral vasoconstriction and a tachycardia and generally appear very different from patients with autonomic dysfunction, who have warm, smooth skin and a fixed heart rate.

POSTURAL HYPOTENSION IN DIABETICS

Postural hypotension is a frequent consequence of diabetes mellitus. It may occur as a result of autonomic neuropathy, decreased plasma volume from renal loss of albumin, or diminished red blood cell volume.

After standing, diastolic blood pressure in normal subjects increases, but blood pressure in diabetics often decreases. Diabetics with disease of very short duration and with no retinopathy may have a normal blood pressure response to standing, but blood pressure in diabetics with disease of long duration usually decreases even though they may have no symptoms of postural dizziness [45]. Although some diabetics have signs of sympathetic denervation without vagal neuropathy [45], the usual course involves deterioration in vagal control of heart rate several years before prominent signs of sympathetic neuropathy appear [18]. This unbalanced loss of parasympathetic function leads to a resting tachycardia and a loss in beat-to-beat variation of the heart rate before there is any change in the rate of urinary secretion of NE and epinephrine (E) [21]. In response to hypoglycemia, a diabetic at this early stage of autonomic neuropathy may still have increased NE and E output but has a defective release of glucagon because glucagon release is mediated through the parasympathetic nervous system [31].

After the parasympathetic nerves deteriorate, sympathetic neuropathy also develops, at which point postural hypotension becomes severe enough to cause symptoms. The defective response of sympathetic nerves in diabetes mellitus is caused by postganglionic lesions in the sympathetic nerves themselves as demonstrated by their lack of response to cholinergic stimulation [30]. Diabetics with persistent or severe autonomic neuropathy have NE levels of less than 20% of normal in their heart and blood vessels. Their E levels are also variably diminished, and dopamine levels are about one half of normal [34]. As expected, patients who have these low tissue levels of NE also have low plasma levels of NE, and on standing, their NE output is much diminished [11] (Figure 6.2). The low circulating levels of NE measured in these subjects represent an even lower rate of secretion of NE from sympathetic nerves since their rate of clearance of NE from plasma is diminished [14]. The decreased capacity of the sympathetic nerves leads to disordered regulation of blood flow. Normally, when the leg is placed in a dependent posture, blood flow to the ankle decreases by 50%. In diabetics with autonomic neuropathy, blood flow to the ankle increases by 25% under the same circumstances [22]. When the diabetic with autonomic neuropathy stands up, blood goes to his legs, not his head, and postural dizziness ensues.

Although extensive neuropathy of the sympathetic nerves alone is adequate to cause postural hypotension, postural hypotension in diabetics can be aggravated by abnormal renin release. Although diabetics usually have normal basal renin and aldosterone levels, renin levels fail to increase in response to stimulation with NE or upright posture [13] or in response to diuretics or vasodilators [29]. Patients with orthostatic hypotension from idiopathic sympathetic neuropathy are capable of releasing renin in response to upright posture, so this defect cannot be attributed to diminished sympathetic nervous stimulation of the juxtaglomerular apparatus. It is due instead to a basic defect that prevents renin release in response to a variety of stimuli, another manifestation of diabetic renal disease which usually coexists with diabetic autonomic neuropathy.

Diabetic autonomic neuropathy causes postural hypotension and other disabling symptoms and is associated with a 50% mortality in 5 years [19]. Half of these patients die from renal failure, but the other half die from diseases that may be related directly to the autonomic neuropathy. Myocardial infarction is unusual in these patients [18,35], but there appears to be a marked increase in the incidence of respiratory arrest and sudden death [20,35].

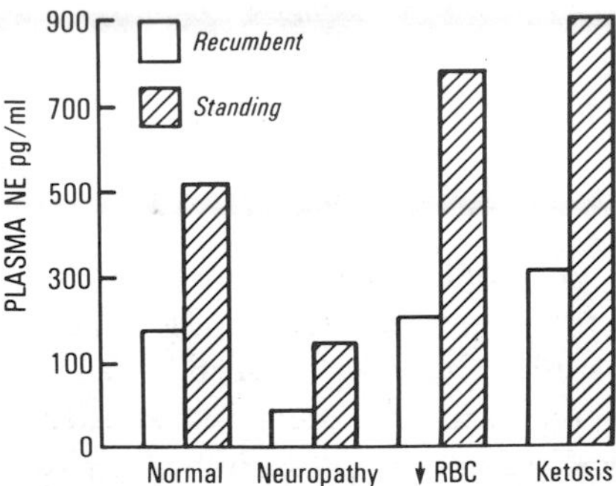

Figure 6.2 Norepinephrine (NE) levels while recumbent and standing in normal subjects and diabetics. Patients with diabetic neuropathy have low NE levels and a blunted NE response to standing. Those with a diminished red blood cell (RBC) volume have normal NE levels while recumbent, but an exaggerated response to standing. Patients in diabetic ketoacidosis have increased NE while recumbent and while standing. (*Data from Bannister et al* [*1*], *Benowitz et al* [*4*], *and Chobanian et al* [*8*].)

Hyperadrenergic Responses in Diabetics

Diabetics with poor metabolic control and ketosis have increased circulating levels of NE while at rest [10], and these NE levels increase greatly after moderate levels of exercise [9] (see Figure 6.2). After these patients are treated with insulin, NE levels decrease to the normal range [12]. The increased NE levels are analogous to other hormonal responses such as growth hormone, glucagon, and cortisol, which are also elevated in uncontrolled diabetes mellitus.

Some patients with well-controlled diabetes and postural hypotension have an exaggerated increase in their NE levels on standing. This type of response is characteristic of patients with decreased blood volume, which is compensated for by an enhanced release of NE from the sympathetic nerves [47]. This type of response is seen in patients with diabetic renal disease and nephrotic syndrome, but is also found in diabetics who have normal plasma volume with decreased red blood cell volume [15] (see Figure 6.2). These patients may have a normal hematocrit, but their total red blood cell volume is diminished, leading to volume contraction. Patients with only a mild degree of sympathetic neuropathy may still have postural hypotension because, even though they may be able to secrete supranormal levels of NE in response to standing, they still lack sufficient noradrenergic response to compensate for diminished blood volume.

Insulin

In normal human beings, intravenous insulin administration increases plasma NE and heart rate and decreases peripheral blood flow [11] (see Chapter 13). In diabetics with sympathetic neuropathy, enhanced NE secretion cannot take place and so blood pressure decreases. This hypotensive effect transpires whether insulin is administered subcutaneously or intravenously, takes place almost immediately after intravenous insulin before blood glucose can fall [36], and occurs even when blood glucose is maintained at normal levels. It is possible to alter the schedule of insulin administration to relieve the severity of postural hypotension [37]. We address specific aspects of the treatment of postural hypotension in diabetics later in this chapter.

THERAPY OF POSTURAL HYPOTENSION

Physical Measures

Blood pools in dependent parts of the body when people stand, so measures that counteract blood pooling are effective in all types of postural hypotension. Most elastic stockings provide too little counterpressure to have any detectable effect, but the Jobst venous pressure gradient support is a special leotard that exerts external pressure. This pressure balances venous hydrostatic pressure by exerting greatest compression at the feet with progressively less compression up to the costal margin. This garment is effective, but an antigravity suit is even more effective although cumbersome and difficult to obtain. These garments are both safe and effective, but patients often refuse to wear them because of discomfort. Patients with postural hypotension from autonomic dysfunction have heat intolerance owing to lack of sweating, so these garments do not work well in warm climates where hyperthermia can lead to vasodilatation and worsening hypotension. When capacitance vessels in the legs fill with blood on standing, a myogenic reflex constricts the veins and returns blood to the heart. Counterpressure garments decrease this myogenic response and must provide enough pressure to replace the effects of the myogenic stretch reflex to be effective. If the garment is loose enough to be comfortable, it is probably ineffective.

Jobst stockings are particularly helpful with sodium-retaining drugs, which tend to cause volume overload and recumbent hypertension. The garment can be donned during the daytime when the patient is up and hypotensive, and then removed at night to allow excess fluid to pool in the legs. Removal at night is particularly effective if the patient keeps his bed tilted head up, as these combined measures promote renin release and fluid retention and diminish nocturia. Although these physical measures are uniformly helpful in patients with postural hypotension, they can be uncomfortable and patient compliance is not uniform. Patients with fluid retention and recumbent hypertension should not lie completely horizontally because the resulting hypertension is asymptomatic but dangerous [40].

Fludrocortisone

Fludrocortisone (Florinef) is the most consistently useful drug in the treatment of postural hypotension. Its sodium-retaining properties provide physiologic therapy for patients who have chronic hypovolemia. Mineralocorticoids such as fludrocortisone decrease postural hypotension through two mechanisms: they sensitize blood vessels to the effects of NE and they retain sodium and expand volume. The sensitization to NE occurs at low dose (0.1 mg/day), which may cause no detectable fluid retention. This effect is present in normal subjects and is especially marked in patients with hyporeninemic hypoaldosteronism where endogenous mineralocorticoid levels are diminished, and in anephric patients with low renin levels who have postural hypotension after the iatrogenic hypovolemia of hemodialysis. Low-dose fludrocortisone therapy is quite safe and usually has a small but marked effect of increasing the blood pressure of postural hypotensive patients while they are standing.

High doses of fludrocortisone do not have much more effect on vascular sensitivity to NE than do low doses, but they do cause sodium retention, increase blood volume, and raise blood pressure in both supine and standing postures. High doses can also cause congestive heart failure, hypokalemia, and supine hypertension. Patients treated with high doses of fludrocortisone have an increased incidence of sudden death, usually at night while they sleep supine. This therapy has both obvious and hidden dangers, but is sometimes the only effective means of treatment for patients with postural hypotension. Patients notice an improvement in their symptoms when supine diastolic blood pressure has increased by 10 mm Hg, at which time they have usually gained from 2 to 5 kg. This requires a dose of from 0.3 to 1.5 mg of fludrocortisone daily and sometimes requires anincrease in dietary salt. The patient can maintain the effect by weighing in daily and adjusting dietary sodium to keep weight elevated but stable. Patients who have postural hypotension as the result of CNS diseases such as the Shy-Drager syndrome seem particularly prone to pulmonary congestion on this fluid-retaining regimen, but patients with isolated autonomic neuropathy have fewer side effects from the drug and live longer. Patients should receive low-dose fludrocortisone and a trial of prostaglandin-synthesis inhibitors, β-blockers, or vasoconstrictors before resorting to high-dose fludrocortisone. However, treatment with sodium-retaining doses of fludrocortisone can sometimes make the difference between a patient who is confined to bed and one who is functional.

Prostaglandin Inhibitors

Indomethacin augments the release of NE following nerve stimulation in vitro [7], can enhance the excretion of NE in rats at rest [26] or during stress [44], and can increase vascular responses to NE [41]. Thus, several lines of evidence indicate that a prostaglandin-synthesis inhibitor might both enhance the release of NE and increase the response of the vasculature to NE. These effects make these drugs ideal candidates for the treatment of postural hypotension, where an enhanced sympathetic nervous response is needed to maintain a patient's blood pressure while standing.

Patients with Bartter's syndrome have abnormally high plasma NE levels and vascular resistance to the effects of NE. Indomethacin restores their vascular sensitivity to NE [41]. Kochar and Itskovitz [28] treated five patients with postural hypotension with indomethacin and noted an increase in blood pressure of 20 to 30 mm Hg. Four of the patients had marked relief of their symptoms, and one patient had return of symptoms 48 hours after stopping the drug. All of these patients had normal levels of urinary catecholamines (CA), metanephrine, and vanillylmandelic acid (VMA), and normal levels of dopamine β-hydroxylase (DBH), suggesting that they had some remaining autonomic nervous activity. Another patient with "patchy autonomic neuropathy" and normal urinary catecholamines had a good response to indomethacin with a marked increase in blood pressure and relief of symptoms [38]. However, Bannister et al [2] reported that three patients with Shy-Drager syndrome whose autonomic function was grossly impaired, had no discernible improvement in their postural hypotension in response to indomethacin. It thus appears that several patients with normal CA output have had considerable relief of their postural hypotension in response to indomethacin. In the authors' experience, patients who have no adrenergic response to standing also fail to respond to treatment with indomethacin. This experience is consistent with the report of Silverberg et al [41], which stated that in patients with Bartter's syndrome, indomethacin restores vascular sensitivity to NE; and with Klein et al [27], who observed that a hyperadrenergic patient with postural hypotension benefited from indomethacin but hypoadrenergic patients did not. Hui and Conolly [24] also reported that indomethacin had no effect in a patient with low plasma NE. These reports suggested that hypotensive patients capable of releasing NE may have enhanced vascular responsiveness and enhanced NE release when treated with indomethacin. Patients incapable of releasing NE receive little or no benefit from the drug. When indomethacin is effective in patients with postural hypotension, its beneficial effects are apparently due to inhibition of prostaglandin synthesis because flurbiprofen and aspirin are also effective in patients who respond to indomethacin [38,43].

β-Receptor Blockers

Although cardiac β-receptors stimulate the heart and raise blood pressure, vascular β-receptors mediate vasodilatation and can lower blood pressure. β-receptor sensitivity decreases after treatment with agonist drugs such as isoproterenol and increases after treatment with β blockers. A hypotensive patient with very low levels of plasma NE had a β-receptor concentration more than twice normal, as well as increased isoproterenol sensitivity [24].

Brevetti et al [5] reported that a patient with "no significant amounts of catecholamines or their metabolites" had a marked symptomatic improvement in his postural hypotension after treatment with propranolol, although this patient did not have well-documented postural hypotension. Chobanian et al [8] reported a thorough study of five patients who had very low circulating levels of CA and denervation supersensitivity to NE. The blood pressure of four of the five patients increased in response to propranolol in both recumbent and standing positions, and orthostatic symptoms decreased. One of the patients had such a marked hypertensive response to propranolol that the drug had to be discontinued. Patients with autonomic neuropathies develop denervation supersensitivity of both their β- and α-receptors. Although their circulating CA levels may be low, they are always detectable. In these patients, blockade of the supersensitive β-receptors can block vasodilatation and allow vasoconstriction in response to α-receptor stimulation.

Although most patients with disorders of the autonomic nervous system and postural hypotension have a fixed heart rate that does not change when they stand, some hypotensive patients have a marked tachycardia on standing. This tachycardia occurs if sympathetic innervation to the heart is spared or if adrenal E is released in response to the stress of hypotension on standing. Patients who secrete E in response to their postural hypotension should have an especially beneficial response to β blockers. Miller et al [32] reported that a woman with marked tachycardia and hypotension on standing experienced an increase in blood pressure and capacity to stand in response to 40 mg of propranolol daily; she even developed occasional supine hypertension on the drug.

Patients with CNS defects, such as the Shy-Drager syndrome, that prevent activation of an otherwise normal SNS, have normal CA levels while recumbent and little increase in their adrenergic-receptor sensitivity. Kochar and Itskovitz [28] reported that four such patients had no response to treatment with propranolol and ephedrine, and all the patients' erect blood pressure increased in response to indomethacin. It thus appears that two groups of patients with postural hypotension have some improvement in their upright blood pressure after treatment with propranolol: patients who have almost complete autonomic denervation and an increase in their β-receptor sensitivity and patients with an inappropriate tachycardia in response to standing. On the other hand, patients with postural hypotension owing to a CNS disease are likely to have a fixed heart rate and normal β-receptor sensitivity and seem not to respond to propranolol therapy. Although there has been no definitive study of which patients will respond to β blockers, it would seem reasonable to try a course of propranolol therapy in patients with denervation supersensitivity from autonomic neuropathy and in patients who have a marked tachycardia on standing.

Pressors

Patients with postural hypotension owing to volume depletion may have a chronic increase in their circulating level of NE and diminished receptor sensitivity. Therapy with pressor agents is unlikely to be effective in increasing blood pressure, but when it is effective, it is likely to be dangerous as it may compromise the blood supply to vital organs. Patients with postural hypotension owing to a CNS disease such as Shy-Drager syndrome have a normal or slightly increased sensitivity to infused NE. They have peripheral neuronal stores of NE, which are not released in adequate amounts when they stand. However, patients with peripheral autonomic neuropathy and decreased NE stores have increased β-adrenergic [14], α-adrenergic [2], and antidiuretic hormone receptor [33] sensitivity. Hypotensive patients thus may have either diminished or increased sensitivity to pressors, depending on the cause of their hypotension.

It is difficult to evaluate the effects of pressor drugs on patients with orthostatic hypotension. Although we use the upright blood pressure measurement as a guide to therapy, the real problem in these patients is not low blood pressure, but low brain perfusion. Because pressor agents may cause a diffuse vasoconstriction, they are capable of increasing blood pressure while simultaneously decreasing blood flow to the brain. When a patient is treated with a vasoconstricting drug, it is as important to question and examine him while standing as it is to follow the blood pressure. For example, patients with familial dysautonomia have postural hypotension from birth and become quite accustomed to it. Some of them develop slurred speech and diminished perception when they stand, yet they say they feel fine.

They may faint abruptly with no subjective symptoms of dizziness. Because postural hypotension may alter the patient's perceptual skills, it is not always reliable to ask a patient how he feels when he stands; it is more reliable to have the patient perform some simple motor and intellectual tests while recumbent and while standing. This is particularly important in evaluating the effects of pressor drugs which can constrict the cerebral vasculature.

Monoamine Oxidase Inhibitors Plus Tyramine

Tyramine is a normal constituent of many foods and is chemically related to NE. It can interfere with storage of NE in nerve terminals and cause a chemical release of the neurotransmitter. It is only effective in patients who have stores of NE to release [47] and is thus more potent in patients with Shy-Drager syndrome than in patients with peripheral autonomic neuropathies. Tyramine is usually metabolized before it can have access to noradrenergic stores, but its action can be greatly prolonged when the enzyme monoamine oxidase (MAO) is inhibited. Even when MAO is effectively inhibited, tyramine needs to be given every 2 hours to maintain its pressor effects. This short duration of action is actually beneficial because the patient can then omit doses when he wants to lie down. Tyramine is not available as a pharmaceutical preparation and has been administered in the form of cheddar cheese, a food which contains large amounts of the amine. Absorption of tyramine from cheese is unreliable, however, and a much more consistent effect can be had when the chemical is administered in capsules. The drug tends to increase blood pressure in the supine posture even more than in standing positions. Some investigators have found it to cause dangerous increases in blood pressure and yet have no detectable effect on hypotensive systems [16]. This regimen has been tried in many variations, including different sources of tyramine, use of L-dopa in place of tyramine, variations in the dose of MAO inhibitor used, and so on. Unfortunately, most of the positive reports have provided anecdotal evidence of improvement without objective measurements of increased function in patients while they were standing. It is clear, however, that the drugs can increase blood pressure to dangerous and occasionally fatal levels.

Adrenergic-Agonist Drugs

A great variety of adrenergic-agonist drugs have been used in the treatment of postural hypotension. The most popular have been ephedrine, phenylephrine, amphetamine, hydroxyamphetamine, and phenylpropanolamine [3]. These drugs may act through stimulation of α- or β-receptors, or through release of NE. Ephedrine combines all three actions. Sensitivity to these agents may be remarkably increased in patients with denervation hypersensitivity; these patients can develop marked hypertension in response to phenylephrine eye drops [39].

Although these adrenergic pressor agents are among the most commonly used drugs for treating postural hypotension, their effect on hypotensive symptoms has not been systematically studied. Kochar and Itskovitz [28] found that 25 mg of ephedrine combined with propranolol had no effect on the blood pressure of patients with Shy-Drager syndrome. However, it is clearly possible to elevate blood pressure with some of these drugs. Davies et al [16] reported that both phenylephrine and ephedrine could cause dangerous levels of supine hypertension, and they therefore discouraged their use. Many of these drugs have central stimulant effects and may elicit subjective reports of improvement in postural dizziness without affecting blood pressure. There is little objective evidence in the literature on which to base a decision as to whether these drugs are actually beneficial. Patients should be kept under close observation when these drugs are first used because hypotensive patients have a wide range of sensitivity to adrenergic agents. The effect of an agent on an individual patient should then be evaluated on the basis of his neurologic and intellectual performance while standing as well as on the basis of relief of symptoms. The agents should not be continued simply because they relieve postural hypotension, because it is quite possible for them to elevate blood pressure and simultaneously decrease blood flow to the brain.

Dihydroergotamine

Dihydroergotamine is an ergot derivative marketed in the United States for parenteral treatment of vascular headache. It is available outside of the United States as a tablet formulation but has low bioavailability. The drug has mixed adrenergic-agonist and antagonist properties, but is able to constrict capacitance veins and thereby decrease venous pooling. Jennings et al [25] found that the drug increased central blood volume and cardiac index in patients with postural hypotension who were tilted upright. He reported that 10 to 40 mg of dihydroergotamine increased recumbent and standing blood pressure in patients with "autonomic insufficiency." Benowitz et al [4] gave 1 mg once daily to a patient with severe autonomic neuropathy; the patient's blood pressure increased while recumbent and while standing. The drug appears to be most useful in patients whose blood volume has been expanded with fludrocortisone, where it prevents pooling of the expanded blood volume. Although experience with this agent in postural hypotension is fairly limited, it appears to have a small beneficial effect when used in conjunction with other drugs.

Therapy of Postural Hypotension in Diabetes

Diabetic neuropathy generally does not lead to total destruction of the SNS and therefore fails to cause the increase in β-adrenergic sensitivity found in total autonomic neuropathy. β-blocking drugs thus should not be effective in these patients and may be hazardous if they block an E response to hypoglycemia. Most diabetics who have progressed to the stage of autonomic neuropathy also have some renal dysfunction, and indomethacin may further diminish their renal clearance. Although aldosterone levels fail to increase in response to upright posture in patients with diabetic autonomic neuropathy, these patients nonetheless have an increase in body sodium content [17]. Because of this, the dose of fludrocortisone needed to cause fluid retention is smaller than usual [23], and beneficial effects have been reported with low doses of this drug [6]. The sensitivity to pressor agents may be somewhat increased in these patients, although pressors may do nothing to remedy the maldistribution of blood flow away from the brain and to the legs when these patients stand up. They seem able to tolerate large drops in blood pressure fairly well, perhaps because their neuropathy and postural hypotension have such a prolonged and slow onset. However, they are frequently placed on hemodialysis for treatment of renal failure, and the associated large shifts in fluid volume then make their postural hypotension much more difficult to control.

APPROACH TO THE PATIENT WITH POSTURAL HYPOTENSION

Once it is established that a patient is suffering from postural hypotension, the first and most appropriate step in devising therapy for the patient is to obtain an adequate diagnosis as to the cause of the poor control of blood pressure. For example, patients with diabetes develop postural hypotension because of low cardiac output, nephrotic syndrome with decreased plasma volume, anemia, diabetic autonomic neuropathy, or cerebrovascular insufficiency with impaired central control of blood pressure. Obviously, the patient with heart failure or nephrotic syndrome should have therapy directed at the disease causing the postural hypotension, not at the postural hypotension itself. Patients who do not have an underlying disease amenable to therapy should then be evaluated to determine if they have central or peripheral neurologic disease, to see if they have an adequate blood volume, and to determine their sympathetic nervous response to standing. All hypotensive patients should have some beneficial response to low-dose fludrocortisone, particularly patients who have low levels of circulating aldosterone. Patients with volume depletion benefit from higher doses of fludrocortisone and salt. Patients who have degeneration of their peripheral autonomic nerves, low levels of circulating CA, and hypersensitive β-receptors are likely to benefit from β-blocking agents. Patients who are still able to produce some NE in response to standing may have their vascular sensitivity to NE enhanced by a prostaglandin-synthesis inhibitor such as indomethacin. All patients with postural hypotension should benefit from wearing a waist-high Jobst leotard or antigravity suit, although some people find these garments intolerably uncomfortable, particularly in hot weather. Frequently, these treatments fail to provide adequate relief of postural hypotensive symptoms, in which case treatment with fluid-retaining doses of fludrocortisone or with pressor agents can be considered.

Both iatrogenic fluid retention and pressor agents can cause supine hypertension in these patients. Although they sometimes die as a result of their hypotension, they much more frequently die from cardiovascular disease and pneumonia. Treatment that can induce hypertension should not be initiated until the patient and physician decide that potential benefits outweigh risks. Patients with Shy-Drager syndrome often have marked postural hypotension, but the main limitation to their mobility may be their parkinsonism and cerebellar disease, in which case relief of postural hypotension will still not allow the patient to walk. Their partial bulbar paralysis makes them particularly susceptible to the effects of pulmonary congestion induced by fluid overload, and relief of postural hypotension in these patients by volume expansion is not always worth the risk incurred. Treatment with volume expansion is usually helpful to relieve postural hypotension, but the patient should sleep with the head of the bed tilted up to avoid supine hypertension. Pressor agents increase blood pressure but may not always increase cerebral blood flow; they need to be evaluated on the basis of their ability to relieve symptoms.

The wide variety of treatments available for postural hypotension attests to the inadequacy of each of them. Postural hypotension is usually one component of more extensive disease, and the decision to treat depends on the patient's overall medical condition. The patient's response to treatment depends on the cause of the hypotension, and an accurate diagnosis can indicate which therapy is likely to succeed.

REFERENCES

1. Bannister R, Davies B, Holly E, Rosenthal T, Sever P. Defective cardiovascular reflexes and supersensitivity to sympathomimetic drugs in autonomic failure. Brain 102:163–176, 1979.
2. Bannister R, Davies B, Sever P. Indomethacin for Shy-Drager syndrome. Lancet i:1312, 1978.
3. Barnett AJ. Idiopathic orthostatic hypotension: A pharmacological study of the action of sympathomimetic drugs. Med J Aust 1:213–216, 1968.
4. Benowitz NL, Byrd R, Schambelan M, Rosenberg J, Roizen MF. Dihydroergotamine treatment for orthostatic hypotension from Vacor rodenticide. Ann Intern Med 92:387–388, 1980.
5. Brevetti G, Chiariello M, Lavecchia G, Rengo F. Effects of propranolol in a case of orthostatic hypotension. Br Heart J 41:245–248, 1979.
6. Campbell IW, Ewing DJ, Clarke BF. Therapeutic experience with fludrocortisone in diabetic postural hypotension. Br Med J 1:872–874, 1976.
7. Chanh PH, Junstad M, Wenmalm A. Augmented noradrenaline release following nerve stimulation after inhibition of prostaglandin synthesis with indomethacin. Acta Physiol Scand 86:563–576, 1972.
8. Chobanian AV, Volicer L, Liang CS, Kershaw G, Tifft C. Use of propranolol in the treatment of idiopathic orthostatic hypotension. Assoc Am Phys Trans 90:324–333, 1977.
9. Christensen NJ. Abnormally high plasma catecholamines at rest and during exercise in ketotic juvenile diabetics. Scand J Clin Lab Invest 26:343–344, 1970.
10. Christensen NJ. Plasma norepinephrine and epinephrine in untreated diabetics during fasting and after insulin administration. Diabetes 23:1–8, 1974.
11. Christensen NJ. Autonomic neuropathy in diabetics: physiology, catecholamines and effects of insulin. Horm Metab Res [suppl.] 9:94–97, 1978.

12. Christensen NJ, Glabo H, Hansen JF, Hesse B, Richter EA, Trap-Jensen J. Catecholamines and exercise. Diabetes 28:58–62, 1979.
13. Christlieb AR, Munichoodappa C, Braaten JT. Decreased response of plasma renin activity to orthostasis in diabetic patients with orthostatic hypotension. Diabetes 23:835–840, 1974.
14. Cordes U, Beyer J, von Ungern-Sternberg A. Plasma catecholamines in long-term diabetes. Horm Metab Res 9:90–93, 1980.
15. Cryer PE. Disorders of sympathetic neural function in human diabetes mellitus: Hypoadrenergic and hyperadrenergic postural hypotension. Metabolism 29:1186–1189, 1980.
16. Davies B, Bannister R, Sever P. Pressor amines and monoamine oxidase inhibitors for treatment of postural hypotension in autonomic failure. Lancet 1:172–175, 1978.
17. de Chatel R, Weidmann P, Flammer J, Ziegler WH, Beretta-Piccoli C, Vetter W, Reubi FC. Sodium, renin, aldosterone, catecholamines and blood pressure in diabetes mellitus. Kidney Int 12:412–421, 1977.
18. Ewing DJ, Campbell IW, Clarke FB. Assessment of cardiovascular effects in diabetic autonomic neuropathy and prognostic implications. Ann Intern Med 92:308–311, 1980.
19. Ewing DJ, Campbell IW, Clarke FB. The natural history of diabetic autonomic neuropathy. Q J Med 49:95–108, 1980.
20. Ewing DJ, Campbell IW, Clarke BF. Heart rate changes in diabetes mellitus. Lancet i:183–186, 1981.
21. Gluck A, Boll H, Weidmann P, Flammer J, Ziegler WH. Evaluation of autonomic neuropathy in diabetes mellitus. Klin Wochenschr 57:457–466, 1979.
22. Hilsted J. Decreased sympathetic vasomotor tone in diabetic orthostatic hypotension. Diabetes 28:970–973, 1979.
23. Hosking DJ, Bennett T, Hampton JR. Diabetic autonomic neuropathy. Diabetes 27:1043–1055, 1978.
24. Hui KK, Conolly ME. Increased numbers of beta receptors in orthostatic hypotension due to autonomic dysfunction. N Engl J Med 304:1473–1476, 1981.
25. Jennings G, Esler M, Holmes R. Treatment of orthostatic hypotension with dihydroergotamine. Br Med J 2:307–309, 1979.
26. Junstad M, Wenmalm W. Increased renal excretion of noradrenaline in rats after treatment with prostaglandin synthesis inhibitor indomethacin. Acta Physiol Scand 85:573–576, 1972.
27. Klein RL, McBaggett J, Thureson Klein A, Langford H. Idiopathic orthostatic hypotension: Circulating noradrenaline and ultrastructure of saphenous vein. J Autonom Nerv Syst 2:205–222, 1980.
28. Kochar MA, Itskovitz HD. Treatment of idiopathic orthostatic hypotension (Shy-Drager syndrome) with indomethacin. Lancet i:1011–1014, 1978.
29. Lefebvre J, Blacker C, Fossati P, Linquette M. Orthostatic hypotension in complicated diabetes mellitus: study of the renin-angiotensin-aldosterone system. Diab Metab 5:11–15, 1979.
30. Leveston SA, Shah SD, Cryer PE. Cholinergic stimulation of norepinephrine release in man. J Clin Invest 64:374–380, 1979.
31. Maher TD, Tanenberg RJ, Greenberg BZ, Hoffman JE, Doe RP, Goetz FC. Lack of glucagon response to hypoglycemia in diabetic autonomic neuropathy. Diabetes 26:196–200, 1976.
32. Miller AJ, Cohen HC, Glick G. Propranolol in the treatment of orthostatic tachycardia associated with orthostatic hypotension. Am Heart J 88:493–495, 1974.

33. Mohring J, Glanzer K, Maciel MA, Dusing R, Kramer JH, Arbogast R, Koch-Weser J. Greatly enhanced pressor response to antidiuretic hormone in patients with impaired cardiovascular reflexes due to idiopathic orthostatic hypotension. J Cardiovasc Pharmacol 2:367–376, 1980.
34. Neubauer B, Christensen NJ. Norepinephrine, epinephrine and dopamine content of the cardiovascular system in long-term diabetics. Diabetes 25:6–10, 1975.
35. Page M, Watkins PJ. Provocation of postural hypotension by insulin in diabetic autonomic neuropathy. Diabetes 25:90–95, 1976.
36. Page M, Watkins PJ. Cardiorespiratory arrest and diabetic autonomic neuropathy. Lancet 1:14–16, 1978.
37. Palmer KT, Perkins CJ, Smith RBW. Insulin-aggravated postural hypotension. Aust NZ J Med 7:161–162, 1977.
38. Perkins CM, Lee MR. Flurbiprofen and fludrocortisone in severe autonomic neuropathy. Lancet ii:1058, 1978.
39. Robertson D. Contraindication to the use of ocular phenylephrine in idiopathic orthostatic hypotension. Am J Ophthalmol 87:918–922, 1979.
40. Schirger A, Thomas SE. Idiopathic orthostatic hypotension: Clinical spectrum prognosis. Cardiology 61(Suppl. 1):144–149, 1976.
41. Silverberg AB, Mennes PA, Cryer PE. Resistance to endogenous norepinephrine in Bartter's syndrome. Am J Med 64:231–235, 1978.
42. Sjostrand T. Regulation of blood distribution in man. Acta Physiol Scand 26:312–327, 1952.
43. Smythies JR, Russell RO. Possible role of prostaglandins in idiopathic orthostatic hypotension. Lancet ii:964, 1974.
44. Stjarne L. Enhancement by indomethacin of cold-induced hypersecretion of noradrenaline in the rat in vivo—by suppression of PGE-mediated feedback control. Acta Physiol Scand 86:388–397, 1972.
45. Sundkvist G, Lilja B, Almer L-O. Abnormal diastolic blood pressure and heart rate reactions to tilting in diabetes mellitus. Diabetologia 19:433–438, 1980.
46. Tibbs PZ, Young B, Ziegler MG, McAllister RG. Studies of experimental cervical cord transsection. J Neurosurg 50:629–632, 1979.
47. Ziegler MG. Postural hypotension. Annu Rev Med 31:329–345, 1980.
48. Ziegler MG, Lake CR, Kopin IJ. Deficient sympathetic nervous response in familial dysautonomia. N Engl J Med 294:630–633, 1976.
49. Ziegler MG, Lake CR, Kopin IJ. The sympathetic nervous system defect in primary orthostatic hypotension. N Engl J Med 296:293–297, 1977.

7

Norepinephrine, Alcohol, and Alcoholism

John A. Ewing
Robert D. Myers

Interest in the role of norepinephrine (NE) in the disease state of alcoholism as well as the biologic effects of alcohol has been aroused for two reasons. First, NE, which serves as both a neurotransmitter and neurohormone, and possibly its precursor dopamine (DA), have been implicated in a number of psychiatric disorders including schizophrenia and depression [24]. Secondly, drugs which act centrally to alter mood and psychic state, such as amphetamines and phenothiazines, are known to exert profound effects on noradrenergic systems in the brain. Even the hedonic mechanisms underlying rewarded behavior and pleasurable experience may be mediated by a specific bundle of noradrenergic pathways arising in the brainstem and projecting to the forebrain [51]. The uniqueness of alcohol rests in its capacity not only to produce euphoria, dysphoria, and other mental states, but also to cause addiction. From the observations made in the last 25 years, it is likely that the processes of both effects may indeed entail noradrenergic mechanisms in the brain and other parts of the nervous system [23,51].

EFFECTS OF ALCOHOL ON BRAIN NOREPINEPHRINE

Several excellent reviews [15,39,41,51] have dealt with the multifaceted actions of alcohol on NE content, metabolism, turnover, and release within the central nervous system (CNS). In the following section, we consider several effects of long-term alcohol use on noradrenergic systems in the brain.

Effects of Chronic Alcohol Administration

In studies in which alcohol is given by intragastric intubation or in the drinking water or liquid diet in the home cage, little if any change in the endogenous level of NE is generally found [39]. Inconsistent results are reported with respect to the synthesis of NE from tyrosine, its use as measured by its disappearance, or its so-called "release" as reflected by the accumulation of the metabolite vanillylmandelic acid (VMA) [51]. Complicating factors in the interpretation of these data involve (1) technique of administering alcohol (i.e., vapor inhalation versus drinking); (2) the consequent blood alcohol levels; (3) duration of exposure to alcohol from less than 3 weeks to up to 12 months; and (4) analytic procedures for amine determination in tissue. Moreover, a study of actual presynaptic release within the brain of the live animal has not been accomplished.

In recent studies, somewhat better controls and relatively advanced methods of biochemical analysis have more realistically portrayed the possible role of NE in the central actions of alcohol. For example, in rats given increasing concentrations of alcohol from the time of weaning to 270 days, the content of NE declined significantly in the limbic system and the level of DA rose. Following withdrawal from alcohol, the content of both amines was significantly reduced at the same time that the rate of tyrosine hydroxylase (TH) formation was increased in the striatum and limbic system [52]. An analysis of the endogenous concentration of catecholamines (CA) in the rat's cerebrum also showed that after 21 days of drinking 15% alcohol, NE as well as DA levels were elevated in the diencephalon and corpus striatum with very little, if any, change in other areas of the brain [59]. After TH inhibition in these animals with α-methyl-p-tyrosine (AMPT), the typical depletion of NE was slowed, indicating a decline in its turnover. Alcohol, however, affected the release of ^{3}H-NE less than the release of acetylcholine from slices of cerebral cortex in the rat made tolerant to alcohol [12].

During the withdrawal period following chronic treatment with alcohol, there may be changes in the level or metabolism of NE in the brain [56]. For example, in rats abruptly withdrawn from alcohol, NE and its metabolites were significantly elevated in the midbrain with a similar pattern observed in the telencephalon and heart [72]. However, in rats that died as a result of alcohol withdrawal, the amount of NE in the brain was significantly reduced, in contrast to the absence of change found in amine levels in the animal "intoxicated" daily with alcohol [3]. In vitro studies also showed that brain tissue taken from a rat soon after withdrawal from alcohol was less sensitive to exogenously applied NE [30].

Drugs which enhance the content of NE in the brain or reduce the content of serotonin (5-hydroxytryptamine; 5-HT) tend to inhibit certain withdrawal signs [13]. On the other hand, the depletion of brain NE, but not DA, by 6-hydroxydopamine (6-OHDA) causes a much more severe withdrawal reaction in the alcohol-dependent rats than in the controls [87]. A threshold shift in the excitability of CNS neurons owing to CA depletion may be responsible, because tolerance to alcohol also develops in rats depleted of brain NE [87].

Evidence exists for a temporally biphasic action of alcohol as a result of chronic exposure. Following 3 months of alcohol drinking by adult rats, not only was the NE level in their hypothalamus twice that of the controls, but an enhanced fluorescence of noradrenergic nerve terminals was also evident [19]. However, both NE content and fluorescence declined substantially when alcohol was administered for 6 to 8 months.

When rats are exposed to alcohol either prenatally or postnatally, the content of NE in the hypothalamus is significantly reduced [20]. Because of the lower specific activity of dopamine-β-hydroxylase (DBH) in the brain of rat pups given alcohol, the rate of NE synthesis probably declines following such exposure. It is interesting that in the same diencephalic region and in the pons-medulla of adult rats given alcohol, 2.0 gm/kg of body weight, the rate of NE turnover was also reduced but no changes occurred in the frontal or parietal cortex or in subcortical tissue [6]. Because a malnourished control group failed to exhibit the decrease in NE turnover, an alteration in CA turnover cannot be attributed to a dietary deficiency with subsequent malnutrition [20]. The effect of early alcohol exposure is prolonged and profound since this change in hypothalamic NE was observed in the rat 26 weeks later [21].

In offspring from pregnant rats maintained on alcohol in a liquid diet during the latter stages of gestation, the synaptosomal uptake of ^{3}H-tyramine and its conversion to ^{3}H-octopamine were significantly enhanced [82]. Because these metabolic changes did not occur when alcohol was administered to the adult rats, it is apparent that the maternal ingestion of alcohol can affect the function of noradrenergic synapses in the developing brain in terms of both the uptake and storage of the neurotransmitter. Corresponding to these results is the finding that the brain of the fetus, obtained from a pregnant rat maintained on an alcohol diet, exhibited an increase in NE level at 18 to 21 days of gestation [75]. The specificity of the effect is not clear because 5-HT, acetylcholine, γ-amino butyric acid (GABA), and glutamate levels also rose in the fetal brain of both alcohol-treated and control rats [75]. Thus again the content of a putative transmitter does not seem to indicate the action of alcohol on the actual CNS kinetics or endogenous activity of the CA at the level of the neuronal synapse [42].

Chronic alcohol exposure does not appear to alter CA receptors. Rats made physically dependent on alcohol either by oral administration or intubation for 3 days exhibit no alteration in α-adrenergic or β-adrenergic receptor binding in CA-rich areas of the brain, including the cerebral cortex, hypothalamus, and hippocampus [38]. Similarly, serotonergic, cholinergic, and GABAergic receptors also do not seem to be affected. However, β-adrenergic receptor density is lower in cortical tissue of inbred mice that are particularly sensitive to alcohol behaviorally (i.e., animals which exhibited "long sleep time") [22].

When rats were treated with alcohol for 13 days, haloperidol binding to DA receptors in mesolimbic areas declined but was unchanged in the striatum [61]. Others also report the lack of change in the affinity of dopaminergic receptors for spiroperidol in striatal homogenate [22,73]. When alcohol was administered to the rats for 3 weeks as the only available fluid, ^{3}H-spiroperidol binding as well as methionine-enkephalin (met-en-kephalin) content in the striatum was selectively elevated [76]. Thus, alcohol dependence could be mediated partially through a dopaminergic as well as noradrenergic mechanism, possibly by way of presynaptic and postsynaptic elements. Opiate receptors located in dopaminergic nerve terminals in the striatum may account for some of the long-term addictive actions of alcohol [77]. Although two strains of rats, inbred for high- or low-alcohol preference, showed little difference in the amount of NE in whole brain [2], there were genetic differences in CA metabolism in the brains of DBA mice (alcohol avoiders) and C57 mice (alcohol preferrers) following an alcohol challenge. Because these differences corresponded to the amount of enkephalinergic influence of DA activity [7], endogenous opioid mechanisms may be involved in central actions of alcohol.

Effects of Acute Alcohol Administration

The results of studies on the action of alcohol on noradrenergic mechanisms in the brain are conflicting. A host of differences in methods of extraction, fluorimetric assay, and other preparative procedures for the CA is presumably responsible for the discrepancies. Other variables include the dose, route of administration, and length of exposure to alcohol.

In many reports, alcohol evoked no ostensible changes in the endogenous level, synthesis, or turnover of NE in the brain [39]. Some investigators found that the level of NE in the brains of mice, rats or rabbits decreased following ingestion of alcohol, but an increase may have occurred in its synthesis [51]. As noted in studies in which alcohol is given over a long period of time, the actual in vivo release of NE in the brain of an unrestrained animal has not been demonstrated. What is termed *release* is physiologically incorrect because a postmortem measure of accumulation of an amine metabolite in tissue clearly may not reflect the presynaptic liberation of the neurotransmitter [62].

It is possible that the activity of NE in noradrenergic pathways in the brain could account for the excitant as well as depressant effects of alcohol. For example, when synaptosomes were isolated from mice brains and then incubated with ^{3}H-NE, a high concentration of alcohol (1–6%) caused release of the uptaken ^{3}H-NE whereas a low concentration (0.1–0.5%) attenuated release [81]. The interpretation that alcohol inhibits NE release from CNS neurons, which is directly related to the depressant effect of alcohol, would seem to be physiologically backwards. That is, NE acts principally in the CNS as an inhibitory transmitter, and its release and postsynaptic action is to suppress the firing rate of the neuron [62].

Specific morphologic structures in the brain are now beginning to be examined for changes in neurochemistry in relation to alcohol exposure. For example, 2.0 gm/kg of alcohol given intraperitoneally to rats reduced NE turnover in the hypothalamus but augmented it in the pons and medulla [6]; no change was evident in the cerebral cortex or other subcortical regions. Because DA turnover is somewhat different, a dissociation may occur in the action of alcohol on these two CA at the cellular level. Recent studies of monoamine metabolism in slices of hippocampus and olfactory tubercle have shown that alcohol reduces CA synthesis from tyrosine, which appears to be related to the dopaminergic innervation of the nerve cells [84]. Thus, the metabolic pathway for NE biosynthesis in other regions of the brain could conceivably be affected by alcohol at the precursor step. In fact, it is probable that alcohol interferes with CA synthesis in the brain at the step involving the conversion of 3, 4-dihydroxyphenylalanine (dopa) to DA [53].

Other metabolic investigations of alcohol's short-term effects have revealed that alcohol can cause an increase in NE in the whole brain, whereas pyrazole, used extensively to elevate the level of systemic alcohol owing to inhibition of alcohol dehydrogenase, may decrease brain NE [9]. When both substances are given together, the steady-state level of NE is unaltered. This suggests that a drug such as pyrazole, used commonly to study alcohol metabolism, apparently has marked side effects independent of its commonly acknowledged pharmacologic properties. Acetaldehyde, alcohol's first metabolic intermediary, may also be partially responsible for some of alcohol's pharmacologic effects because the short-term injection of acetaldehyde, but not alcohol, causes a substantial change in the pattern of NE metabolites, indicating enhanced turnover of the amine [83]. Initially, however, alcohol augments the release and reduces the uptake of the amine.

A time-dependent biphasic effect on NE metabolites in the rat's brainstem occurred after a low 1.0 gm/kg dose of alcohol [71]. It is unlikely that the initial behavioral hyperactivity induced by alcohol was due to increased synthesis and release of the monoamine, once again because NE is an inhibitory, not excitatory, transmitter in the CNS. In this connection, when the rat was deprived of forebrain NE following a 6-OHDA lesion, the locomotor stimulation produced by a low dose of alcohol was unaffected, but the typical sedation following a slightly larger dose was diminished or absent [55].

At the membrane level, accumulating evidence suggests that the interaction between alcohol and NE occurs via the α-adrenergic receptor system [74]. In combination, alcohol and CA exert an effect via the ($Na^+ + K^+$)-adenosine triphosphatase (ATPase) enzyme mechanism in the rat brain [43]. In terms of this action, alcohol induces a direct and dose-dependent, biphasic modification of ligand binding to α-adrenergic receptors in the rat brain and, in fact, produces a decline in the overall receptor population [11].

Peripherally, alcohol can enhance the spontaneous release of NE from the vas deferens of rats [18] and can inhibit the evoked release of the CA from terminal sympathetic nerves in isolated rabbit hearts [35]. The sample of tissue examined, the techniques for biochemical analysis, and the dose of alcohol given are important determinants for the outcome of such experiments. Nevertheless, it is apparent that the short-term exposure of noradrenergic neurons to alcohol and to other lipophilic drugs, including anesthetics, serves to alter the cellular activity of this amine in vivo.

Finally, another aspect of alcohol's potential long-term action concerns the integrity of the blood-brain barrier, particularly with respect to entry of amine metabolites into the CNS [58,63]. Of importance is the observation that a relatively low dose of alcohol increases permeability of the rat's blood-brain barrier to dopa [25]. The availability of amine substrate to transiently formed aldehyde could favor the biosynthesis in the brain of an alkaloid product which may possess addictive properties.

HUMAN STUDIES

The majority of human studies on the relationship of NE and ethanol are performed with patient populations, but occasionally healthy subjects are used. The states of intoxication and withdrawal are dealt with separately in this section.

Intoxication

Perman [70] gave alcohol to healthy subjects in doses ranging from 0.25 to 0.54 gm/kg, achieving peak blood alcohol levels of from 15 to 80 mg/dl. Although excretion of urinary epinephrine (E) increased significantly following alcohol administration, there was no consistent change in urinary NE; the increased E excretion may have been due to adrenal medullary stimulation.

In 16 male alcoholic patients given alcohol at least 1 week after recovery from acute alcohol intoxication and withdrawal in a hospital setting, the 24-hour excretion of urinary CA showed no alterations compared with the values of 12 healthy subjects [33]. Subjects either drank brandy or wine or received intravenous infusions of ethanol to an average of 2.3 gm/kg for approximately 5 hours. The peak blood alcohol concentrations varied between 150 and 330 mg/dl. The levels of urinary CA were determined at 24-hour intervals before, during, and after intoxication. Excretion of urinary NE and E were similar in the alcoholics and the healthy controls. Even in the subjects receiving the higher doses of intravenous ethanol, the urinary NE and E levels did not increase. These authors [33] concluded that previously demonstrated increases in urinary CA seem to be related to a longer lasting abuse of alcohol than was the case in this experiment. In fact, as is presented later in this section, the increased CA levels they had previously demonstrated in urine were associated with the withdrawal state.

In another study with healthy young men [5], alcohol was diluted with orange juice and given in a dose of 0.71 gm/kg, and the control subjects drank only orange juice. An average increase in urinary excretion of all the CA and their metabolites was observed in the experimental group, but reached significance only in the case of NE, DA, and metanephrine (M).

Ogata et al [69] studied four healthy male alcoholics who had been abstinent for at least 7 days. In the first experiment, each patient was given a measured amount of alcohol for 20 days so that mean blood alcohol concentration reached 86 mg/dl. In a second experiment, free drinking was permitted for 20 days, and the blood alcohol concentration averaged 192 mg/dl. Urinary excretion of NE rose in a dose-related manner during both experiments. The authors concluded that prolonged alcohol ingestion is associated with both stimulation of adrenergic activity and alterations in the pathways of CA catabolism.

After ^{14}C-labeled NE was administered intravenously to normal men, the metabolic alteration induced by the ingestion of 60 ml of ethanol was determined [14]. Alcohol ingestion caused a decrease in the excretion of ^{14}C-VMA but an enhanced excretion of ^{14}C-3-methoxy-4-hydroxyphenylglycol (MHPG). No alteration was found in the pattern of excretion of ^{14}C-NE, normetanephrine (NM), 3,4-dihydroxymandelic acid, or 3,4-dihydroxyphenylglycol (DHPG). Although the altered metabolism of NE following alcohol probably occurs peripherally, inasmuch as NE does not penetrate the blood-brain barrier to a notable degree, Davis et al [14] surmised that a similar alteration in the metabolism of endogeneous NE may take place within the CNS. They suggested that the observed alteration of NE metabolism from the usual oxidative to the reductive pathway is due in part to the increased NADH/NAD ratio, resulting from ethanol metabolism or from competitive inhibition by acetaldehyde formed from the metabolism of alcohol.

Central NE metabolism during alcohol intoxication in both the addict and healthy volunteer was investigated by Borg et al [8], who examined the concentrations of the major NE metabolite, MHPG, in cerebrospinal fluid (CSF) obtained by lumbar puncture. In the alcoholic patient, the level of MHPG was markedly elevated during intoxication but declined successively during 1 and 3 weeks of abstinence. A correlation was also found between the concentration of MHPG in CSF and the blood-alcohol concentration. Healthy volunteers who received 80 gm of ethanol also showed significant increases in MHPG concentrations in CSF. Borg et al [8] concluded that alcohol administration markedly stimulates NE metabolism in human CNS, possibly by increasing unit impulse activity of central noradrenergic neurons.

In a human experimental study, healthy volunteers were treated on a double-blind basis with AMPT at two dose levels or with placebo [1]. The subjects then drank a fixed amount of alcohol, and measures were made of mood and performance. Pretreatment with AMPT caused a reduction of ethanol-induced stimulation and euphoria. Because AMPT inhibits the conversion of tyrosine to DA, it was believed that this experiment supported the concept that central CA may be involved in ethanol-induced stimulation and euphoria in human beings. However, the AMPT alone produced feelings of fatigue and dysphoria, which may have influenced the results.

Withdrawal

The clinical picture of alcohol withdrawal in humans suggests a hyperadrenergic state. Patients display tremor, tachycardia, hypertension, sweating, and complain of anxiety symptoms. In addition, one study [32] noted that the urinary NE and E levels in patients who were experiencing delirium tremens and other conditions were elevated even after blood alcohol levels returned to zero. Only the increase in blood pressure correlated closely with the clinical signs. Thus, the high excretion of urinary CA may reflect the sympathetic hyperactivity which is observed clinically.

Sellers et al [79] concluded that the hyperadrenergic state of alcohol withdrawal is principally due to increased central autonomic outflow. They showed that centrally acting drugs such as chlordiazepoxide and propranolol decreased urinary and plasma CA.

In alcoholics on an inpatient ward from whom all medications were withdrawn, a lumbar puncture was performed at the end of 1 week of hospitalization and repeated during the third or fourth week in some cases [44]. The levels of 5-hydroxyindoleacetic acid (5-HIAA) and homovanillic acid (HVA) in CSF were determined. For control purposes, CSF was also obtained from 30 neurologic patients having no history of alcoholism. Although the CSF concentration of 5-HIAA was not significantly different between the alcoholics and controls, the level of HVA in the alcoholics was significantly lower than in the controls. This was particularly exaggerated in those alcoholics exhibiting withdrawal symptoms, but the low values were not evident at 4 weeks. In the same study, patients with delirium tremens and several with other withdrawal symptoms had significantly elevated levels of serum DBH activity, which may have reflected increased sympathetic activity. These authors [44] concluded that withdrawal symptoms involve aberrations in both 5-HT and DA metabolism.

Hawley et al [36] also examined CSF in patients experiencing acute alcohol-withdrawal and found that the NE concentration in CSF was higher than in controls with neurologic disease. During recovery, the NE concentration in CSF decreased. Although these findings may help to explain the adrenergic signs observed during alcohol withdrawal, CSF levels of other neurohormones will have to be determined simultaneously to ensure the specificity of noradrenergic involvement.

Ethanol Sensitivity in Orientals

Wolff [86] was one of the first to describe the phenomenon of sensitivity of the Oriental individual to alcohol. Studies in our human research laboratory led to our recognition of the similarity between this phenomenon and the disulfiram–ethanol reaction [29]. Later we demonstrated that acetaldehyde toxicity is indeed a key part of the phenomenon [26]. Fukui and Wakasugi [31] have shown that an atypical or "Oriental" form of liver alcohol dehydrogenase (LADH) is found much more frequently in Oriental than in non-Oriental people. In the presence of this active LADH, the initial metabolism of absorbed ethanol may occur very rapidly until rate limitation is invoked by the reduction of NAD. Goedde et al [34] also demonstrated that a rapidly acting type of aldehyde dehydrogenase (ALDH) is frequently absent or deficient in Orientals. Thus, the phenomenon may involve the more rapid production of acetaldehyde during the early stage of alcohol metabolism, an impairment in the metabolism of acetaldehyde, or both.

The phenomenon of Oriental sensitivity appears to be frequently associated with skin flushing; subjects may also complain of tachycardia, pounding in the head, and other unpleasant reactions. In subjects with and without the Oriental type of alcohol sensitivity, alcohol ingestion by the "flushing" group caused significant elevations of urinary E and NE excretion [48]. Only the latter is significantly increased in the "nonflushing" group. In a similar study by Mizoi et al [60], urinary excretion of E and NE after alcohol drinking was increased above the baseline in the "flushing" group but not in the "nonflushing" group. The mean baseline values in the two groups were similar. Both groups showed significant reduction in urinary VMA excretion following alcohol ingestion, but the increase in urinary excretion of MHPG was nearly double in the "flushing" group and approximately 30% in the "nonflushing" group. The authors [60] believed that the increased excretion of MHPG reflected a predominant influence of acetaldehyde. The decline in urinary VMA excretion might be the product of the increased NADH/NAD ratio.

No significant differences were found between "flushing" and "nonflushing" groups in terms of mean maximum blood alcohol levels following ingestion of alcohol [40]. In the "flushing" group, alcohol led to a significant increase in urinary E and NE. It was concluded that heart palpitations and peripheral vessel dilation were caused by the accumulation of acetaldehyde or CA in the blood during alcohol metabolism.

Dopamine-β-Hydroxylase

Both animal studies and clinical observations suggest that ethanol ingestion is associated with sympathetic nervous system (SNS) stimulation. We attempted, therefore, to use plasma levels of DBH activity as an index of the SNS in some experiments with humans [28]. In a series of three initial experiments, healthy subjects whose prior levels of DBH were in the upper quartile of our values had different responses compared with those whose values fell in the lower quartile. No actual changes in DBH activity occurred following ethanol administration in any studies we have done involving short-term administration of ethanol. However, those with the higher levels of DBH rated themselves as feeling more euphoric, less intoxicated, and less sick than those with lower levels. In a further study in which subjects were invited to drink on a self-selected basis, those whose DBH levels were above the group mean drank almost twice as many drinks and reached blood alcohol levels twice as high as those whose DBH activity was below the mean [27]. These studies indicated a relationship between DBH activity and subjective response to ethanol and possibly the desire to drink alcoholic beverages. However, the relationship is a relatively weak one. In some further studies in which our subjects were exposed to considerable social forces (they drank in the presence of a spouse or a close friend), the former relationship between DBH activity and response to alcohol drinking was not demonstrated.

Disulfiram

Because disulfiram (Antabuse) is used to deter alcoholic patients from drinking, the relationship between it and NE warrants mention. Lake et al [49] showed that small but significant increases in plasma NE and blood pressure were found in patients receiving 500 mg per day of disulfiram. This increase was not demonstrated in patients receiving 250 mg per day or placebo, nor did either dose significantly affect the plasma DBH activity. In a clinical study of healthy young men receiving disulfiram, we were also unable to demonstrate plasma DBH inhibition [80]. Lake et al [49] concluded that patients receiving high doses of disulfiram should have their blood pressure monitored and that the dose should be decreased to 250 mg per day when possible.

CENTRAL NERVOUS SYSTEM NOREPINEPHRINE AND VOLUNTARY ALCOHOL DRINKING

In 1968, it was suggested that an aberration in monoamine activity in the brain could affect experimental animals' voluntary drinking of alcohol [68]. However, 5-HT rather than NE was thought to underlie the animals' preference for alcohol. In rats, *p*-chlorophenylalanine, an inhibitor of tryptophan hydroxylase, exerts a far more potent effect on alcohol preference than AMPT, a TH inhibitor that causes a depletion of CA in the brain. AMPT produced only a relatively small and transitory suppressant effect on the self-selection of alcohol offered to the rat in a range of concentrations from 3 to 30% [85].

One study took a more direct approach to the role of NE and 5-HT in alcohol drinking involving the differential lesioning of noradrenergic or serotonergic pathways in the brain by 6-OHDA or a serotonergic neurotoxin (5,6-dihydroxytryptamine; 5,6-DHT), both infused directly into the cerebral ventricle of the animal [66]. In this study, 6-OHDA depletion of CNS CA significantly reduced alcohol intake, whereas 5,6-DHT increased intake [66]. The effect of central NE reduction on alcohol drinking could be genetically linked, since alcohol preference in Sprague-Dawley and Long-Evans rats is greatly affected, whereas the neurotoxin has little or no effect on the preference for alcohol in Wistar and Holtzman strains [57].

In a similar study [78], the effect of intracerebroventricular (ICV) 6-OHDA on the free choice of alcohol was confirmed. However, 6-hydroxydopa, which destroys noradrenergic neurons without affecting dopaminergic cells, reportedly failed to alter alcohol preference in Sprague-Dawley rats. This result suggested that DA is also involved in the shift in voluntary drinking of alcohol.

When 6-OHDA is infused directly into the ascending noradrenergic fiber bundle, forebrain NE is depleted with little effect on the central level of DA. In this instance, Wistar rats rejected a 15% alcohol solution persistently but the injected controls did not [54]. A related study reported that a lesion of the ascending dopaminergic pathway with 6-OHDA did not affect the voluntary intake of a 10% solution of alcohol [46]. However, a decrease in alcohol drinking following a 6-OHDA lesion of the dorsal noradrenergic pathway was not observed. In fact, a transient increase in alcohol intake reportedly occurred 3 to 6 weeks following the 6-OHDA injection [45,47]. When an ICV infusion of 6-OHDA was preceded by desmethylimipramine (DMI) to protect NE-containing neurons from the neurotoxin's effect, alcohol consumption of rats was not significantly attenuated [10]. The latter result suggests that NE may play a more important role than DA in the voluntary drinking of alcohol by experimental animals.

Other experimental studies employing the peripheral administration of an amine-depleting agent provide ample support for the theory of the role of NE in self-selection of alcohol. For example, in rats, self-injection of alcohol was diminished by drugs that interfered with the brain's synthesis of NE, but not DA [16]. Results with the DBH inhibitor, FLA-57, further support the view that NE may be involved in the positive reinforcing property of alcohol drinking in this species [4]. FLA-57 suppressed the intragastric self-delivery of 25 mg/kg doses of alcohol at the same time that the content of NE in the brain was reduced by 47% without any notable alteration in the amount of DA or 5-HT [17].

Concerning genetic differences, it is interesting that C57B mice, which will drink certain concentrations of alcohol, and DBA mice, nondrinking animals, failed to show any difference in content or uptake of NE in samples of whole brain [37]. Nevertheless, subtle differences reportedly may arise in CA content in the brain of so-called alcohol-preferring and nonpreferring rats [50]. It is unlikely that a simple measure of neurotransmitter quantity in the whole or even a part of the brain of an animal reflects any functional significance to the phenomenon of alcohol self-selection or to other complex behavioral processes involving dynamic events in individual transmitter pathways [42,62].

Finally, the validity of lesioning and other studies in which a single concentration of alcohol is used as the main dependent variable is questionable [45,67]. The design of these studies violates a cardinal pharmacologic principle: namely, a range of doses (i.e., concentrations) is required for the analysis of self-administration of any centrally active compound [64].

CONCLUSIONS

The role of NE and its multiple functions in both the central and peripheral nervous systems in relation to alcohol are not fully understood. Clinically, it is impossible to examine the in vivo activity of NE in the brain of the alcoholic patient. Promising leads, however, are presently being followed through postmortem study of brain tissue and by analysis of CSF from alcoholic patients in several laboratories in the United States, Sweden, and Japan. Both strategies are limited by the need to uncover in vivo the ongoing activity of this CA in specific NE-containing cells of the nervous system.

In the experimental animal, an equally large number of unanswered questions punctuate the issue of alcohol's effect on NE's intricate function. Interpretative difficulties are often caused by limitations in experimental procedures, and problems may occur when using a single concentration of alcohol in studies of voluntary drinking. Postmortem analysis of whole brain tissue does not recognize the anatomically distinct "circuits" of NE neurons which underlie quite different aspects of the control of behavioral, motor, and vegetative processes. In vivo studies with live animals can now be undertaken in which the brain is assayed during different stages of alcohol induction, "intoxication," dependence, and withdrawal. In addition to CSF analysis, perfusate collected from discrete noradrenergic fiber bundles in the brain can reveal the kinetics of NE release under different conditions of alcohol exposure.

The relationship of NE to other monoamines, neuroactive peptides, and other endogenous factors should be considered in view of the likelihood of their reciprocal interaction. By illustration, it is already known that 5-HT and NE may function in opposition to one another with regard to alcohol drinking and withdrawal. Similarly, the influence of acetaldehyde as well as the amine-aldehyde metabolites is not yet understood with respect to their potential importance in alcohol's pharmacologic actions. Interestingly, the NE-aldehyde condensation products examined thus far do not appear to be nearly as biologically active as the alkaloid products derived from DA and 5-HT [65].

Finally, experimental controls for alcohol's pharmacologic specificity are continually required. The effects of anesthetics, sedatives, or other lipophilic substances as well as other alcohols on NE activity should be compared with ethyl alcohol. Although the potency of such substances may differ from ethyl alcohol, the direction of effect on NE in nerve tissue may be the same. Progress in these areas will permit further in vivo elucidation of the functional importance of NE in the manifestations of alcohol's remarkable behavioral, pharmacologic, and physiologic actions.

REFERENCES

1. Ahlenius S, Carlsson A, Engel J, Svensson T, Södersten P. Antagonism by alpha methyltyrosine of the ethanol-induced stimulation and euphoria in man. Clin Pharmacol Ther 14:586–591, 1973.
2. Ahtee L, Eriksson K. Dopamine and noradrenaline content in the brain of rat strains selected for their alcohol intake. Acta Physiol Scand 93:563–565, 1975.
3. Ahtee L, Svartström-Fraser M. Effect of ethanol dependence and withdrawal on the catecholamines in rat brain and heart. Acta Pharmacol Toxicol 36:289–298, 1975.
4. Amit Z, Brown ZW, Levitan DE, Ögren S-O. Noradrenergic mediation of the positive reinforcing properties of ethanol: 1. Suppression of ethanol consumption in laboratory rats following dopamine-beta-hydroxylase inhibition. Arch Int Pharmacodyn Ther 230:65–75, 1977.
5. Anton AH. Ethanol and urinary catecholamines in man. Clin Pharmacol Ther 6:462–469, 1965.
6. Bacopoulos NG, Bhatnagar RK, Van Orden LS, III. The effects of subhypnotic doses of ethanol on regional catecholamine turnover. J Pharmacol Exp Ther 204:1–10, 1978.
7. Barbaccia ML, Reggiani A, Spano PF, Trabucchi M. Ethanol effects on dopaminergic function: modulation by the endogenous opioid system. Pharmacol Biochem Behav 13:303–306, 1980.
8. Borg S, Kvande H, Sedvall G. Central norepinephrine metabolism during alcohol intoxication in addicts and healthy volunteers. Science 213:1135–1137, 1981.
9. Brown FC, Zawad J, Harralson JD. Interactions of pyrazole and ethanol on norepinephrine metabolism in rat brain. J Pharmacol Exp Ther 206:75–80, 1978.

10. Brown ZW, Amit Z. The effects of selective catecholamine depletions by 6-hydroxydopamine on ethanol preference in rats. Neurosci Lett 5:333–336, 1977.
11. Ciofalo FR. Ethanol and α-adrenergic receptors. Proc West Pharmacol Soc 21:267–269, 1978.
12. Clark JW, Kalant H, Carmichael FJ. Effect of ethanol tolerance on release of acetylcholine and norepinephrine by rat cerebral cortex slices. Can J Physiol Pharmacol 55:758–768, 1977.
13. Collier HOJ, Hammond MD, Schneider C. Biogenic amines and head twitches in mice during ethanol withdrawal. Br J Pharmacol 51:310–311, 1974.
14. Davis VE, Brown H, Huff JA, Cashaw JL. Ethanol-induced alterations of norepinephrine metabolism in man. J Lab Clin Med 69:787–799, 1967.
15. Davis VE, Walsh MJ. Effect of Ethanol on Neuroamine Metabolism. In Biological Basis of Alcoholism, Y Israel and J Mardones (eds), 73–97. New York: Wiley Interscience, 1971.
16. Davis WM, Smith SG, Werner TE. Noradrenergic role in the self-administration of ethanol. Pharmacol Biochem Behav 9:369–374, 1978.
17. Davis WM, Werner TE, Smith SG. Reinforcement with intragastric infusions of ethanol: Blocking effect of FLA 47. Pharmacol Biochem Behav 11:545–548, 1979.
18. Degani NC, Sellers EM, Kadzielawa K. Ethanol-induced spontaneous norepinephrine release from the rat vas deferens. J Pharmacol Exp Ther 210:22–26, 1979.
19. Denisenko PP, Konstantinova MS, Naimova TG. Effects of acute and chronic alcohol-poisoning on the norepinephrine content in the rat hypothalamus. Farmakol Toksikol 41:618–620, 1978.
20. Detering N, Collins RM, Jr, Hawkins RL, Ozand PT, Karahasan A. Comparative effects of ethanol and malnutrition on the development of catecholamine neurons: Changes in norepinephrine turnover. J Neurochem 34:1788–1791, 1980.
21. Detering N, Collins RM, Jr, Hawkins RL, Ozand PT, Karahasan A. Comparative effects of ethanol and malnutrition on the development of catecholamine neurons: A long-lasting effect in the hypothalamus. J Neurochem 36:2094–2096, 1981.
22. Dibner MD, Zahniser NR, Wolfe BB, Rabin RA, Molinoff PD. Brain neurotransmitter receptor systems in mice genetically selected for differences in sensitivity to ethanol. Pharmacol Biochem Behav 12:509–513, 1980.
23. Engel J. Neurochemical aspects of the euphoria induced by dependence-producing drugs. Excerpta Med 407:16–22, 1977.
24. Engel J, Carlsson A. Catecholamines and Behavior. In Current Developments in Psychopharmacology, L Valzelli and WB Essman (eds), vol. 4, 1–32. New York: Spectrum Publications, 1977.
25. Eriksson T, Liljequist S, Carlsson A. Ethanol-induced increase in the penetration of exogenously administered L-dopa through the blood-brain barrier. J Pharm Pharmacol 31:636, 1979.
26. Ewing JA, Rouse BA, Aderhold RM. Studies of the Mechanism of Oriental Hypersensitivity to Alcohol. In Currents in Alcoholism, M Galanter (ed), vol. 5, 45–52. New York: Grune and Stratton, 1979.
27. Ewing JA, Rouse BA, Mills KC, Mueller RA. Dopamine beta-hydroxylase activity as a predictor of response to alcohol. Jpn J Stud Alcohol 10:61–69, 1975.
28. Ewing JA, Rouse BA, Mueller RA. Alcohol susceptibility and plasma dopamine β-hydroxylase activity. Res Commun Chem Pathol Pharmacol 8:551–554, 1974.
29. Ewing JA, Rouse BA, Pellizzari ED. Alcohol sensitivity and ethnic background. Am J Psychiatry 131:206–210, 1974.

30. French SW, Palmer DS, Narod ME, Reid PE, Ramey CW. Noradrenergic sensitivity of the cerebral cortex after chronic ethanol ingestion and withdrawal. J Pharmacol Exp Ther 194:319–326, 1975.
31. Fukui M, Wakasugi C. Liver alcohol dehydrogenase in a Japanese population. Jpn J Legal Med 26:46–51, 1972.
32. Giacobini E, Izikowitz S, Wegmann A. Urinary norepinephrine and epinephrine excretion in delirium tremens. Arch Gen Psychiatry 3:289–296, 1960.
33. Giacobini E, Izikowitz S, Wegmann A. The urinary excretion of noradrenaline and adrenaline during acute alcohol intoxication in alcoholic addicts. Experientia 16:467, 1960.
34. Goedde HW, Harada S, Agarwal DP. Racial differences in alcohol sensitivity: a newhypothesis. Hum Genet 51:331–334, 1979.
35. Göthert M, Dührsen U, Rieckesmann J-M. Ethanol, anaesthetics and other lipophilic drugs preferentially inhibit 5-hydroxytryptamine- and acetylcholine-induced noradrenaline release from sympathetic nerves. Arch Int Pharmacodyn 242:196–209, 1979.
36. Hawley RJ, Major LF, Schulman EA, Lake CR. CSF levels of norepinephrine during alcohol withdrawal. Arch Neurol 38:289–292, 1981.
37. Ho AKS, Tsai CS, Kissin B. Neurochemical correlates of alcohol preference in inbred strains of mice. Pharmacol Biochem Behav 3:1073–1076, 1975.
38. Hunt WA, Dalton TK. Neurotransmitter-receptor binding in various brain regions in ethanol-dependent rats. Pharmacol Biochem Behav 14:733–739, 1981.
39. Hunt WA, Majchrowicz E. Alterations in Neurotransmitter Function after Acute and Chronic Treatment with Ethanol. In Biochemistry and Pharmacology of Ethanol, E Majchrowicz and EP Noble (eds), vol 2, 167–185. New York: Plenum Publishing Corporation, 1979.
40. Ijiri I. Studies on the relationship between the concentrations of blood acetaldehyde and urinary catecholamine and the symptoms after drinking alcohol. Jpn J Stud Alcohol 9:35–59, 1974.
41. Israel Y, Carmichael FJ, Macdonald JA. Effects of ethanol on electrolyte metabolism and neurotransmitter release in the CNS. In Alcohol Intoxication and Withdrawal, MM Gross (ed), 55–64. New York: Plenum Publishing Corporation, 1975.
42. Kalant H. Direct effects of ethanol on the nervous system. Fed Proc 34:1930–1941, 1975.
43. Kalant H, Rangaraj N. Interaction of catecholamines and ethanol on the kinetics of rat brain ($Na^+ + K^+$)-ATPase. Eur J Pharmacol 70:157–166, 1981.
44. Kato N, Takahashi S, Tani N, Iwase N, Odani K. Changes in the metabolism of biogenic amines in alcoholism—especially regarding CSF monoamine metabolites and serum DBH activity. Alcohol Clin Exp Res 3:24–27, 1979.
45. Kiianmaa K. Alcohol intake and ethanol intoxication in the rat: Effect of a 6-OHDA-induced lesion of the ascending noradrenaline pathways. Eur J Pharmacol 64:9–19, 1980.
46. Kiianmaa K, Andersson K, Fuxe K. On the role of ascending dopamine systems in the control of voluntary ethanol intake and ethanol intoxication. Pharmacol Biochem Behav 10:603–608, 1979.
47. Kiianmaa K, Fuxe K, Jonsson G, Ahtee L. Evidence for involvement of central NA neurones in alcohol intake. Increased alcohol consumption after degeneration of the NA pathway to the cortex cerebri. Neurosci Lett 1:41–45, 1975.
48. Kijima T. Alcohol sensitivity and urinary catecholamines. Jpn J Stud Alcohol 14:101–117, 1979.

49. Lake CR, Major LF, Ziegler MG, Kopin IJ. Increased sympathetic nervous system activity in alcoholic patients treated with disulfiram. Am J Psychiatry 134:1411–1414, 1977.
50. Li T-K, Lumeng L, McBride WJ, Waller MB. Progress toward a voluntary oral consumption model of alcoholism. Drug Alcohol Depend 4:45–60, 1979.
51. Liljequist S. Behavioural and Biochemical Effects of Chronic Ethanol Administration, 1–43. Sweden: University of Goteborg, 1979.
52. Liljequist S, Ahlenius S, Engel J. The effect of chronic ethanol treatment onbehaviour and central monoamines in the rat. Naunyn Schmiedebergs Arch Pharmacol 300:205–216, 1977.
53. Liljequist S, Carlsson A. Alteration of central catecholamine metabolism following acute administration of ethanol. J Pharm Pharmacol 30:728–730, 1978.
54. Mason ST, Corcoran ME, Fibiger HC. Noradrenaline and ethanol intake in the rat. Neurosci Lett 12:137–142, 1979.
55. Mason ST, Corcoran ME, Fibiger HC. Noradrenergic processes involved in the locomotor effects of ethanol. Eur J Pharmacol 54:383–387, 1979.
56. Mazur M, Szmigielski A. The effect of prolonged ethanol administration and its withdrawal on catecholamine turnover in the rat brain. Acta Physiol Pol 27:281–286, 1976.
57. Melchior CL, Myers RD. Genetic differences in ethanol drinking of the rat following injection of 6-OHDA, 5,6-DHT or 5,7-DHT into the cerebral ventricles. Pharmacol Biochem Behav 5:63–72, 1976.
58. Melchior CL, Myers RD. Preference for alcohol evoked by tetrahydropapaveroline (THP) chronically infused in the cerebral ventricle of the rat. Pharmacol Biochem Behav 7:19–35, 1977.
59. Mena MA, Herrera E. Monoamine metabolism in rat brain regions following long term alcohol treatment. J Neural Transm 47:227–236, 1980.
60. Mizoi Y, Hishida S, Ijiri I, Maruyama J, Asakura S, Kijima T, Okada T, Adachi J. Individual differences in blood and breath acetaldehyde levels and urinary excretion of catecholamines after alcohol intake. Alcohol Clin Exp Res 4:354–360, 1980.
61. Muller P, Britton RS, Seeman P. The effects of long-term ethanol on brain receptors for dopamine, acetylcholine, serotonin and noradrenaline. Eur J Pharmacol 65:31–37, 1980.
62. Myers RD. Handbook of Drug and Chemical Stimulation of the Brain. New York: Van Nostrand Reinhold, 1974.
63. Myers RD. Tetrahydroisoquinolines in the brain: the basis of an animal model of alcoholism. Alcohol Clin Exp Res 2.145–154, 1978.
64. Myers RD. Psychopharmacology of alcohol. Annu Rev Pharmacol Toxicol 18:125–144, 1978.
65. Myers RD. Pharmacological effects of Amine-aldehyde Condensation Products. In Alcohol Tolerance and Dependence, H Rigter and J Crabbe (eds), 339–370. Holland: Elsevier, 1980.
66. Myers RD, Melchior CL. Alcohol drinking in the rat after destruction of serotonergic and catecholaminergic neurons in the brain. Res Comm Chem Pathol Pharmacol 10:363–378, 1975.
67. Myers RD, Melchior CL. Alcohol and Alcoholism: Role of Serotonin. In Serotonin in Health and Disease, WB Essman (ed), vol. 2, 373–430. New York: Spectrum, 1977.
68. Myers RD, Veale WL. Alcohol preference in the rat: Reduction following depletion of brain serotonin. Science 160:1469–1471, 1968.

69. Ogata M, Mendelson JH, Mello NK, Majchrowicz E. Adrenal function and alcoholism. II. Catecholamines. Psychosom Med 33:159–180, 1971.
70. Perman EA. The effect of ethyl alcohol on the secretion from the adrenal medulla in man. Acta Physiol Scand 44:241–247, 1958.
71. Pohorecky LA, Jaffe LS. Noradrenergic involvement in the acute effects of ethanol. Res Comm Chem Pathol Pharmacol 12:433–447, 1975.
72. Pohorecky LA, Jaffe LS, Berkeley HA. Ethanol withdrawal in the rat: Involvement of noradrenergic neurons. Life Sci 15:427–437, 1974.
73. Rabin RA, Wolfe BB, Dibner MD, Zahniser NR, Melchior C, Molinoff PB. Effects of ethanol administration and withdrawal on neurotransmitter receptor systems in C57 mice. J Pharmacol Exp Ther 213:491–496, 1980.
74. Rangaraj N, Kalant H. Alpha adrenoreceptor mediated alteration of ethanol effects on ($Na^+ + K^+$)-ATPase of rat neuronal membranes. Can J Physiol Pharmacol 58:1342–1346, 1980.
75. Rawat AK. Developmental changes in the brain levels of neurotransmitters as influenced by maternal ethanol consumption in the rat. J Neurochem 28:1175–1182, 1977.
76. Reggiani A, Barbaccia ML, Spano PF, Trabucchi M. Dopamine metabolism and receptor function after acute and chronic ethanol. J Neurochem 35:34–37, 1980.
77. Reggiani A, Barbaccia ML, Spano PF, Trabucchi M. Role of dopaminergic-enkephalinergic interactions in the neurochemical effects of ethanol. Subst Alcohol Act Misuse 1:151–158, 1980.
78. Richardson JS, Novakovski DM. Brain monoamines and free choice ethanol consumption in rats. Drug Alcohol Depend 3:253–264, 1978.
79. Sellers EM, Degani N, Cohen LB, Zilm DH, Sellers EA. Central and Peripheral Adrenergic Components in Alcohol Withdrawal. In Currents in Alcoholism, F Seixas (ed), vol 3, 191–202. New York: Grune and Stratton, 1978.
80. Silver DF, Ewing JA, Rouse BA, Mueller RA. Responses to disulfiram in healthy men. J Stud Alcohol 40:1003–1013, 1979.
81. Sun AY. Alcohol-membrane interaction in the brain: norepinephrine release. Res Comm Chem Path Pharmacol 15:705–719, 1976.
82. Thadani PV, Lau C, Slotkin TA, Schanberg SM. Effects of maternal ethanol ingestion on amine uptake into synaptosomes of fetal and neonatal rat brain. J Pharmacol Exp Ther 200:292–297, 1977.
83. Thadani PV, Truitt EB, Jr. Effect of acute ethanol or acetaldehyde administration on the uptake, release, metabolism and turnover rate of norepinephrine in rat brain. Biochem Pharmacol 26:1147–1150, 1977.
84. Umezu K, Bustos G, Roth RH. Regional inhibitory effect of ethanol on monoamine synthesis regulation within the brain. Biochem Pharmacol 29:2477–2483, 1980.
85. Veale WL, Myers RD. Decrease in ethanol intake in rats following administration of ρ-chlorophenylalanine. Neuropharmacology 9:317–326, 1970.
86. Wolff PH. Ethnic differences in alcohol sensitivity. Science 175:449–450, 1972.
87. Wood JM, Laverty R. Effect of depletion of brain catecholamines on ethanol tolerance and dependence. Eur J Pharmacol 58:285–293, 1979.

8

Catecholamine Metabolism in Anorexia Nervosa

Walter H. Kaye
Michael H. Ebert
Howard A. Gross
C. Raymond Lake

Anorexia nervosa is a disorder that most commonly occurs in young women and is characterized by a distorted attitude toward food, a relentless pursuit of thinness, and obsessive thoughts of being too fat. Patients with anorexia nervosa often exhibit a drive for increased physical activity [15]. Symptoms of depression and anxiety may precede or accompany the weight loss and continue after weight recovery [3]. Amenorrhea may precede weight loss [11], but it inevitably follows extreme loss of weight. Underweight anorectic patients have alterations in multiple endocrine systems, abnormal thermoregulation, bradycardia, and hypotension [30].

Many of the abnormalities seen in underweight anorectic patients are secondary to weight loss and caloric deprivation and seem to disappear with weight restoration. However, many patients with anorexia nervosa have a chronic condition, and attempts at weight restoration fail repeatedly. Some patients with anorexia nervosa may attain normal weight and return to menstruation, but continue to have some degree of disordered attitude toward food and weight [21]. It is possible that a primary dysfunction of hypothalamic regulatory centers may exist in some patients with anorexia nervosa. This dysfunction may produce anorexia nervosa symptoms and weight loss and account for continued symptoms in some patients after weight recovery. Such abnormalities may be reflected in changes in catecholamine (CA) metabolism.

Brain CA are important modulators of all the systems disturbed in anorexia nervosa: appetite, mood, and activity as well as endocrine, autonomic, and metabolic systems [4]. Norepinephrine (NE) and its agonists, when injected into the medial hypothalamus, stimulated feeding in animals [17,25]. Dopaminergic or β_2 agonists injected into the lateral hypothalamus suppressed feeding in rats [17]. Disordered central nervous system (CNS) CA function has been hypothesized in affective disorders [24]. CA analogues such as amphetamine produce stereotypic and increased locomotor activity [5]. Monoamines participate in the modulation of neuroendocrine, thermoregulatory, and peripheral autonomic function. CA have an important role in metabolic regulation [16]. CA are capable of stimulating oxygen and glucose consumption in multiple tissues in the body [10].

PERIPHERAL CATECHOLAMINE METABOLISM IN ANOREXIA NERVOSA

There have been few studies of CA in anorexia nervosa. Four studies [1,6,7,9] have found decreases in the urinary excretion of 3-methoxy-4-hydroxyphenylglycol (MHPG) in underweight anorectic patients. Three of these studies reported increases in MHPG with weight restoration. One study investigated levels of urinary normetanephrine (NM) and metanephrine (M) [9], and another study investigated levels of urinary homovanillic acid (HVA) [7]. Both of the investigations of plasma CA [7,29] reported decreases at low weight. We have recently completed measurements of cerebrospinal fluid (CSF) HVA and NE [12]. The results of this study are described in this chapter.

Urinary Metabolites

Halmi et al [9] were one of the first to report decreases in 24-hour urinary concentrations of MHPG in underweight anorectic patients (Table 8.1). Twenty-five anorectic patients with a mean admission weight of 36.7 kg had a mean urinary concentration of MHPG of 796 μg/24 hr. After weight restoration to a mean weight of 44.7 kg, the anorectic patients had a significant increase of urinary MHPG to 951 μg/24 hr. Halmi et al found that urinary MHPG excretion after weight gain remained significantly lower than the 1196 μg/24 hr MHPG excretion found in their group of normal controls.

Gross et al [7] found that ten underweight anorectic patients (mean 32.5 kg) had a mean 24-hour urinary concentration of MHPG of 789 μg/24 hr. After weight restoration to a mean of 43.3 kg, these patients had a significant increase in 24-hour urinary MHPG to 951 μg/24 hr. This level was similar to normal controls' urinary MHPG concentration of 1044 μg/24 hr. Gerner and Gwirtsman [6] reported that 11 patients with anorexia nervosa at less than 80% of ideal body weight had a mean 24-hour urinary concentration of MHPG of 663 μg/kg. Urinary MHPG was not measured after weight restoration. Abraham et al [1] reported 18 underweight anorectic patients (35.3 kg) had a mean 24-hour urinary MHPG concentration of 641 μg/24 hr. Sixteen anorectic patients, after weight restoration (47.1 kg), had an increase of urinary MHPG concentration to 1073 μg/24 hrs. Abraham collected multiple MHPG urine specimens during the process of weight restoration and found a positive correlation between ideal body weight and urinary MHPG concentration.

Only the studies of Halmi et al [9] and Gross et al [7] included normal

Table 8.1 Urinary Metabolites

	Underweight Anorectic Patients			After Weight Restoration			Controls		
	n	*kg*	*μg/24 hr*	*n*	*kg*	*μg/24 hr*	*n*	*kg*	*μg/24 hr*
MHPG									
Halmi et al [9]	25	35.7	796	25	44.7	951	15	51.1	1196
Gross et al [7]	10	32.5 ± 1.1	789 ± 102	10	43.3 ± 1.9	951 ± 111	9	54.4	1044 ± 125
Gerner and Gwirtsman [6]	11	< 80% ideal body weight	663 ± 53	—	—	—	—	—	—
Abraham et al [1]	18	35.3 ± 3.8	641 ± 130	16	47.1 ± 6.8	1073 ± 232	—	—	—
NM									
Halmi et al [9]	25	35.7	83.03	25	44.7	114.79	15	51.1	116.41
M									
Halmi et al [9]	25	35.7	67.55	25	44.7	86.31	15	51.1	63.41
HVA									
Gross et al [7]	10	32.5 ± 1.1	4022 ± 253	10	43.3 ± 69	5223 ± 197	9	54.5	5332 ± 231

n = number of subjects; MHPG = 3-methoxy-4 hydroxyphenylglycol; NM = normetanephrine; M = metanephrine; HVA = homovanillic acid.

control collection of urine for MHPG determination. All studies supported the finding that urinary MHPG excretion is low in underweight patients with anorexia nervosa and increases with weight restoration. The weight-recovered patients in these studies had similar values of MHPG. The issue of whether these values normalize appears to be determined by the different values of their normal controls.

It is unclear whether factors other than weight contribute to the concentrations of MHPG. Halmi found a significant correlation between change in urinary MHPG concentration before and after weight restoration and depression. Both the Gross [7] and Abraham [1] groups failed to find a correlation between MHPG and depression in their studies. Gwirtsman and Gerner [8] found a relationship between low urine MHPG and a failure to suppress cortisol release to dexamethasone, and also found a high percentage of relatives with either primary affective

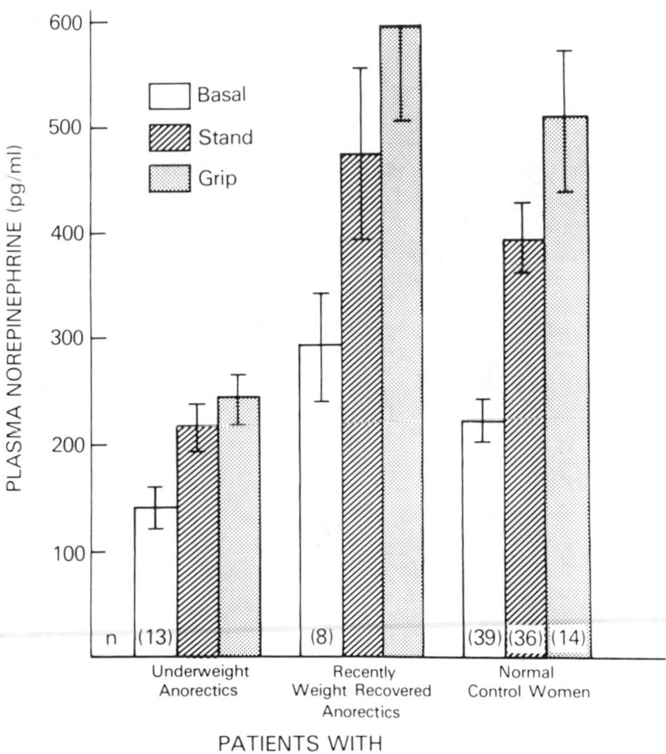

Figure 8.1 Plasma norepinephrine concentrations measured during a basal state, after standing for 5 minutes, and after using an isometric handgrip for 5 minutes. The subjects are underweight anorexia nervosa patients, the same patients after immediate weight restoration, and normal controls.

disorder or alcoholism. They did not report a specific analysis of depression in their anorectic patients.

Halmi et al [9] found that MHPG was not related to activity. Gerner and Gwirtsman [6] found no difference in MHPG concentration between high- and low-activity anorectic patients. Patients remained at bed rest during the Abraham study so that activity was constant for their collections.

Few other urinary CA metabolites have been measured in anorexia nervosa. Gross et al [7] found that urinary excretion of HVA was lower in underweight patients with anorexia than in normal controls (see Table 8.1). Weight gain was attended by an increase in HVA excretion in all patients to levels similar to normal controls. Halmi et al [9] (see Table 8.1) found that levels of urinary M were comparable to control values when patients were underweight and elevated after weight restoration. Underweight anorectic patients had 24-hour urinary concentrations of NM that were less than controls and became normalized appreciably with weight restoration.

Plasma Catecholamines

Plasma NE, plasma tyrosine (the precursor amino acid), and plasma dopamine β-hydroxylase (DBH) were studied by Gross et al [7]. They found that levels of plasma tyrosine and DBH were normal in anorectic patients before and after weight gain. Plasma levels of NE were significantly lower in underweight anorectic patients than in the weight-recovered patients or normal controls (Figure 8.1). Plasma levels of NE in the weight-restored patients were similar to the normal controls. Van Loon [29] reported significant decreases in plasma concentrations of dopamine (DA), NE, and epinephrine (E) in three underweight patients with anorexia compared with six normal women.

CEREBRAL CATECHOLAMINE METABOLISM IN ANOREXIA NERVOSA

We have authored one of the only studies in the literature of central monoamine metabolism in anorexia nervosa [12]. Measuring levels of neurochemicals in CSF is one of the few techniques available for looking directly at brain metabolism. One problem with interpreting results is that CSF levels of neurochemicals are the sum of individual systems and somewhat dependent on their proximity to the ventricles.

Most physiologic studies of anorexia nervosa have been done during weight loss or immediately after weight gain. Consequently, it has been difficult to separate what biologic changes are a consequence of weight loss or rapid weight gain and what biologic abnormalities might be caused by a primary CNS dysfunction. To control for this factor, we studied patients with anorexia nervosa at various stages of the disorder. We hypothesized that if there was a trait-related neurochemical abnormality, it might still be apparent after weight recovery. Patients were studied during three phases of illness: (1) one group was studied after six months or longer at less than 75% of ideal body weight (underweight anorexia nervosa); (2) the same group of underweight anorectics were restudied three to four weeks after correction of weight loss (recently weight recovered); and (3) a separate group of women were studied who, in the past, had been underweight with anorexia nervosa but who at the time of the present study had been weight recovered for a mean of 20 months (long-term weight recovered.)

These long-term weight recovered subjects had similar criteria of the *Diagnostic and Statistical Manual of Mental Disorders* (3rd ed.) [5] for anorexia nervosa in the past, but currently had a stable (± standard error of the mean [SEM]) weight for at least 6 months prior to the study. Most had been anorexia nervosa inpatients on our ward in previous years. These women had similar histories to the anorectic patients currently underweight (Table 8.2). All had some degree of continuing anorexia nervosa symptoms including distorted body image, peculiar eating habits, and aberrations of appetite.

All subjects were hospitalized in clinical research units of the National Institutes of Health Clinical Center, National Institute of Mental Health and gave informed consent for the study; each was diagnosed by two of the authors as meeting DSM III criteria for anorexia nervosa. Eight normal women of similar age were recruited to serve as controls. None had notable current or past psychiatric or medical diseases. All had normal menstrual cycles.

Lumbar punctures were performed at 8:00 AM during the first 7 days of the follicular phase in those women having normal menstrual cycles. Patients fasted

Table 8.2 Physiologic Studies of Patients with Anorexia Nervosa and Controls*

	Underweight	*Recent Weight Recovery*	*Long-Term Weight Recovery*	*Control Women*
Number	8	8	8	8
Age at study (years)	24.5 ± 1.9	—	22.0 ± 1.4	25.6 ± 1.0
Weight at study (kg)	33.4 ± 1.3	44.2 ± 1.2	49.3 ± 2.0	53.6 ± 1.1
Height (cm)	167.9 ± 1.9	—	160 ± 2.3	162 ± 1.9
Situational Discomfort Scale	42.0 ± 6.8	23.3 ± 4.7	21.3 ± 4.3	9.1 ± 1.5
Age at onset of anorexia (years)	18.5 ± 0.8	—	16.9 ± 1.4	
Lowest weight patient had ever been (kg)	29.6 ± 1.1	—	35.3 ± 1.0	
Months weight stable at time of study		<1	20.1 ± 6.6	

* Data are shown as mean ± standard error of the mean (SEM).
SOURCE: Kaye et al [12].

for 12 hours before the study and were allowed out of bed only to go to the bathroom.

Because in anorexia nervosa there is a limitation of dietary intake and often vomiting and laxative abuse, it is important to determine any effect nutritional status might have on essential amino acids involved in CA metabolism. These amino acids include phenylalanine and tyrosine.

The mean plasma tyrosine level for underweight anorectic patients was 3.9 ± 0.3 μmoles/100 ml. Tyrosine levels for the long-term weight-restored group were 4.9 ± 0.4 and for the control group, 4.4 ± 0.2. Plasma tyrosine was significantly elevated in short-term weight-restored anorectic patients compared with levels at their lowest weight (paired t test, $p < 0.02$). There were no differences between any other groups. Mean plasma phenylalanine levels were similar for all four groups of subjects.

Plasma tyrosine values correlated positively with CSF HVA values for the underweight condition ($p < 0.01$) and for controls ($p < 0.05$). There was no

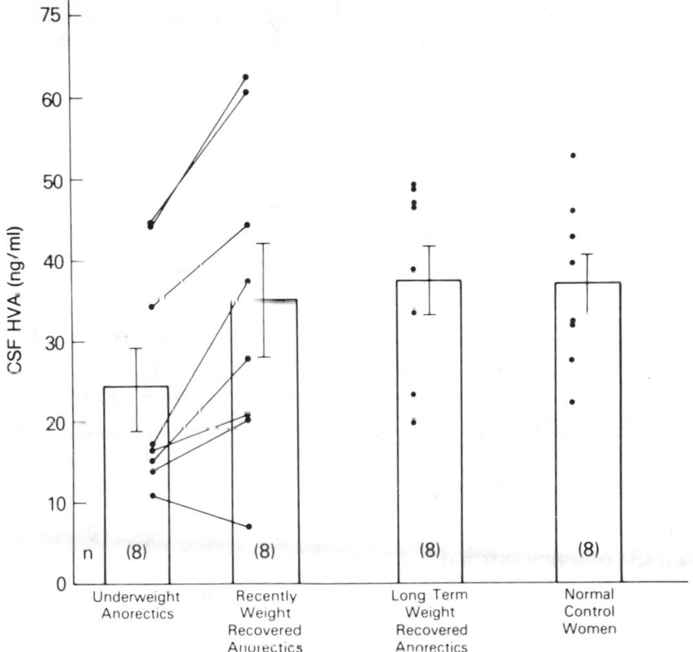

Figure 8.2 Cerebrospinal fluid (CSF) homovanillic acid (HVA) concentrations in underweight anorexia nervosa patients; the same patients after recent weight restoration; a group of long-term weight-recovered patients with a history of weight loss from anorexia nervosa; and normal control women. Underweight anorectic patients had significantly lower levels of CSF HVA ($p < 0.01$) compared with levels after weight restoration.

significant correlation between blood tyrosine values and CSF HVA values for short- or long-term weight-recovered anorectic patients. Plasma tyrosine values correlated positively with CSF NE values for only the underweight conditions ($p < 0.05$). It has been proposed that all neutral amino acids compete for one transport site in the blood-brain barrier. Therefore, the quantity of tyrosine transported to brain from blood is dependent on the amounts of the other neutral amino acids: phenylalanine, tryptophan, valine, leucine, and isoleucine [31,32]. The ratio of plasma tyrosine values to the other neutral plasma amino acids was within normal values for underweight anorectic patients and correlated with CSF HVA values for underweight anorectic patients ($p < 0.02$) and control ($p < 0.05$) conditions.

Seven of eight patients studied as underweight anorectics showed an increase in CSF HVA (Figure 8.2) after weight recovery ($t = 3.77$, $p < .01$). Group means for CSF HVA were otherwise similar.

In contrast to the CSF HVA, CSF NE concentrations (Figure 8.3) demonstrated no consistent pattern of change between underweight anorectics and the same patients after weight recovery. Long-term weight-recovered patients had significantly lower concentrations of CSF NE than the normal controls ($t = 2.60$, $p < .05$) and underweight anorectics ($t = 3.01$, $p < .02$) and demonstrated a similar trend as the recently weight-recovered anorectics ($t = 2.09$, $p < .1$).

CONCLUSIONS

Although it is difficult to make generalizations from such limited data, there are certain consistent trends (Table 8.3). Four studies found approximately a 30% decrease in urinary MHPG excretion in underweight anorectic patients. Some urinary MHPG (20–40%) may be derived from the metabolism of brain NE [14, 18,19]. The other studies of NE metabolism in anorexia tend to support the possibility that the decreased MHPG excretion in urine primarily reflects a decrease in turnover of NE in the periphery. Plasma levels of NE are decreased approximately 50% in underweight anorectic patients, and CSF levels of NE are normal. Urinary NM, which originates from CA pools outside the CNS, is decreased approximately 30% in underweight anorectic patients. However, urinary M, which also originates outside the CNS, remains normal.

What factors might be responsible for decreases in peripheral adrenergic metabolism in underweight anorectics? There is no clear agreement about the contribution of depression or motor activity to the decrease in peripheral NE metabolism. It is unlikely that the decrease in peripheral NE metabolism is a consequence of a limited quantity of amino acid precursors, as other studies [7,26] agree that underweight anorectic patients have normal levels of CA amino acid precursors. Urinary MHPG, NM, M, and plasma NE all increase with weight gain.

Peripheral sympathetic nervous system (SNS) activity and NE metabolism are known to decrease with reduction in food intake. Starvation in human beings

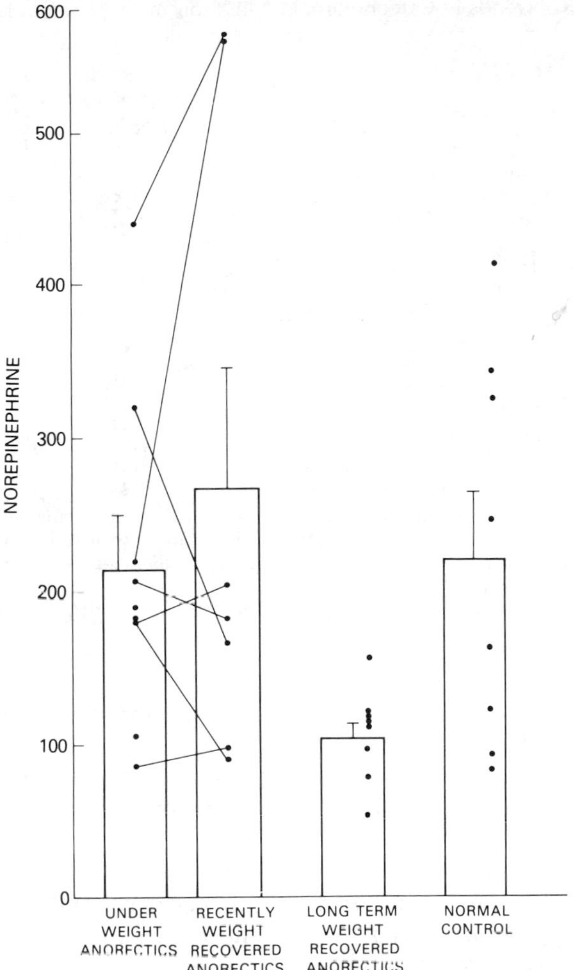

Figure 8.3 Cerebrospinal fluid (CSF) norepinephrine (NE) concentrations in underweight anorexia nervosa patients; the same patients after recent weight restoration; a group of long-term weight-recovered patients with a history of weight loss from anorexia nervosa; and normal control women. Long-term weight recovered anorectic patients had lower CSF NE levels compared with underweight anorectics ($p < 0.05$) or controls ($p < 0.05$).

Table 8.3 Trends in Catecholamine Metabolism in Anorexia Nervosa

	Underweight	*Recent Weight Recovery*	*Long-Term Weight Recovery*
NE Metabolism			
Urinary M	NL	↑ 35%	—
Urinary NM	↓ 30%	NL	—
Urinary MHPG	↓ 30%	? NL or ↓	
Plasma tyrosine	NL	NL	NL
Plasma NE	↓ 50%	NL	—
Plasma DBH	NL	NL	NL
CSF NE	NL	NL	↓ 50%
DA Metabolism			
Urinary HVA	↓ 25%	NL	—
CSF HVA	↓ 30%	NL	NL

NE = norepinephrine; M = metanephrine; NM = normetanephrine; MHPG = 3-methoxy-4-hydroxyphenylglycol; DBH = dopamine β-hydroxylase; CSF = cerebrospinal fluid; DA = dopamine; HVA = homovanillic acid; NL = normal; ↓ = decrease; ↑ = increase.

SOURCE: Gross et al [7], Halmi et al [9], Gernier et al [6], and Abraham et al [1].

is attended by bradycardia, hypotension, and decreased metabolic rate [13,27]. Fasting in rats, even for a relatively short interval, diminishes the turnover rate in NE in the sympathetic nerves of the heart [34] as well as in other organs [33]. Landsberg and Young [16] found that obese women put on a low carbohydrate diet have a reduction of plasma NE. Landsberg and Young hypothesized that suppression of sympathetic activity during fasting conserves calories by diminishing metabolism and heat production. It is most likely that the diminished peripheral adrenergic activity found in underweight anorectic patients is related to loss of body weight and alteration in caloric intake. The normalization of peripheral adrenergic activity found after short-term weight recovery is also probably related to increased caloric intake and increased weight.

Underweight anorectic patients also have approximately a 25% decrease in urinary HVA excretion and approximately a 30% decrease in CSF HVA concentrations (see Table 8.3). A large proportion (approximately one half) of urinary HVA originates from the metabolism of brain DA [14] so the decrease in urinary HVA is consistent with a deficiency of dopaminergic function in the brain in underweight anorectic patients. We have also found approximately a 20% decrease in CSF 5-hydroxyindoleacetic acid (5-HIAA; a serotonin metabolite) in the underweight anorectic patients with return to normal control values after weight recovery [12].

The monoamine metabolites and NE levels in CSF are thought to be the sum of contributions of various brain regions. There is no present method of relating changes in CSF monoamine levels to any specific brain area. It is known that both DA and serotonin (5-hydroxytryptamine; 5-HT) contribute to modulation of appetite, weight, mood, motor activity, central endocrine function, and temperature regulation. It appears that decreases in CSF levels of DA and 5-HT metabolites are associated with weight loss and return to normal levels with weight restoration. It is possible to hypothesize that some of the disturbances seen in anorexia nervosa after weight loss, such as endocrine dysfunction, hypothermia, as well as severe distortions of body image and appetite, might be related to alteration of DA and 5-HT function.

In contrast to other monoamine findings, we demonstrated that underweight anorectics had CSF concentrations of NE that were similar to normal controls and that there was no change in mean CSF NE concentrations with weight recovery. Peripheral adrenergic levels were not obtained in these patients.

Most studies of underweight anorectics were completed soon after their admission. It may be that, on admission, anorectic patients often have fluid and electrolyte abnormalities, are nutritionally compromised, and are stressed. These factors may contribute to decreased adrenergic metabolism. Prior to our CSF study [12], anorectic patients were medically stablized for 2 to 4 weeks. The difference in time after admission may account for differences among studies.

Findings of low levels of NE in the CSF of long-term weight-recovered anorexia nervosa patients raises a possibility that CNS NE metabolism may play a vital role in anorexia nervosa. This speculation is particularly interesting in light of data from animal studies suggesting NE has a major role in CNS appetite regulation. Liebowitz [17] has reviewed the literature, which indicates that NE applied directly by cannula to the medial hypothalamus of several species evokes feeding in a satiated animal and that α antagonists block the facilitating effects of NE. Both NE and clonidine can stimulate feeding in rats when given intraventricularly [25]. Studies with push-pull cannula perfusion have found that NE is released in vivo within the hypothalamus of food deprived animals as they feed [20,28]. Furthermore, McCaleb et al [20] have found that the release of NE from specific hypothalamic nuclei was suppressed by the addition of glucose and enhanced by the addition of insulin or 2-deoxy-D-glucose (which would produce a relative hypoglycemia). Recent work has found that nutrients infused directly into a rat's duodenum directly alter the pattern of NE release within the hypothalamus [22].

The medial and lateral hypothalamic regions are implicated as circuits controlling feeding and satiety [17]. The medial hypothalamus has connections with sympathetic centers in the brainstem [2], and diminished sympathetic activity after destruction of the medial hypothalamus has been inferred from alterations of peripheral lipolytic response [23].

A medial hypothalamus–SNS complex may be an important part of the mechanism in the brain that links food intake to metabolic rate. NE appears to be critical to the function of both of these systems. The disturbance of CNS NE metabolism apparent after long-term weight recovery would suggest that trait-related abnormalities of feeding behavior and metabolism might occur in anorexia nervosa. Further investigations, however, will be necessary to answer questions raised by these data.

The meaning of low levels of CSF NE in each of the long-term weight-recovered anorectic patients is unknown. These patients continued to have anorectic symptoms and behavior. It is possible that low CSF NE in long-term weight-recovered patients identifies (1) a primary abnormality in brain modulation of appetite and weight in anorexia nervosa that is obscured by state-dependent changes at low weight or immediately after rapid weight restoration; (2) a group of good outcome anorectic patients; or (3) compensatory changes in adrenergic function allowing recovery in anorexia. Further studies are necessary to answer questions raised by these data.

There is currently no rationale for use of NE or NE metabolite values in clinical treatment of anorexia. However, the finding of low values in long-term weight-recovered anorectic patients make some speculations feasible. If further studies determine that NE concentrations identify anorectic patients who have good or poor prognoses or that alterations in adrenergic metabolism are associated with recovery, then adrenergic measurements might be clinically helpful.

REFERENCES

1. Abraham SF, Beaumont PJV, Cobbin DM. Catecholamine metabolism and body weight in anorexia nervosa. Br J Psychiatry 138:244–247, 1981.
2. Ban T. Fiber connections in the hypothalamus and some autonomic functions. Pharmacol Biochem Behav 3[Suppl. 1]:3–13, 1975.
3. Cantwell DP, Sturzenberger KS, Burroughs J, Salkin B, Green JK. Anorexia nervosa, an affective disorder. Arch Gen Psychiatry 34:1087–1093, 1977.
4. Cooper JR, Bloom FE, Roth DH. The Biochemical Basis of Neuropharmacology (3rd ed.). New York: Oxford University Press, 1978.
5. Diagnostic and Statistical Manual of Mental Disorders (3rd ed.). American Psychiatric Association, Washington, DC, 1980.
6. Gerner RH, Gwirtsman HE. Abnormalities of dexamethasone suppression test and urinary MHPG in anorexia nervosa. Am J Psychiatry 138:650–653, 1981.
7. Gross HA, Lake CR, Ebert MH, Ziegler MG, Kopin IJ. Catecholamine metabolism in primary anorexia nervosa. J Clin Endocrinol Metab 49:805–809, 1979.
8. Gwirtsman HE, Gerner RH. Neurochemical abnormalities in anorexia nervosa: similarities to affective disorders. Biol Psychiatry 16:991–995, 1981.
9. Halmi KA, Dekirmenjian H, Davis JM, Casper R, Goldberg S. Catecholamine metabolism in anorexia nervosa. Arch Gen Psychiatry 35:458–460, 1978.
10. Himms-Gagen J. Sympathetic regulation of metabolism. Pharmacol Rev 19:367–461, 1967.
11. Kay D, Leigh D. The natural history, treatment, and prognosis of anorexia nervosa, based on a study of 38 patients. J Ment Sci 100:411–431, 1954.
12. Kaye WH, Ebert MH, Lake CR, Raleigh M. CSF monoamine metabolism in anorexia nervosa. Arch Gen Psychiatry 41:350–355, 1984.
13. Keys A, Henschel A, Taylor HL. The size and function of the human heart at rest, in semi-starvation and in subsequent rehabilitation. Am J Physiol 150:153, 1947.
14. Kopin IJ. Measuring Turnover of Neurotransmitter in Human Brain. In Psychopharmacology: A Generation of Progress, MA Lipton, A DiMascio, and KF Killiam (eds), 933–942. New York: Raven Press, 1978.

15. Kron L, Katz JL, Gorzynski G, Weiner H. Hyperactivity in anorexia nervosa: a fundamental clinical feature. Compr Psychiatry 19:433–440, 1978.
16. Landsberg L, Young JB. Fasting, feeding and regulation of the sympathetic nervous system. N Engl J Med 298:1295–1301, 1978.
17. Leibowitz SF. Neurochemical Systems of the Hypothalamus. In Handbook of the Hypothalamus, PJ Morgane, J Pansepp (eds), vol. 3, part A, 299–437. New York: Marcel Dekker, 1980.
18. Maas JW, Dekirmenjian H, Garver D, Redmond DE, Jr, Landis DH. Excretion of catecholamine metabolites following intraventricular injection of 6-hydroxydopamine in the macaca speciosa. Eur J Pharmacol 23:121–130, 1973.
19. Maas JW, Landis DH. The metabolism of circulating norepinephrine by human subjects. J Pharmacol Exp Ther 177:600–612, 1971.
20. McCaleb ML, Myers RD, Singer G, Willis G. Hypothalamic norepinephrine in the rat during feeding and push-pull perfusion with glucose, 2-dg, or insulin. Am J Physiol 236:R312–R321, 1979.
21. Morgan H, Russell G. Value of family background and clinical features as predictors of long-term outcome in anorexia nervosa: four year follow-up study of 41 patients. Psychol Med 5:355–371, 1975.
22. Myers RD, McCaleb ML. Feeding: satiety signal from intestine triggers brain's noradrenergic mechanism. Science 209:1035–1037, 1980.
23. Nishizawa Y, Bray GA. Ventromedial hypothalamic lesions and the mobilization of fatty acids. J Clin Invest 61:714–721, 1978.
24. Prange AJ, Jr. The use of drugs in depression: its theoretical and practical basis. Psychiatry Annu 3:56, 1973.
25. Ritter S, Wise CD, Stein L. Neurochemical regulation of feeding in the rat. J Comp Physiol Psychol 88:778–784, 1975.
26. Russell GFM. The nutritional disorder in anorexia nervosa. J Psychosom Res 11:141–149, 1967.
27. Simonson EA, Henschel A, Keys A. The electrocardiogram of man in semi-starvation and subsequent rehabilitation. Am Heart J 35:584–602, 1948.
28. Van der Gugsten J, Slangen JL. Release of endogenous catecholamines from rat hypothalamus in vivo related to feeding and other behaviors. Pharmacol Biochem Behav 7:211–219, 1977.
29. Van Loon GR. Abnormal catecholamine mechanisms in hypothalamic-pituitary disorders. Metabolism XXIX, 11[Suppl 1]:1198–1202, 1980.
30. Vigersky RA, Loriaux DL. Anorexia Nervosa as a Model of Hypothalamic Dysfunction. In Anorexia Nervosa, RA Vigersky (ed), 109–121. New York: Raven Press, 1977.
31. Wurtman RJ. Effects of Nutrients and Circulating Precursors on the Synthesis of Brain Neurotransmitters. In Central Mechanisms of Anorectic Drugs, S Garattini, and R Samanin (eds), 267–294. New York: Raven Press, 1978.
32. Wurtman RJ, Fernstrom JD. Control of brain monoamine synthesis by diet and plasma amino acids. Am J Clin Nutr 28:638–647, 1975.
33. Young J, Landsberg L. Pancreatic norepinephrine (NE) turnover in the rat: a method of assessing the sympathetic regulation of the endocrine pancreas. Diabetes [Suppl. 1] 25:391, 1976.
34. Young J, Landsberg L. Suppression of sympathetic nervous system during fasting. Science 195:1473–1475, 1977.

III

Pediatric Disorders and the Catecholamines

9

Overview of Norepinephrine in Selected Pediatric Disorders

Alan Zametkin
Mary Elizabeth Smith
Judith L. Rapoport

A few disorders such as Down's syndrome cause clear, consistent alterations in monoamines, suggesting that altered catecholamine (CA) metabolism, at least in some individuals, is a primary component of the condition. In other disorders, either monoamine disturbance has not been consistently demonstrated (migraine, childhood schizophrenia) or alterations of CA or metabolites are probably secondary to the disease process, as with anorexia nervosa (see Chapter 8) or muscular dystrophy (see Chapter 5).

A variety of studies have indirectly examined CA in pediatric disorders, inferring a role from pharmacologic manipulation. We have not reviewed those disorders in which there has been little direct evidence of an intrinsic association between CA alteration and the underlying disease. For example, although amphetamine is said to exacerbate Sydenham's chorea [53], we found no direct study of CA metabolism in Sydenham's chorea for pediatric populations, and so the disorder is not covered in this review.

Several studies provide valuable information about individual differences among normal children of such measures as dopamine β-hydroxylase (DBH), urinary CA, and metabolites as related to age, sex, and emotional state. These studies provide a useful framework for evaluating CA alteration in specific illnesses.

One infant study [71] examined plasma DBH in 193 normal newborns. The enzyme was correlated significantly with behavioral items suggesting "difficult" temperament at age 5 months. DBH activity also showed a slight but significant correlation with a newborn score of minor physical anomalies thought to reflect subtle toxic influences early in pregnancy. More recently, urinary CA measurements in newborns and age groups from 1 to 80 years revealed significant increases during the first year of life but minimal changes after the first year [69]. Individual variability was large precluding additional significant findings. Another study of urinary CA and CA metabolites found adult values were reached by 2.5 years of life

[30]. However, when CA excretion rate is correlated with body surface area, no significant increases are observed from infancy to adulthood [69].

A few studies of CA excretion in older children have established useful parameters [50,51]. Large samples of grade-school children were examined during passive (film watching) and active (mathematics test) conditions. No sex differences were found during the passive condition, but during work, boys excreted more epinephrine (E) than did girls. Moreover, children who had increased E excretion during the mathematics test performed better on the test. Positive correlations were found between E and norepinephrine (NE) excretion and teachers' ratings of good social adjustment and emotional stability. Other studies have documented increased E and NE during physical exercise [7], but more for older than for younger players. In that study, minimal exercise (bicycle riding) did not increase CA excretion. Winkel and Slob [93] have related urinary CA in adolescent boys to aggression and emotional disturbances, although the methodology was not completely described.

In all of these studies, E is more responsive than NE to stress-related situations (see Chapters 1 and 3). Stress produces an increase of approximately 20% in boys. A study of CA excretion in children in connection with various types of dental treatment, such as extraction, shows that anticipation of treatment produces as great an increase in E and NE excretion as the painful procedures themselves, suggesting a complex interaction between CA excretion and psychological variables.

These findings emphasize the need to use controls for psychological variables, such as short- or long-term stress, when comparing NE or E metabolism. It is clear that additional controls, such as patients with other chronic illnesses, should be included, and the stress of measurement procedures should be assessed and related to levels of NE, E, and their metabolites.

CHILDHOOD SCHIZOPHRENIA AND INFANTILE AUTISM

During the past 10 to 15 years, CA metabolism in childhood schizophrenia and infantile autism has been studied through measurements of CA, metabolites, and enzymes in blood, urine, and cerebrospinal fluid (CSF), as well as indirectly through pharmacologic manipulation.

The new American Psychiatric Association diagnostic nomenclature, *Diagnostic and Statistical Manual of Mental Disorders* (third edition) (*DSM-III*), clearly distinguishes infantile autism from childhood schizophrenia. The descriptions of these disorders in *DSM-III* will make future research more precise, but this does not clarify the confusion concerning diagnoses and criteria in previous research. Only a few studies, such as Cohen et al [17], have provided a clear description of the disorder. A comprehensive review of biochemical studies of children with autism, childhood schizophrenia, and related developmental disabilities is recommended [46,70,73].

Childhood Schizophrenia

Owing to the diagnostic overlap previously mentioned, descriptions of biochemical studies in "pure childhood schizophrenia" are rare. Several studies which seem to differentiate autistic children from schizophrenic, nonautistic children are reviewed briefly in the following sections.

Catecholamines and Metabolites

Cohen et al [15,17] studied homovanillic acid (HVA) and 5-hydroxyindoleacetic acid (5-HIAA) in the CSF of neuropsychiatrically disabled children. Their results showed significant increases in CSF HVA and 5-HIAA levels in autistic versus epileptic patients, although there were no differences between autistic and "atypical psychotic but nonautistic" patients. In the latter study [15], four groups were described: "primary childhood autism"; "central processing disturbance"; "nonautistic psychosis of early childhood"; and "primary childhood aphasia." These groups were compared with "pediatric contrast patients." Using the probenecid-loading technique for examining CSF, statistical analysis revealed that CSF 5-HIAA levels were significantly lower in autistic compared with nonautistic psychotic groups. There were no other significant differences in metabolite concentrations in the other groups. For a more complete review see Cohen et al [18].

Serotonin

One study found that children with schizophrenia have been reported to have decreased serotonin (5-hydroxytryptamine; 5-HT) uptake in platelets [78], while others [11,63] have reported no difference between child schizophrenics and controls. Campbell et al [11] reported that 5-HT blood concentrations in psychotic children were not significantly different from the comparison cases but were related inversely to levels of intellectual functioning, confirming a previous report but inconsistent with the work of Ritvo [73]. Campbell [12] reported normal platelet monoamine oxidase (MAO) activity for 21 schizophrenic children compared with 18 age-matched controls.

Several studies have used drug trials in indirect attempts to shed light on CA mechanisms. However, results do not permit clear inference about mechanisms, and the drugs of choice at this time for true childhood schizophrenia appear to be antipsychotic medication. For this reason, the dopaminergic system is a major area of research into the pathophysiology of childhood schizophrenia.

Infantile Autism

Catecholamines and Metabolites

Lake et al [59], in a rare study with clearly defined patient criteria, found elevated plasma NE levels in 11 autistic children and their families compared with controls.

The specificity of this finding is uncertain, however, as stress may have mediated the elevation. Young et al [96], studying childhood autism in five subjects, reported a decreased 24-hour urine 3-methoxy-4-hydroxyphenylglycol (MHPG), the metabolic breakdown product of NE.

Cohen et al [17] measured CSF levels of HVA and 5-HIAA after probenecid administration in autistic children and found significantly lower 5-HIAA levels than in nonautistic psychotic children. In a later study [18], some autistic children with lower 5-HIAA CSF levels also had elevated HVA CSF levels. These patients appeared to be the most deviant clinically with increased stereotypy and hyperactivity.

Enzyme Studies

Coleman et al [22] found no differences in DBH activity between autistic children, schizophrenic children and controls. Lake et al [59] reported that plasma DBH activity is significantly lower in autistic patients and their healthy relatives than in control groups, and earlier, Goldstein et al [41] reported that plasma DBH was lower for 78 autistic children compared with 78 age- and sex-matched controls. The autistics' significantly increased plasma NE levels [59] seem inconsistent with the decreased DBH. The finding of decreased DBH in autism by two independent groups warrants further exploration. Cohen et al [20] reported no differences in platelet MAO activity between autistic and normal children. MAO decreased with age, however, in the autistic children, and there was a trend toward greater platelet MAO activity in prepubertal and pubertal male autistic children relative to normal males.

Platelet and Blood Serotonin

Much attention has been focused on platelet and blood 5-HT levels since the original report by Schain and Freedman [79] demonstrating that children with Kannerian autism, as diagnosed by the criteria of Kanner, have elevated levels of whole blood 5-HT. Ritvo et al [73] replicated this finding and also demonstrated that both 5-HT levels and platelet counts are significantly higher in autistic children than in age-matched controls. The mean 5-HT per platelet value was not significantly different between the groups, however. Boullin et al [9] confirmed the findings of elevated platelet counts in a survey of autistic children. The studies of Takahashi et al [86] further supported the findings of increased blood 5-HT levels in autistics. However, Campbell et al [11] were unable to replicate the findings of increased 5-HT concentration in psychotic children. Studies of platelet uptake and efflux of 5-HT are confused by different diagnostic criteria. Earlier reports of increased platelet 5-HT efflux in the study of Boullin et al [9] were not replicated by Yuwiler's group [97] using different diagnostic criteria.

Attempts to regulate 5-HT levels by administering tryptophan or L-dopa for modulation of dopaminergic systems have been inconclusive [46]. Schain and Freedman [79] gave 1 gm of tryptophan to children with autism and other disorders and found no changes in blood 5-HIAA levels or blood 5-HT levels. Similarly, they found no change in the excretion of 5-HIAA after tryptophan loading. Hanley et al [47] reported that L-tryptophan (3 gm/day for 3 days) administered to hyperserotonemic autistics, nonhyperserotonemic autistics, and normal controls produced marked increase in 5-HIAA excretion in all three groups and an increase in urinary 5-HT excretion in the hyperserotonemic autistic children. However, he found the opposite effect, i.e., a decrease in urinary 5-HT excretion, in the mildly retarded group. To theorize that a metabolic defect in 5-HT or tryptophan metabolism is the underlying pathophysiology of infantile autism seems premature.

Certainly no study conclusively documents an improved clinical outcome using L-tryptophan. Ritvo [74] administered L-dopa to four hospitalized boys for 6 months with no improvement. Blood 5-HT concentration decreased significantly in the three youngest patients, but no clinical change was apparent. Similarly, Campbell et al [10] reported the use of L-dopa in children who could not be clearly defined as either schizophrenic or autistic. Nine hundred to 2250 mg/day of L-dopa stimulated play energy, motor initiation (in hypoactive children), language behavior, and effective responsiveness. In the same study, L-amphetamine yielded poor results.

In summary, although considerable research has been done to uncover a metabolic defect that would account for the extensive symptomotology of childhood schizophrenia and infantile autism, no clearly reproducible data have emerged during the past several decades.

CHILDHOOD ENURESIS

Numerous studies have documented the short-term efficacy of tricyclic antidepressants in controlling nocturnal enuresis [67]. These studies suggest that enuresis may result from a neurotransmitter abnormality. Noradrenergic mechanisms are probably involved, because methscopolamine, a peripheral anticholinergic agent, is not an effective treatment [6]. However, no direct evidence for neurotransmitter abnormalities in enuresis has been demonstrated.

GILLES DE LA TOURETTE'S SYNDROME

Gilles de la Tourette's syndrome is an illness beginning in childhood and characterized by multiform involuntary movements, noises, and other stereotypic actions. Because haloperidol causes remission and stimulants cause exacerbation, there is a strong basis for theorizing dopaminergic involvement in the pathophysiology of this disorder. Studies of CA in Gilles de la Tourette's syndrome are not as extensive as studies of CA in childhood schizophrenia or infantile autism. Cohen et al [16] investigated CSF acid monoamine metabolites after probenecid administration in six children and found reduced accumulation of 5-HIAA in patients with muscle tics compared with normal controls. The degree of reduction of 5-HIAA relative to HVA appeared to be associated with the severity of the tic disorder. Placed on D-amphetamine, tic symptoms worsened, CSF HVA levels decreased, and CSF 5-HIAA concentrations increased. CSF HVA was lower in children with multiple tics than in normal children.

Lake et al [58] assessed plasma NE levels in an older patient group (average age, 18 years) and found that NE levels did not differ from the control subjects in basal, postural, or exercise stress states. Lake's group found no difference in DBH activity between unrelated age-matched controls and a control group consisting of nonaffected family members, a finding consistent with the work of Cohen et al [16]. Similarly, platelet MAO, plasma MAO, and erythrocyte catechol-O-methyltransferase (COMT) activities of Tourette's syndrome patients did not differ from either control group. Patients taking haloperidol had DBH activities no different from those of the drug-free patients, leading Lake's group to conclude that there may be no generalized disorder of NE metabolism in patients with Gilles de la Tourette's syndrome. This is consistent with another adult study [35] in which plasma DBH and NE were the same as controls.

Giller et al [39] examined MAO and COMT activities in cultured fibroblasts and blood cells from children with autism, children with Gilles de la Tourette's syndrome, and controls. The enzyme activities were similar for patients and matched controls. However, in both disorders there was a significant positive correlation between clinical severity and levels of type-A MAO activity, the enzyme principally responsible for degradation of 5-HT, dopamine (DA), and NE.

Extensive clinical use of haloperidol, as mentioned, suggests dopaminergic pathophysiology. In contrast to this widely known phenomenon, Cohen et al [19] reported an amelioration of symptoms of Tourette's syndrome in eight haloperidol-resistant children treated with clonidine, an α-adrenergic agonist. The primary action of clonidine may be on noradrenergic, dopaminergic, or serotonergic systems; its most likely action, however, is on the locus coeruleus (LC). Because of the conflicting data, it is not yet clear that haloperidol is the only treatment and that dopaminergic dysfunction is the only explanation of the pathophysiology of this syndrome.

LESCH-NYHAN SYNDROME

Lesch-Nyhan syndrome is an X-linked disorder of purine metabolism, characterized by automutilation, aggressive and compulsive self-destructive behavior, choreoathetoid cerebral palsy, marked hypertonicity, athetoid dysarthria, and dysphasia. As in the case of dystonia musculorum deformans, in which there is increased DBH activity and increased concentrations of NE, Lesch-Nyhan patients also seem to have components of hypertonicity and involuntary dyskinetic movements. For this reason, Lake and Ziegler [56] measured plasma DBH activity to assess sympathetic responses to stress and posture in 14 children with Lesch-Nyhan syndrome (mean age 14 years). DBH activity of Lesch-Nyhan patients was significantly lower than that of 14 volunteers. Plasma NE in upright patients did not differ. However, the plasma NE increase on standing was significantly blunted in Lesch-Nyhan patients. In summarizing their data, Lake and Ziegler argued that absence of elevated plasma NE after venipuncture, diminished increment in NE on postural change, and low plasma DBH activities support the notion of diminished autonomic responsivity in Lesch-Nyhan syndrome. This may be secondary to disuse, though, and not a primary defect of the disorder.

One may hypothesize that along with the basic enzymatic deficiency of hypoxanthine phosphoribosyltransferase and enzymes, the activities of which are normally highest in the basal ganglia, abnormalities might also exist in CA input or control over these brain structures. Edelstein et al [34] studied MAO activity in fibroblasts of normal and Lesch-Nyhan children. The study demonstrated that MAO activity is low in fibroblasts from typical Lesch-Nyhan patients and that the severity of the neurologic symptoms correlates with MAO activity. The study raised very interesting ideas about the relationship between purine and CA enzymes.

JUVENILE DIABETES

The literature on plasma CA in juvenile diabetes is limited. Christensen's review [14] tested the suppositions that plasma NE levels are elevated in untreated ketotic juvenile diabetics and reduced in well-treated long-term diabetics. In a study of only three patients, he demonstrated that plasma E levels were elevated twentyfold preceding diabetic pre-coma, whereas plasma NE showed a fourfold increase. In the long-term diabetic with neuropathy, total plasma CA concentrations were reduced at rest when compared with controls, but on standing, CA levels were within normal limits.

DYSTONIA MUSCULORUM DEFORMANS

Dystonia musculorum deformans is a rare, genetically transmitted group of illnesses characterized by the development of dystonic movements and postures without dementia or other organ system disease. Although no anatomic pathology of the brain has been noted [98], other diseases producing similar dystonias (e.g., Huntington's chorea, Parkinson's disease, Wilson's disease) are associated with basal ganglia pathology [65]. Moreover, certain drugs which alter brain monoamines, including the phenothiazines and L-dopa, have provoked dystonic spasms and postures. Indirectly, then, there is evidence of a defect in striatal amine metabolism. L-dopa is perhaps the most controversial agent studied; some researchers note that it improves dystonia [2,13,21,64], while others find that it exacerbates muscle spasms and dystonic posturing [3,24].

Enzymes important in DA metabolism are the subject of more recent studies. Raised levels of DBH are found in patients with autosomal dominant [33,94] and autosomal recessive forms of the disease as well as in some of the unaffected members of the same families. Because DBH is released from sympathetic nerves along with NE, the increased DBH may indicate, among other things, overactivity of the sympathetic nervous system (SNS) owing to the stress of the disease; a receptor insensitivity causing increased synthesis of neurotransmitter [26]; an abnormality in central control of DBH production [68]; or slower clearing or inactivation of DBH [94]. Other studies have found that CSF monoamine metabolites are normal or low in selected dystonic patients [25,26].

At this point it is still unclear if there is a primary disorder of CA metabolism in dystonia musculorum deformans.

FAMILIAL DYSAUTONOMIA

Familial dysautonomia (Riley-Day syndrome) is an autosomal recessive disease of altered sympathetic function [72]. Some of the associated abnormalities include reduced or absent tearing, episodic hypertension, postural hypotension, excessive perspiration, disturbed swallowing, absent or hypoactive deep tendon reflexes, relative indifference to pain and temperature, emotional lability, absence of fungiform and circumvallate papillae, and poor taste discrimination [31,32]. Affected patients may have defects in both cholinergic and adrenergic systems [31].

On infusion of methacholine, a drug with actions similar to acetylcholine, several improvements may be noted: overflow tearing, increased deep tendon reflexes, and a return of taste discrimination. The patients also exhibit an increased sensitivity to infused NE, with skin blotching and extreme hypertension. Dysautonomic patients experience these responses spontaneously, suggesting a supersensitivity to, and perhaps insufficiency of, endogenous NE [83,84]. Examination of tissues from these subjects [95] reveals an increase in adrenal CA, perhaps owing to a deficiency of CA release. E secretion in response to hypoglycemia, however, is normal.

CA metabolites including vanillylmandelic acid (VMA) and HVA are not consistently altered. VMA has been reported normal [43,44] and low [40,83,90], and HVA has been found high [40,83,90] and normal [40,44].

DBH in dysautonomic patients is decreased [89,99]. These patients have normal NE levels and blood pressures while supine, but do not show an increase in plasma NE, DBH, pulse rate, and blood pressure normally when they stand up [99]. Apparently, the autonomic nervous system functions fairly well in a supine resting condition, but reacts poorly to change or stress (e.g., position changes, exercise). One might postulate that the primary defect in the regulation of the SNS is centrally located, as suggested by some researchers [54,68,99].

DUCHENNE TYPE MUSCULAR DYSTROPHY

The pathogenesis of human muscular dystrophy remains unclear; theories include abnormal neural influence on muscle, abnormal microvascular supply of muscle, or genetic fault in muscle surface membrane. No major evidence has accumulated for any theory. Because CA are strong vasoactive agents able to induce muscle ischemia, their role in muscular dystrophy has been suggested [29]. However, urinary studies of CA in humans conflict [66]. In a more thorough study, Dalmaz et al [29] examined urinary CA and metabolites in 20 patients with Duchenne type muscular dystrophy and 7 patients with other forms of genetic myopathy. A control group of 21 age- and sex-matched children was included. There was an increase in urinary amines (NE, normetanephrine and DA) in Duchenne patients only, and only in those children who were severely afflicted. These increases, therefore, seem secondary to the disease process. In their discussion, the authors speculated either that altered oxidative pathways in muscle change CA excretion or CA increases in view of the increased role of E and NE for thermogenesis. These children use CA for thermogenesis because they are unable to pursue normal activities or shiver adequately, or both.

CYSTIC FIBROSIS

Previous studies of cystic fibrosis patients show that their leukocytes produce less cyclic adenosine 3′5′-monophosphate (cAMP) in response to isoproterenol than do controls. One possible explanation for this finding is that elevated levels of circulating CA desensitized the cystic fibrosis leukocytes to isoproterenol effects. Earlier studies showed elevated CA in the urine and in adrenal medullae at autopsy [9]. Because of these findings, Lake et al [55] measured plasma NE and DBH in cystic fibrosis patients and found no difference from age- and sex-matched controls, although patients with cystic fibrosis had lower BP. Curiously, plasma sodium and chloride were slightly but significantly lower in these patients compared with controls, which might explain the findings. Thus, no primary CA abnormality is indicated and the previous findings were probably secondary to other disease processes.

REYE'S SYNDROME

Encephalopathy with fatty degeneration of the viscera, or Reye's syndrome, has become increasingly recognized as a distinct, clinical, and pathologic entity in children. Brain edema is a major aspect of the disorder. As part of a study monitoring intraventricular fluid in the management of Reye's syndrome, Shaywitz et al [81] measured 5-HIAA and HVA. They found markedly increased concentrations of HVA but not of 5-HIAA. Monoamine metabolites did not correlate significantly with intracranial pressure or with mortality or morbidity. Previous reports suggested that octopamine (the β-hydroxylated derivative of tyramine and a possible false neurotransmitter in mammalian brain) is elevated in Reye's syndrome [60]. The elevated HVA found by Shaywitz et al [81] supports the idea that brain monoaminergic systems may be involved in the genesis of this disorder. Within a larger framework, however, other studies of coma also find elevated monoamines, suggesting that elevated CSF amines are secondary to ischemia or similar metabolic insult

[88]. CA metabolism for additional disorders, such as head injury, has not been selectively studied for children and so is not reviewed here.

DOWN'S SYNDROME

Down's syndrome results from an abnormality in the twenty-first chromosome. Approximately 90% of patients with Down's syndrome have trisomy 21. As mental retardation is the major disability associated with Down's syndrome, the possibility arises for neurotransmitter abnormalities. Although 5-HIAA levels are normal in CSF, 5-HT levels are low in blood and platelets of patients with trisomic Down's syndrome [22,61,62,75,87]. Shaywitz et al [80] cite several other studies of CSF 5-HIAA, which are also consistent with these studies. To date, these studies have little practical value because treatment of Down's syndrome patients with 5-hydroxytryptophan has not been clinically useful [23].

A few studies address CA metabolism in this disorder. Urinary levels of NE are low [52], but fluorometric techniques do not find abnormal levels of plasma NE or E. COMT levels are high in children with Down's syndrome and other retarded children [45], and several investigators document low levels of DBH in Down's syndrome [23,37,42,91,92]. Lake et al [57] show that Down's patients actually have higher standing and supine plasma NE levels than controls, although systolic BP is lower. Plasma DBH is also diminished, in keeping with other studies previously cited. The interesting point in Lake's group's study is that patients may have normal or increased NE despite low DBH levels. The altered DBH is thought therefore to relate more specifically to the chromosomal abnormality. An alternative view is that decreased levels may reflect a general immaturity of the nervous system, as DBH is low at birth and in early years. Similarly, retarded subjects may be more anxious than normal subjects during the venipuncture, and psychological stress may produce the higher levels.

Platelet MAO [4] is significantly lower in children with Down's syndrome compared to age- and sex-matched controls. Because the main pathway for breakdown of 5-HT is catalyzed by MAO, the low concentration of blood 5-HT in Down's syndrome is not due to enhanced rate of 5-HT breakdown.

MIGRAINE

Migraine is a disorder of the autonomic nervous system present in approximately 5% of school-aged children [5,38]. Researchers describe three phases in most migraines: vasoconstriction, vasodilation, and recovery [36]. Because vascular changes apparently play a large role in the development and resolution of a migraine attack, much attention focuses on vasoactive substances. 5-HT, a vasoconstrictor of scalp vessels in human beings, is interesting because a decrease in levels may be responsible for a vasodilation of vessels, similar to the second phase (headache phase) of the migraine. Several studies with conflicting results focus on the relationship of 5-

HT and 5-HIAA to attacks. Some researchers [82] find increased urinary levels of 5-HIAA during attacks, but the majority [1,49,76] report either decreased blood and platelet 5-HIAA or decreased 5-HT. Reserpine, which depletes nerve endings of NE and 5-HT, may cause attacks in susceptible individuals [1].

More recent investigations point to the possibility that during attacks, arteries become hyperpermeable, allowing escape of vasoactive substances and causing development of a local inflammatory reaction involving platelets [27,28]. Although the platelets' exact involvement is still unknown, they are the primary source of blood 5-HT, and changes in 5-HT levels during attacks may merely reflect a change in platelet activity.

Agents used for treatment and prophylaxis of migraines, including ergotamine, dihydroergotamine, and methysergide, are all active vasoconstrictors, a fact which provides more indirect evidence that vasoactive agents are a key to the better understanding of migraine attacks. In fact, the venoconstrictor effects of 5-HT are apparently potentiated by small doses of the ergot alkaloids, which is probably the reason these agents are effective treatments for migraine.

Tyramine appears to trigger migraines, as does phenylethylamine; both are present in foodstuffs commonly accused of initiating attacks. In addition, a defect in MAO activity with respect to tyramine and phenylethylamine is reported [48,77].

Studies of urinary VMA in adults are inconsistent and so are not included here.

REFERENCES

1. Anthony M, Hinterberger H, Lance JW. Plasma serotonin in migraine and stress. Arch Neurol 16:544–552, 1967.
2. Barbeau A. Rationale for the use of L-dopa in the torsion dystonias. Neurology (Minneap) 20:96–102, 1970.
3. Barrett RE, Yahr MD, Duvoisin RC. Torsion dystonia and spasmodic torticollis—results of treatment with L-dopa. Neurology (Minneap) 20:107–113, 1970.
4. Benson P, Southgate J. Diminished activity of platelet monoamine oxidase in Down's syndrome. Am J Hum Genet 23:211–214, 1971.
5. Bille B. Migraine in school children. Acta Paediatr Scand 51:14–29, 1962.
6. Blackwell B, Currah J. The Psychopharmacology of Nocturnal Enuresis. In Bladder Control and Enuresis, I. Kolvin and MR Meadows (eds), 231–251. Philadelphia: JB Lippincott, 1973.
7. Blinkie C, Cunningham D, Leung F. Urinary catecholamine excretion during competition in 11 to 23 year old hockey players. Sports 10:188–193, 1978.
8. Bongiovanni A, Takouae W, Steiker D. Study of adrenal glands in childhood: hormonal content correlated with morphologic characteristics. Lab Invest 10:956, 1961.
9. Boullin D, Coleman M, O'Brien R. Abnormalities in platelet 5-hydroxytryptamine efflux in patients with infantile autism. Nature 226:371–372, 1970.
10. Campbell M, Collins PJ, Friedman E, David R, Genieser N. Levodopa and levoamphetamine: a cross-over study in young schizophrenic children. Curr Ther Res 1:70–86, 1976.

11. Campbell M, Friedman E, Devoto E, Greenspan L, Collins P. Blood serotonin in psychotic and brain damaged children. J Autism Child Schiz 4:33–41, 1974.
12. Campbell M, Friedman E, Green WA, Burdoc E. Blood platelets, monoamine oxidase activity in schizophrenic children and their families: a preliminary study. Neuropsychobiology 2:239–246, 1976.
13. Chase TN. Biochemical and pharmacologic studies of dystonia. Neurology (Minneap) 20:122–130, 1970.
14. Christensen NJ. Plasma catecholamines in juvenile diabetics. Scand J Clin Lab Invest 27:227–231, 1971.
15. Cohen DJ, Caparulo BK, Shaywitz BA, Bowers MH. Dopamine and serotonin metabolism in neuropsychiatrically disturbed children. Arch Gen Psychiatry 34:545–550, 1977.
16. Cohen DJ, Shaywitz BA, Caparulo B, Young JG, Bowers MB. Chronic, multiple tics of Gilles de la Tourette's disease. Arch Gen Psychiatry 35:245–250, 1978.
17. Cohen DJ, Shaywitz BA, Johnson W, Bowen M. Biogenic amine in autistic atypical children: cerebrospinal fluid measures of homovanillic acid and 5-hydroxyindoleacetic acid. Arch Gen Psychiatry 31:845–853, 1974.
18. Cohen DJ, Shaywitz BA, Young JG, Bowers M. Cerebrospinal Fluid Monoamine Metabolites in Neuropsychiatric Disorders of Childhood. In Neurobiology of Cerebrospinal Fluid, JH Wood (ed), vol. 1, 665–683. New York: Plenum Press, 1980.
19. Cohen DJ, Young JG, Nathanson JA, Shaywitz BA. Clonidine in Tourette's syndrome. Lancet 2:551–553, 1979.
20. Cohen DJ, Young JG, Roth JA. Platelet monoamine oxidase in early childhood autism. Arch Gen Psychiatry 34:534–537, 1977.
21. Coleman M. Preliminary remarks on the L-dopa therapy of dystonia. Neurology (Minneap) 20:114–121, 1970.
22. Coleman M, Campbell M, Freedman LS, Roffman M, Ebstein R, Goldstein M. Serum dopamine-beta-hydroxylase levels in Down's syndrome. Clin Genet 5:312–315, 1974.
23. Coleman M, Steinberg L. A Double-Blind Trial of 5-Hydroxytryptophan in Trisomy-21 Patients. In Serotonin in Down's Syndrome, M Coleman (ed), 43–60. New York: American Elsevier Publishing Co., 1973.
24. Cooper IS. Levodopa-induced dystonia. Lancet 2:1317–1318, 1972.
25. Curzon G. Involuntary movements other than parkinsonism. Biochemical aspects. Proc R Soc Med 55:873–876, 1973.
26. Dairman W, Udenfriend S. Increased conversion of tyrosine to catecholamines in the intact rat following elevation of tissue tyrosine hydroxylase levels by administered phenoxybenzamine. Mol Pharmacol 6:350–356, 1970.
27. Dalessio DJ. Mechanisms of headache. Med Clin North Am 62:429–442, 1978.
28. Dalessio DJ, Otis S, Smith R. Vasomotor phenomena, platelet antagonism and migraine therapy. Research and clinical studies. Headache 6:34–40, 1978.
29. Dalmaz Y, Pegrin L, Mamelle J, Tuil D, Gilly R, Cier J. The pattern of urinary catecholamines and their metabolites in Duchenne myopathy in relation to disease evolution. J Neural Transm 46:17–34, 1979.
30. Dalmaz Y, Pegrin L, Sann L, Dutruge J. Age related changes in catecholamine metabolites of human urine from birth to adulthood. J Neural Transm 46:153–174, 1979.
31. Dancis J, Smith AA. Current concepts: familial dysautonomia. N Engl J Med 274:207–209, 1966.
32. Dancis J. Altered drug response in familial dysautonomia. Ann NY Acad Sci 151:876–879, 1968.
33. Ebstein RP, Freedman LS, Lieberman A, Park DH, Pasternack B, Goldstein M, Cole-

man M. A familial study in serum dopamine-β-hydroxylase levels in torsion dystonia. Neurology (Minneap) 24:684–687, 1974.

34. Edelstein SB, Castiglione CM, Breakfield XO. Monoamine oxidase activity in normal and Lesch-Nyhan fibroblasts. J Neurochem 31:1247–1254, 1978.
35. Eldridge R, Sweet R, Lake R, Ziegler M, Shapiro AK. Gilles de la Tourette's syndrome: clinical, genetic, psychologic, biological aspects in 21 selected families. Neurology (Minneap) 27:115–124, 1977.
36. Fenichel GM. Migraine in childhood: brief review of this inherited disorder which strikes five per cent of school-age children. Clin Pediatr 7:192–194, 1968.
37. Freedman L, Goldstein M, Coleman M. Serum dopamine-beta-hydroxylase activity in Down's syndrome: a familial study. Res Commun Chem Pathol Pharmacol 81:543–549, 1974.
38. Friedman AP. Headache. In Clinical Neurology 2, AB Baker, (ed). Hagerstown, PA: Harper and Row, 1980.
39. Giller EL, Young JG, Breakfield XO, Carbonari C, Braverman M, Cohen DJ. Monoamine oxidase in catechol-O-methyltransferase activities in cultured fibroblasts and blood cells from children with autism and the Gilles de la Tourette's syndrome. Psychiatry Res 2:187–197, 1980.
40. Gitlow SE, Bertani LM, Wilk E, Li BL, Dziedzic S. Excretion of catecholamine metabolites by children with familial dysautonomia. Pediatrics 46:513–522, 1970.
41. Goldstein M. Dopamine-beta-hydroxylase and Endogenous Total 5-Hydroxyindole Levels in Autistic Patients and Controls: Dopamine-beta-hydroxylase Studies. In The Autistic Syndromes, M Coleman (ed), 57–59. Amsterdam: North Holland, 1976.
42. Goldstein M, Freedman L, Ebstein R, Park D. Studies on dopamine-beta-hydroxylase in mental disorders. J Psychiatr Res 11:205–210, 1974.
43. Goodall J, Shinebourne E, Lake BD. Early diagnosis of familial dysautonomia: case report with special reference to primary pathophysiological findings. Arch Dis Child 43:455–458, 1968.
44. Green M, Williams M. The sympathetic neurohormones in pheochromocytoma, neuroblastoma and dysautonomia. Trans Am Neurol Assoc 88:223–224, 1963.
45. Gustavson KH, Wetterberg L, Backstrom M, Ross SB. Catechol-O-methyltransferase activity in erythrocytes in Down's syndrome. Clin Genet 4:279–280, 1973.
46. Guthrie RD, Wyatt RJ. Biochemistry and schizophrenia 3: a review of childhood psychosis. Schiz Bull 12:19–32, 1975.
47. Hanley HC, Stahl SM, Freedman DX. Hyperserotonemia and amine metabolites in autistic and retarded children. Arch Gen Psychiatry 34:521–531, 1977.
48. Hannington E, Horn M, Wilkinson M. Further Observations on the Effects of Tyramine. In Background to Migraine: Third Migraine Symposium, AL Cochrane (ed). New York: Springer Verlag, 1970.
49. Hilton BP, Cumings JN. 5-Hydroxytryptamine levels and platelet aggregation responses in subjects with acute migraine headache. J Neurol Neurosurg Psychiatry 35:505–509, 1972.
50. Johansson G. Sex differences in the catecholamine output of children. Acta Physiol Scand 85:569–572, 1972.
51. Johansson G, Frankenhauser M, Machusson D. Catecholamine output in school children as related to performance and adjustment. Scand J Psychol 14:20–28, 1973.
52. Keele DK, Richards C, Brown J, Marshall J. Catecholamine metabolism in Down's syndrome. Am J Ment Defic 74:125–129, 1969.

53. Klawans H, Weiner A. The effect of *d*-amphetamine on choreiform movement disorders. Neurology (Minneap) 24:312–318, 1974.
54. Kopin IJ. Catecholamine metabolism (and the biochemical assessment of sympathetic activity) J Clin Endocrinol Metab 6:525–549, 1977.
55. Lake CR, Davis P, Ziegler MG, Kopin IJ. Electrolytes and norepinephrine levels in blood of patients with cystic fibrosis. Clin Chim Acta 92:141–146, 1979.
56. Lake CR, Ziegler MG. Lesch-Nyhan syndrome: low dopamine-beta-hydroxylase activity and diminished sympathetic response to stress and posture. Science 196:905–906, 1977.
57. Lake CR, Ziegler MG, Coleman M, Kopin IJ. Evaluation of the sympathetic nervous system in trisomy-21 (Down's syndrome). J Psychiatr Res 15:1–6, 1979.
58. Lake CR, Ziegler MG, Eldridge R, Murphy DL. Catecholamine metabolism in Gilles de la Tourette's syndrome. Am J Psychiatry 134:257–260, 1977.
59. Lake CR, Ziegler MG, Murphy DL. Increased norepinephrine levels and decreased dopamine-beta-hydroxylase activity in primary autism. Arch Gen Psychiatry 34:553–556, 1977.
60. Lloyd K, Davidson K, Price HJ. Catecholamine and octopamine concentrations in brains of patients with Reye syndrome. Neurology (Minneap) 27:985–988, 1977.
61. Lott I, Chase T, Murphy D. Down's syndrome: transport, storage and metabolism of serotonin in blood platelets. Pediatr Res 6:730–735, 1972.
62. Lott I, Murphy D, Chase T. Down's syndrome, central monoamine turnover in patients with diminished platelet serotonin. Neurology (Minneap) 22:967–972, 1972.
63. Lucas A, Warner K, Gottlieb J. Biological studies in childhood schizophrenia: serotonin uptake by platelets. Biol Psychiatry 3:123–128, 1971.
64. Mandell S. The treatment of dystonia with L-dopa and haloperidol. Neurology (NY) 20:103–106, 1970.
65. Marsden CD, Harrison MJ. Idiopathic torsion dystonia (dystonia musculorum deformans): a review of forty-two patients. Brain 97:793–810, 1974.
66. Mendell J, Murphy D, Engel W, Chase T, Gordon E. Catecholamines and indoleamines in patients with Duchenne muscular dystrophy. Arch Neurol 27:518–520, 1972.
67. Mikkelson EJ, Rapoport JR, Nee LE, Grunenau C, Mendelson GC. Childhood enuresis. Arch Gen Psychiatry 37:1139–1144, 1980.
68. Molinoff PB, Brimijoin S, Weinshilboum R, Axelrod J. Neurally mediated increase in dopamine-beta-hydroxylase activity. Proc Natl Acad Sci USA 66:453–458, 1970.
69. Nakai T, Yamada R. Urinary catecholamine excretion by various age groups with special reference to clinical value of measuring catecholamines in newborns. Pediatr Res 17:456–460, 1983.
70. Piggott LR. Overview of selected basic research in autism. J Autism Dev Disord 9:199–218, 1979.
71. Rapoport J, Prandoni C, Renfield M, Lake CR, Ziegler M. Newborn dopamine-beta-hydroxylase, minor physical anomalies and infant temperament. Am J Psychiatry 134:676–679, 1977.
72. Riley CM, Day RL, Greeley DM, Langford WS. Central autonomic dysfunction with defective lacrimation: report of five cases. Pediatrics 3:468–478, 1949.
73. Ritvo ER. Biochemical studies of children with a syndrome of autism, childhood schizophrenia, and related developmental disabilities: a review. J Child Psychol Psychiatry 18:373–379, 1976.
74. Ritvo E, Yuwiler A, Geller E, Kales A, Rashkins S, Schico A, Plotkin S, Axelrod R, Howard C. Effects of L-dopa in autism. J Autism Child Schiz 1:190–205, 1971.

75. Rosner EM, Ong B, Paine RS, Mahanand D. Blood-serotonin activity in trisomic and translocation Down's syndrome. Lancet 1:1191–1193, 1965.
76. Rydzewski W. Serotonin (5-HT) in migraine: levels in whole blood in and between attacks. Headache 16:16–19, 1976.
77. Sandler M, Youdim MBH, Hannington E. A phenylethylamine oxidizing defect in migraine. Nature 250:335–337, 1974.
78. Sankar DVS. Biogenic amine uptake by blood platelets and RBC in childhood schizophrenia. Acta Paedopsychiatr (Basel) 37:174–183, 1970.
79. Schain R, Freedman D. Studies on 5-hydroxyindole metabolism in autistic and other mentally retarded children. J Pediatr 58:315–328, 1961.
80. Shaywitz BA, Cohen DJ, Bowers MB. Cerebrospinal Fluid Monoamine Metabolites. In Neurological Disorders of Childhood, JH Wood (ed), 219–236. New York: Plenum, 1980.
81. Shaywitz B, Venes J, Cohen D, Bovers M. Reye syndrome: monoamine metabolites in ventricular fluid. Neurology (NY) 29:467–472, 1979.
82. Sicuteri F, Testi A, Anselmi B. Biochemical investigations in headache: increase in the hydroxyindoleacetic acid excretion during migraine attacks. Int Arch Allergy Appl Immunol 19:55–58, 1961.
83. Smith AA, Dancis J. Exaggerated response to infused norepinephrine in familial dysautonomia. N Engl J Med 270:704–707, 1964.
84. Smith AA, Dancis J. Catecholamine release in familial dysautonomia. N Engl J Med 227:61–64, 1967.
85. Tabaddor K, Wolfson LI, Sharpless NS. Diminished ventricular fluid dopamine metabolite in adult-outset dystonia. Neurology (Minneap) 28:1254–1258, 1978.
86. Takahashi S, Kanai H, Miyamoto Y. Reassessment of elevated serotonin levels in blood platelets in early infantile autism. J Autism Child Schiz 6:317–326, 1976.
87. Tu J, Zellweger H. Blood-serotonin deficiency in Down's syndrome. Lancet 2:715–716, 1965.
88. Vecht C, van Woerkom T, Teelken A, Minderhaud J. Homovanillic acid and 5-hydroxyindoleacetic acid cerebrospinal fluid levels. Arch Neurol 32:792–797, 1975.
89. Weinshilboum RM, Axelrod J. Reduced plasma dopamine-beta-hydroxylase activity in familial dysautonomia. N Engl J Med 285:938–942, 1971.
90. Westlake RJ, Kopin IJ, Gordon EK. Catecholamine metabolite excretion by patients with familial dysautonomia and their mothers. Clin Res 13:336, 1965.
91. Wetterberg L, Aberg H, Ross SB, Froden O. Plasma dopamine-beta-hydroxylase in hypertension and various neuropsychiatric disorders. Scand J Clin Lab Invest 30:283–289, 1972.
92. Wetterberg L, Gustavson K, Backstrom M, Ross SB, Fruden O. Low dopamine-beta-hydroxylase activity in Down's syndrome. Clin Genet 3:152–153, 1972a.
93. Winkel P, Slob A. Catecholamine excretion of normal male adolescents during various periods of the day cycle. Clin Chim Acta 45:113–118, 1973.
94. Wooten GF, Eldridge R, Axelrod J, Stern RS. Elevated plasma dopamine-beta-hydroxylase activity in autosomal dominant torsion dystonia. N Engl J Med 288:284–287, 1973.
95. Yatsu F, Zussman W. Familial dysautonomia (Riley-Day syndrome): a case report with post mortem findings of a patient at age 31. Arch Neurol 10:459–463, 1964.
96. Young JG, Cohen DJ, Caparulo BK, Brown S, Maas JW. Decreased 24-hour urine MHPG in childhood autism. Am J Psychiatry 136:1055–1057, 1979.
97. Yuwiler A, Ritvo E, Geller E, Glossman R, Schneiderman G, Matsuno D. Uptake

and efflux of serotonin from platelets of autistic and non-autistic children. J Autism Child Schiz 5:83–98, 1975.
98. Zeman W, Dyken P. Dystonia Musculorum Deformans: diseases of the Basal Ganglia. In Handbook of Clinical Neurology, PJ Vinken and GW Bruyn (eds), vol. 6, 284–287. Amsterdam: North Holland Publishing Co., 1968.
99. Ziegler MG, Lake CR, Kopin IJ. Deficient nervous response in familial dysautonomia. N Engl J Med 294:630–633, 1976.

10

Catecholamine Metabolism in Hyperactive Children

Gerald L. Brown
Michael H. Ebert

There have been a number of hypotheses relating disorders of catecholamine (CA) metabolism and hyperactivity in children. Kornetsky [64] raised the possibility of an overly active catecholaminergic system in his discussion of the mechanisms of psychoactive drug action in immature organisms. Wender [121,122] proposed a functional deficiency of CA in hyperactive children with the greater focus on the possibility of a functional dopamine (DA) rather than norepinephrine (NE) deficiency. Wender based his hypothesis on (1) possible decreased functioning of the reward-system median forebrain bundle; (2) behavior in children with Economo's encephalitis, which causes DA deficiency; (3) action of amphetamine and its cyclized derivative, methylphenidate, both of which release NE and DA among other pharmacologic actions; and (4) specificity of biochemical pharmacologic interactions such as the proposed differences in the mode of action of D-amphetamine and L-amphetamine. This latter distinction was taken to indicate that DA deficiency might be of more importance than NE deficiency [121,122], based on the hypothesis that D-amphetamine is a more potent reuptake blocker of NE than L-amphetamine. Whereas D-amphetamine also was thought to be more potent in releasing NE at the synapse, L-amphetamine appeared to affect DA and NE equally [37,72,104–106]. However, a number of other studies question whether the differential effects of D-amphetamine and L-amphetamine can be used to distinguish NE and DA metabolism [3,26,48,65,79,95,105,108,112,113]. Other biochemical alterations, particularly involving serotonin (5-hydroxytryptamine; 5-HT) [11,29,51–53,88,120], have been proposed; but such hypotheses are discussed minimally in this chapter and only to the extent that they may be associated with or clarify the role of CA.

DIRECT BIOCHEMICAL STUDIES

Direct biochemical studies in hyperactive children involve cerebrospinal fluid (CSF), blood, and urine.

Cerebrospinal Fluid Studies

CSF studies involve both homovanillic acid (HVA), a metabolite of DA, and 5-hydroxyindoleacetic acid (5-HIAA), a metabolite of 5-HT. Shetty and Chase [103] found no differences in hyperactive children versus normal children on baseline and probenecid-induced accumulations of HVA and 5-HIAA. Clinical improvement in hyperactive children following D-amphetamine was, however, accompanied by a significant elevation of HVA and a nonsignificant elevation of 5-HIAA. Shaywitz et al [96,97] also reported no difference between baseline CSF HVA and 5-HIAA in hyperactive children versus normal children, but when postprobenecid HVA levels were corrected for the level of CSF probenecid, hyperactive children did have low CSF HVA. The correction was based on a significant correlation between CSF HVA and CSF probenecid; thus, the low HVA must be interpreted with caution. However, a group of children with "central processing disturbance—similar to severe hyperactive children" versus a pediatric control group with minimal behavior symptoms showed no differences in CSF HVA and 5-HIAA [27].

Blood Studies

Plasma NE has been measured in hyperactive children versus age-matched normal children with no difference in levels observed [74]. Within the hyperactive group, a positive correlation existed between the Abbreviated Conners Teacher Rating Scale (ABCTRS) [31,33] and the supine baseline NE; furthermore, a positive correlation also existed between a ten-point behavioral-anxiety scale and supine baseline NE [74]. These children also showed a higher mean intrasubject coefficient of variation (CV) than that noted in normal adults studied with the same assay (Table 10.1). Thus, plasma NE may reflect a state variable for behavior more than it indicates a trait variable in comparing hyperactive children with normal children. Hyperactive children, often impulsive, show greater and more frequent fluctuations of behavior than normal children. However, the intrasubject NE variation may reflect a less well-regulated NE system as a trait variable. Furthermore, a later study by Langer et al [67] has shown that 9:00 AM plasma NE levels are unaffected by 2 weeks of D-amphetamine (0.75 mg/kg of body weight) versus 2 weeks of placebo in the same group of hyperactive children.

Some of the enzymes that regulate NE metabolism have been studied in hyperactive children. Rapoport et al [87] showed that hyperactive children are no different from normal children with regard to plasma dopamine β-hydroxylase (DBH). However, a recent report by Rogeness et al [90] has indicated that undersocialized children with conduct disorders in combination with attention-deficit disorders have lower levels of DBH. Whether biochemical differences between groups subdivided by such clinical descriptions are meaningful is open to question. Mikkelsen et al [74] also showed no difference in DBH between hyperactive children versus normal children (see Table 10.1). Shekim et al [98] have recently reported in a pilot study that platelet monoamine oxidase (MAO) is lower in hyperactive

Table 10.1 Intrasubject Variation in Supine Norepinephrine and Dopamine β-hydroxylase Values* in Hyperactive Children

	NE (pg/ml)				DBH (units)†			
Subject No.	*No. of Values*	$\overline{X}$	*SD*	*CV(%)*	*No. of Values*	$\overline{X}$	*SD*	*CV(%)*
1	4	475	44	9	4	35	20	55
2	4	324	94	29	4	376	46	12
3	4	201	50	25	4	639	80	13
4	5	259	18	7	5	569	166	29
5	4	358	22	6	4	825	30	4
6	5	134	40	30	4	133	54	41
7	4	100	36	35	4	1003	340	34
Mean coefficient of variation				20%				27%

NE = norepinephrine; DBH = dopamine β-hydroxylase; $\overline{X}$ = mean; SD = standard deviation; CV = coefficient of variation.

* Supine values when subject was either medication-free or on placebo.

† One unit of DBH activity is one nanomole of phenylethylamine converted to phenylethanolamine per milliliter of plasma per hour of incubation time.

SOURCE: Mikkelsen et al [74].

children versus normal children. Catechol-O-methyltransferase (COMT) levels in psychotic aggressive children, neurotic children, or both are higher than those seen in schizophrenic children; however, the diagnostic criteria and lack of a normal control group make this study difficult to evaluate [117]. Studies measuring the indoleamines include two that report low platelet 5-HT in hyperactive children [29,120], two that report no differences between hyperactive and normal children [47,88], and others that find plasma 5-HIAA low in hyperactive children [30,31,53].

Urine Studies

The most frequently studied body fluid in hyperactive children is urine. Rapoport et al [84] initially studied NE and epinephrine (E) in hyperactive children and found that D-amphetamine decreased the level of playroom activity; predrug NE values predicted that decrease. In a second study, Rapoport et al [85] observed that urinary NE values before D-amphetamine did not predict a decrease in behavioral activity on the drug. Wender et al [123] subsequently studied the excretion of NE, E, normetanephrine, (NM), metanephrine (M), 3-methoxy-4-hydroxyphenylglycol (MHPG), vanillylmandelic acid (VMA), HVA, and 5-HIAA in hyperactive children versus normal children, both at baseline and after D-amphetamine. They found no baseline differences between hyperactive children and normal children, but after at least 1 week of D-amphetamine, both M and E were significantly increased. The second study by Rapoport et al [85] reported higher NE in hyperactive children versus normal children, but no differences with regard to E, MHPG, DA, or HVA; further increased E after single-dose D-amphetamine was noted in normal children, but not in the hyperactive children. Khan and Dekirmenjian [59] reported no differences in NM, M, or MHPG in hyperactive children versus normal children. Shekim et al [99–102] in several studies also measured NM, M, MHPG, and HVA in hyperactive children and demonstrated both lower MHPG in hyperactive children versus normal children and a further decrease following 2 weeks of D-amphetamine. They found no differences in HVA levels in hyperactive children versus normal children or in hyperactive children following D-amphetamine. Brown et al [14] conducted a study of hyperactive children which considered diet, motor activity, diurnal variation, gender, and age, as well as dose, absorption-elimination, and length of treatment interval of D-amphetamine. This report showed variability of MHPG and HVA in repeated placebo conditions (coefficients of variation [CV] = 28 percent and 21 percent, respectively). There were no significant day–night (9:00 AM to 9:00 PM, 9:00 PM to 9:00 AM) diurnal variations, though the lower nighttime MHPG might be consistent with the diurnal variation reported in adult depressed patients [119]. D-amphetamine did not alter the relationships between daytime and nighttime excretion, nor did the metabolites correlate with each other in any condition. Daytime motor activity, measured by an activity monitor [28], does not correlate with daytime excretion of MHPG or HVA. Absorption-elimination data [16,18] determined from serial plasma levels following a single dose of D-amphetamine show small interindividual variations. Neither individual peak plasma levels nor apparent elimination half-life periods are related to MHPG or HVA excretion. A significant difference by analysis of variance exists among placebo, 3-day, and 8-day MHPG excretion; no significant difference is observed in HVA excretion. MHPG excretion shows a nonsignificant decrease at 3 days and a significant decrease at 8 days versus placebo (see Figure 10.1); HVA excretion at both 3 and 8 days is not significantly altered versus placebo. All of these studies include the expression of metabolite in relationship to creatinine excretion. In general, creatinine is measured both to assess constancy of kidney function and to index degree of completeness of urine collection. Mean values from subject to subject differ significantly; however, individual CVs are quite similar. Thus, using creatinine as an index of excretion may be more problematic when comparing one population with another than when using subjects as their own controls. Variables known to affect creatinine excretion as it relates to children were briefly reviewed by Brown et al [14]. All studies on hyperactive children reporting the effect of D-amphetamine on MHPG excretion suggest a progressive decrease in MHPG excretion with duration of treatment through 14 days. Although the measurement of MHPG by gas chromatography–mass spectrometry (GCMS) showed the most consistent results in two independent studies [14,19], measurement of MHPG by gas liquid chromatography in other studies also showed similar results [59,99–102,123]. The similarities and differences in these studies are summarized in Table 10.2. Of therapeutic interest, the only child with an increase in MHPG excretion in the initial Brown et al [14] study showed no change at all in ABCTRS score.

The second study by Brown et al [19] essentially replicated the MHPG and

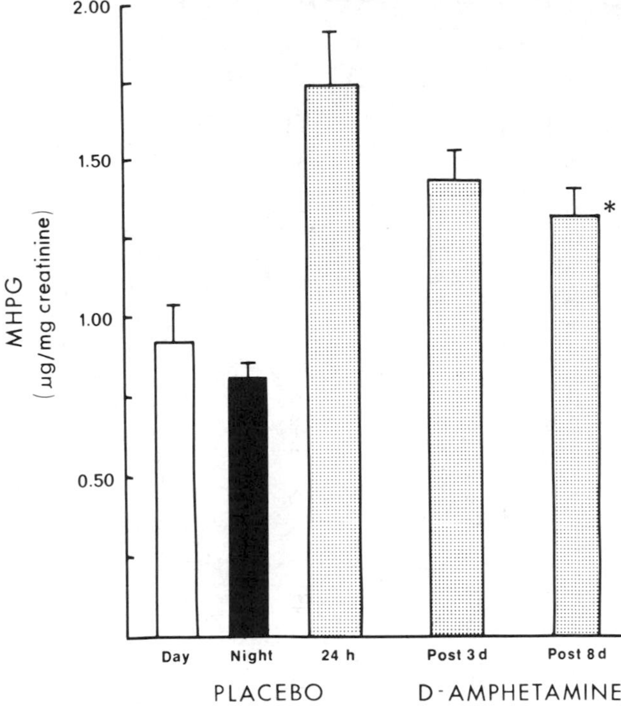

Figure 10.1 The differential excretion of 3-methoxy-4-hydroxyphenylglycol (MHPG) from daytime and nighttime urine collections and the effect of a course of D-amphetamine treatment in eight hyperactive boys. (Significant decrease in MHPG excretion after 8 days of D-amphetamine: two-tailed t test; $N = 7$; $t = 2.77$; $^{*}p < 0.05$.)

HVA findings, both with respect to effects of D-amphetamine and a possible relationship between clinical response and decrease in MHPG excretion. In addition, this second D-amphetamine study, a double-blind, placebo-controlled, counterbalanced crossover at 14 days (no order effect), showed nonsignificant decreases in NE and its metabolites, NM and VMA; no significant effects on DA excretion nor on its metabolites, 3,4-dihydroxyphenylacetic acid (DOPAC) and 3-methoxytyramine (3-MT); and a significant decrease in tyramine (TRM) and its metabolite, *p*-hydroxyphenylacetic acid (PHPA) (Figure 10.2). Further studies on the same group of subjects show that phenylethylamine (PEA) excretion is increased following D-amphetamine, but its metabolite, phenylacetic acid (PAA), is unchanged [124]. Although lower PEA has been reported in hyperactive children versus normal children, this difference is not consistent [125]. PEA has a chemical structure identical to that of amphetamine except that PEA lacks the alpha methyl side

Table 10.2 Comparison of D-Amphetamine–induced Changes in MHPG Excretion[a] in Independent Groups of Boys with the Hyperactive Syndrome

Study	*Assay Method*	*Diet*	*N*	*Age*[b]	*D-Amphetamine Dose (mg/day)*	*Baseline*	*No. of Days on D-Amphetamine* 1	3	7[c]	8	14
Wender et al [123]	GLC	LMA	9[d]	9.3 (range 7–13)	10–20	1.43 ± .66			1.30 ± .58		
Rapoport et al [85]	GCMS	LMA	15	9.4 ± 2.1	16.1 ± 4.6	1.69 ± .31	1.41 ± .48				
Shekim et al [101]	GLC	Not controlled	21	9.5 ± 1.6	13.8 ± 2.7	1.20 ± .47					0.83 ± .29[e]
Brown et al [14]	GCMS	LMA	8	7.3 ± 0.9	16.2 ± 2.7	1.74 ± .49		1.42 ± .27		1.31 ± .22[f]	
Brown et al [19]	GCMS	LMA	12	9.3 ± 0.4	15–20	1.82 ± .64					1.55 ± .43[f]

MHPG = 3-methoxy-4-hydroxyphenylglycol; N = number of subjects; GLC = gas liquid chromatography; LMA = low monoamine diet; GCMS = gas chromatography–mass spectrometry.

[a] Mean micrograms per milligram creatinine ± standard deviation.

[b] Mean years ± standard deviation.

[c] At least one week.

[d] Eight boys, one girl.

[e] $p < 0.01$ (paired two-tailed t test).

[f] $p < 0.05$ (paired two-tailed t test); $F(2, 10) = 4.10$; $p = 0.05$ (ANOVA).

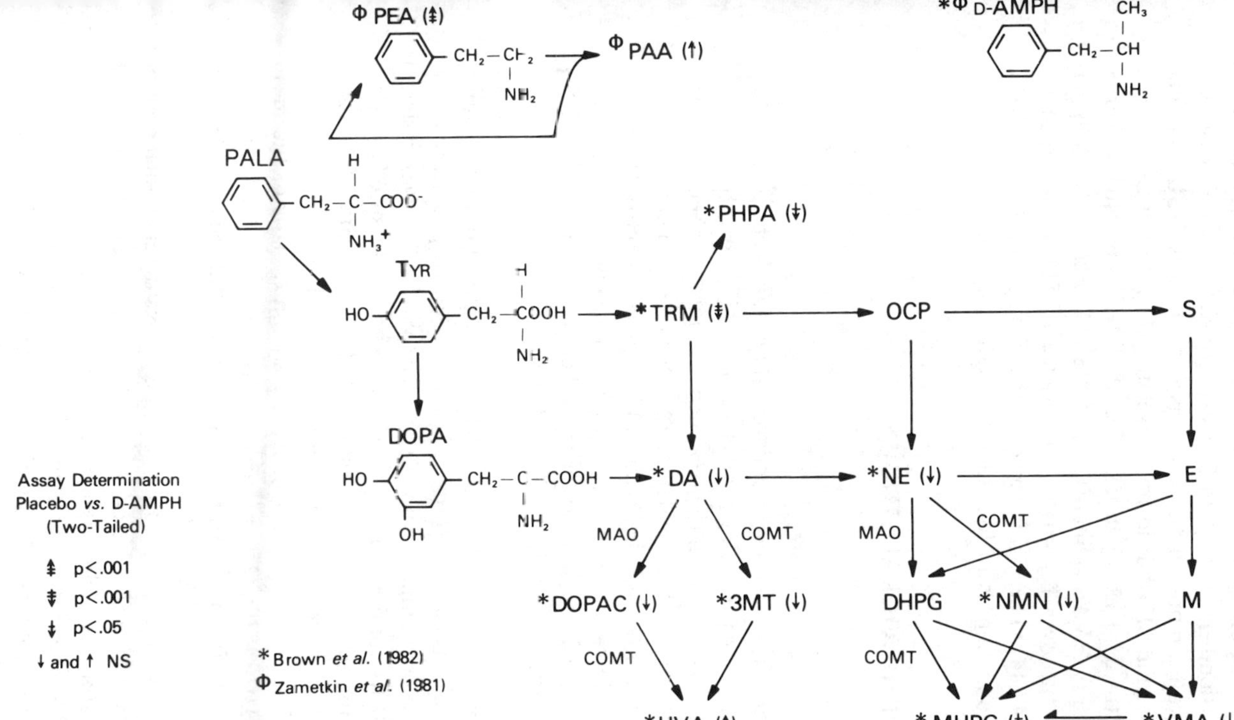

Figure 10.2 Effect of 2 weeks of D-amphetamine on phenylethylamine (PEA), tyramine (TRM), dopamine (DA), and norepinephrine (NE) and respective metabolites phenylacetic acid (PAA), para-hydroxyphenylacetic acid (PHPA), 3-methoxytyramine (3-MT), 3,4 dihydroxyphenylacetic acid (DOPAC), homovanillic acid (HVA), normetanephrine (NM), 3-methoxy-4-hydroxyphenylglycol (MHPG), and vanillylmandelic acid (VMA) in 12 hyperactive boys. (D-AMPH = D-amphetamine; PALA = phenylalanine; TYR = tyrosine; OCP = octopamine; S = synephrine; E = epinephrine; COMT = catechol-O-methyltransferase; DHPG = 3,4-dihydroxyphenylglycol.)

chain of amphetamine. Recent research on the brain's "amphetamine receptor" could well lead to a further elucidation of amphetamine's robust effect on excretion of PEA in hyperactive children [56,81].

MHPG is thought to be the major central nervous system (CNS) metabolite of NE [40,41,70,71,93]. Blombery et al [5,6], however, reported that at least 50% of plasma MHPG, before excretion in the urine, is converted to VMA; plasma-free MHPG and urinary total MHPG do not correlate [111]. Although excretion of HVA is less frequently used as an index of CNS DA, Kopin [63] reported greater than 50% of urinary HVA originates from CNS DA. Plasma HVA apparently reflects CNS DA turnover [2]; urinary clearance of HVA may relate to plasma turnover rates [43,44]. The significance of the changes in TRM, PHPA, and PEA following D-amphetamine in hyperactive children is unclear.

PHARMACOKINETIC-BEHAVIORAL STUDIES

Amphetamine

A number of drug studies in hyperactive children show involvement of CA in the mediation of therapeutic pharmacologic effects. Since 1937, when Bradley [8,9] reported the efficacy of amphetamines in the treatment of aggressive behavior disorders in children, amphetamine has been widely used in the management of hyperactive children [4,9,22,32,42,49,60,76,77]. Double-blind, placebo-controlled studies of the effects of D-amphetamine on hyperactive children have confirmed its efficacy and its use as a standard for comparison in pharmacotherapeutic trials [1,34,53,57]. Understanding the clinical pharmacokinetics [54] of D-amphetamine in hyperactive children can have practical theoretic implications. Changes in absorption, protein-binding, first-pass metabolism, excretion, and altered metabolism of amphetamine may result in differences in response in some children. An initial pharmacokinetic study of a single oral dose of D-amphetamine in hyperactive children was designed to document the serial behavioral and motor activity responses to specific plasma levels as they change during absorption and elimination of the medication [12,16,18]. Serial plasma D-amphetamine levels in nanograms per milliliter were obtained during a 30-hour period after a single oral mean ($\pm$ standard error of the mean [SEM]) dose of 0.45 $\pm$ 0.02 mg/kg. The group ($N = 16$) mean ($\pm$ SEM) apparent half-life was 6.8 $\pm$ 0.5 hours (Figure 10.3). Both hyperactive children and depressed adults [39], after a single similar dose of D-amphetamine, attain peak levels and maximal behavioral response at the same time, despite a considerably longer elimination phase of D-amphetamine for the adults (19.4 $\pm$ 4.6 hours). To study the reliability of both laboratory and clinical methodology, six of the children were studied a second time with seven intervening drug-free days. Each received identical doses on both study days (0.49 $\pm$ 0.03 mg/kg). The mean ($\pm$ SEM) apparent elimination half-life of the first study day was 6.7 $\pm$ 0.6 hours and 6.0 $\pm$ 0.8 hours for the second study day. Intraclass correlation coefficients (ICC) of serial plasma D-amphetamine levels on the first and second days were significant in all

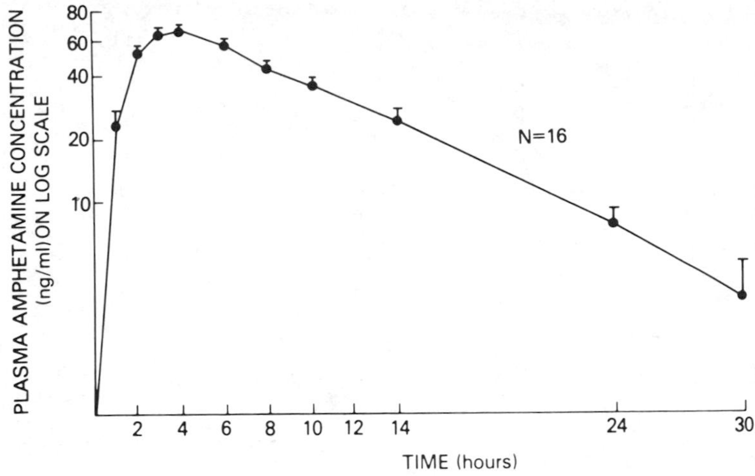

Figure 10.3 Plasma amphetamine levels over time. Serial plasma D-amphetamine levels in nanograms per milliliter were obtained over a 30-hour period after a single oral mean (± standard error of the mean [SEM]) dose of 0.45 ± 0.02 mg/kg. All children (male) were admitted for a history of impulsive, maladaptive social behavior, hyperactivity, and learning disability. The group (N = 16) mean (± SEM) apparent half-life was 6.8 ± 0.5 hours. The absorption-elimination time relationships are shown.

six children (ICC range: 0.77–0.93); a chi-square test indicated that the ICC's did not differ significantly from one another; the pooled ICC was 0.88. Serial behavior rating (ABCTRS) and motor activity measurements [12,18] during the first 6 hours after the dose of D-amphetamine show that significant drug responses were restricted to hours 1 through 4, a time during which amphetamine absorption exceeds its elimination and just prior to its peak plasma level between hours 3 and 4 (Figures 10.4 and 10.5).

To test the hypothesis that sustained-release capsules of D-amphetamine would provide a prolonged clinical response in hyperactive children, a pharmacokinetic and therapeutic response study of this preparation was undertaken [17]. With regard to absorption-elimination, the sustained-release preparation (dose, 0.48 mg/kg) has a slower rate of absorption than the elixir (dose, 0.5 mg/kg) (Figure 10.6), with the rate of absorption for the tablet preparation (dose, 0.49 mg/kg) falling between the elixir and the sustained-release preparation (Figures 10.6 and 10.7). Rate of absorption for the elixir is clearly dose-dependent (see Figure 10.6). Half-lives are not significantly different, though that of the sustained-release capsule is more variable, as might be expected. With regard to behavioral and motor activity effects, the only significant effects are at 2 hours, despite a peak plasma level that plateaus during the 3- through 8-hour interval as compared to the 3- to 4-hour interval for the tablet.

Brown et al [13] followed these studies with a second series of pharmacokinetic

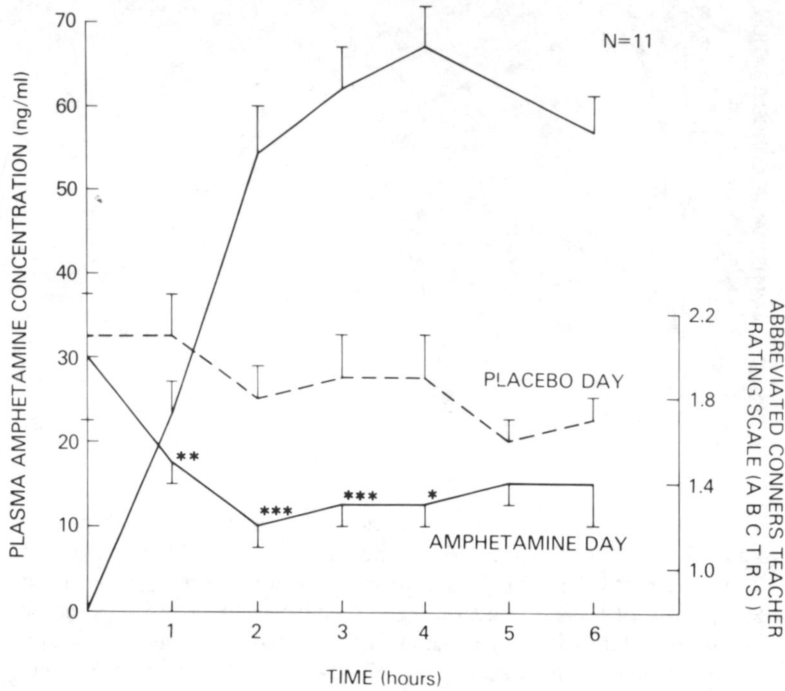

Figure 10.4 Amphetamine blood levels and behavior. Hyperactive children (N = 11) were given a single oral mean (± standard error of the mean [SEM]) dose of 0.45 ± 0.02 mg/kg of D-amphetamine. The resulting mean (± SEM) plasma levels are shown. Differences between behavioral ratings on Abbreviated Conners Teacher Rating Scale (ABCTRS) after placebo and after D-amphetamine were analyzed by one-tailed paired *t* tests. (*$p < 0.025$; **$p < 0.01$; ***$p < 0.005$.)

studies in which refinements in food intake prior to single-dose D-amphetamine and matched placebo yielded essentially the same results with regard to behavioral and motor activity effects. Test-retest reliability and dose response were also assessed. High reliability of the 0.5 mg/kg dose was observed, but 1.0 mg/kg was less effective than the 0.5 mg/kg dose. During the D-amphetamine absorption phase in this second group of D-amphetamine pharmacokinetic studies, the changes in plasma D-amphetamine and supine plasma NE levels correlated significantly [74]. Both pulse rate and blood pressure significantly increased after amphetamine and during the absorption phase. A 1.0 mg/kg dose increased plasma NE significantly, having its greatest effect at hour 1 with a decreasing, but significant, effect through hour 3; the 0.5 mg/kg dose has its least, but significant, effect at hour 1 with an increasing effect through hour 3 (Figure 10.8). These data are consistent with the nearly twofold increase in plasma levels of D-amphetamine during the absorption phase when the 1.0 mg/kg dose is compared to the 0.5 mg/kg dose

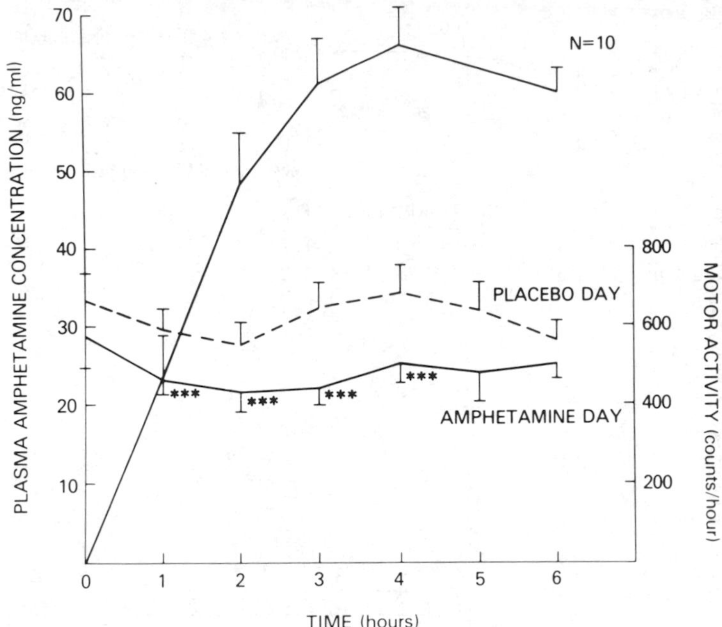

Figure 10.5 Amphetamine blood levels and motor activity. Hyperactive children (N = 10) were given a single oral mean (± standard error of the mean [SEM]) dose of 0.43 ± 0.02 mg/kg of D-amphetamine. The resulting mean (± SEM) plasma levels are shown. Differences between motor activity as determined by an ambulatory motor monitor after placebo and after D-amphetamine were analyzed by one-tailed paired *t* tests. (***$p < 0.005$.)

(see Figure 10.6); this twofold difference in plasma levels of D-amphetamine persists through 8 hours. The 1.0 mg/kg dose produces an increase in plasma NE two times greater than the 0.5 mg/kg dose at 1 hour, but at 3 hours, plasma NE is at the same level of increase for both doses. Thus, other than a greater release of NE at 1 hour, there would appear to be no advantage to using the higher dose because the therapeutic effect is not greater, but, indeed, somewhat less at the higher dose; a disadvantage is the potential for more potent cardiovascular effects.

In a similar series of single-dose amphetamine studies done in the same setting, Nurnberger et al [80] found that normal monozygotic twins experienced concordant behavioral excitation, reproducible in individuals over time; the behavioral excitation was uncorrelated with plasma D-amphetamine levels. All measures of behavior were made only in the early absorption phase at a time when the rate of change in plasma D-amphetamine was maximal. In addition, D-amphetamine–induced excitation was predicted by high plasma baseline MHPG in the normal twins and low plasma baseline MHPG in patients with affective disorders. For all single-

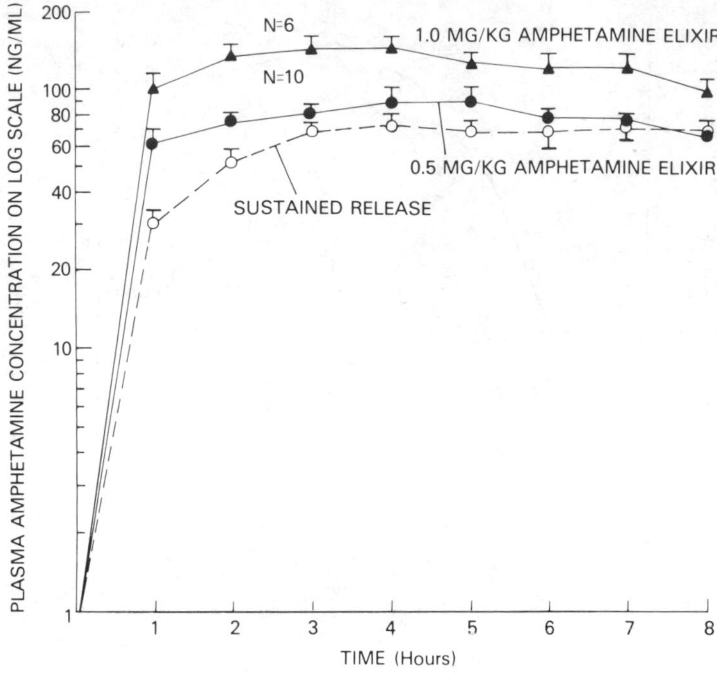

Figure 10.6 Plasma amphetamine levels over time. Serial plasma D-amphetamine levels in nanograms per milliliter were obtained over an 8-hour period after single oral doses (elixir) of 0.5 mg/kg ($N = 10$) and 1.0 mg/kg in six hyperactive children with at least three intervening drug-free days. These same children were also studied after a single oral (mean ± standard error of the mean [SEM]) dose of 0.48 ± .03 mg/kg of a sustained-release preparation. The rate of absorption for the low-dose elixir D-amphetamine was greater than that for the similar dose of sustained-release D-amphetamine as indicated by a significantly higher level of plasma D-amphetamine at hours 1, 2, and 3 on the elixir study day when analyzed by one-tailed paired t tests ($^{**}p < 0.01$; $^{*}p < 0.025$). The plasma levels obtained from 1.0 mg/kg elixir were twofold greater than those obtained from the 0.5 mg/kg dose.

dose amphetamine studies described, intraassay and interassay CVs are small; radioimmunoassay is comparable to GCMS [83].

Prior to these D-amphetamine pharmacokinetic studies, Epstein et al [45] reported that more organically impaired hyperactive children (determined by psychiatric anamnesis and brief neurologic examination) excreted D-amphetamine more rapidly and had a greater therapeutic response. However, frequency of neurologic "soft signs" in a group of hyperactive children appears to be significantly determined by age as well as by the disorder itself [73]. In a subsequent study by Rapoport

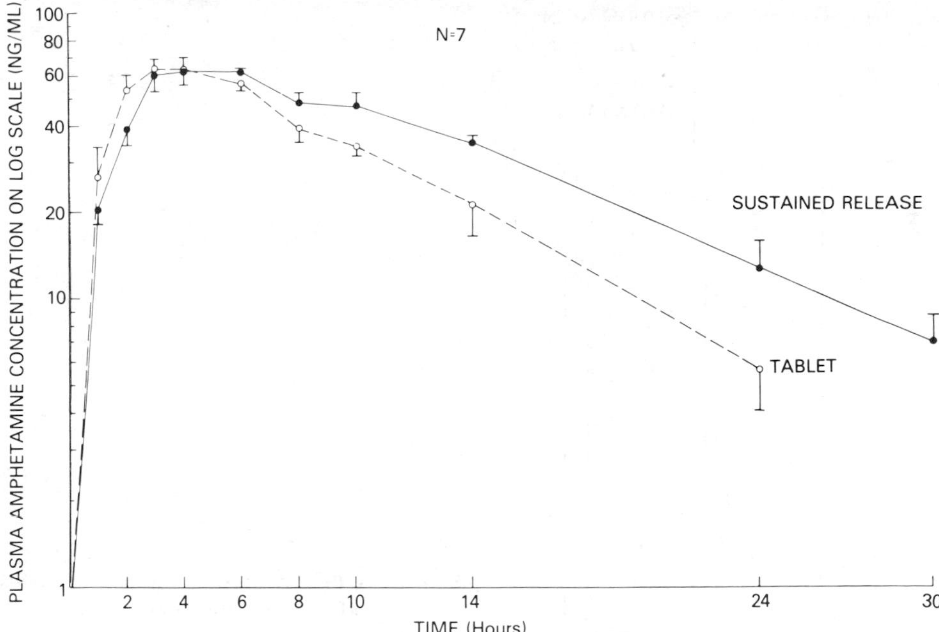

Figure 10.7 Plasma amphetamine levels over time after sustained-release preparation versus tablet. Serial plasma D-amphetamine levels in nanograms per milliliter were obtained over a 30-hour period after identical single oral mean (± standard error of the mean [SEM]) doses of 0.49 ± 0.4 mg/kg in seven hyperactive children with at least 7 intervening drug-free days. On one study day the child received a tablet preparation and on the other a sustained-release preparation. The mean (± SEM) apparent half-lives were not significantly different (6.6 ± 0.5 and 8.4 ± 1.2 hours, respectively) when a least-squares linear regression analysis of the plasma disappearance curve of each individual was calculated on the 2 study days. For the tablet, less than half of the values at 30 hours were obtained and no mean was calculated.

et al [85], hyperactive children excreted D-amphetamine more rapidly than normal children. The "organic status" of the hyperactive children or their prior use of D-amphetamine does not seem to account for large interindividual variations in urinary excretion of D-amphetamine nor for its absorption in the plasma [12,18] of these children.

Studies of the effect of methamphetamine on NE metabolism and behavior in rats demonstrated that methamphetamine (5.0 mg/kg) inhibits reuptake and increases NM levels in the first few hours after the drug is administered. In these experiments, increases in NM, a metabolite that reflects extraneuronal metabolism of NE, correlated highly with the behavioral response to methamphetamine [35]. When rhesus monkeys were assessed behaviorally after single oral doses of D-amphetamine (0.32 and 2.0 mg/kg), maximal behavioral effects were seen prior to the peak plasma level of amphetamine at times when the plasma level was

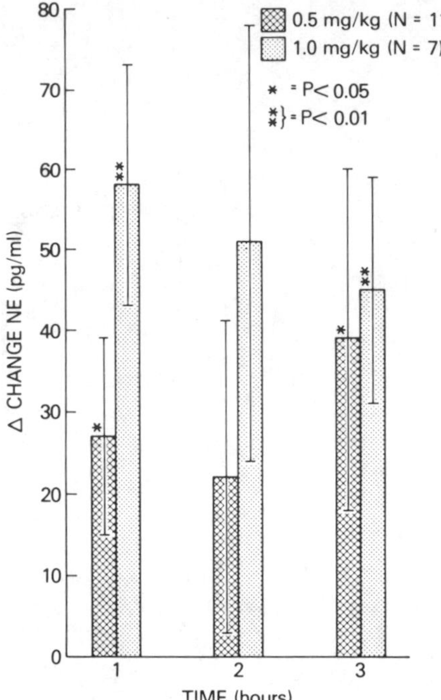

Figure 10.8. Differences among changes at 1, 2, and 3 hours after D-amphetamine (2 doses) versus after placebo for supine plasma norepinephrine (NE).

half that of the subsequent peak level attained [38]. The mechanism of the decreased response to later similar levels of D-amphetamine (from a single dose) in plasma may be related to the depletion of CA stores, to replacement of a "false neurotransmitter" metabolite of amphetamine [61,62], or to alteration in receptor sensitivity [20,21,23].

Methylphenidate

Effects of D-amphetamine on the excretion of CA metabolites and pharmacokinetic aspects of D-amphetamine are reviewed in the previous sections. The other most common pharmacologic intervention for hyperactive children is methylphenidate. The mechanisms of action of the two drugs are similar, but some differences exist. D-amphetamine seems to release DA from extravesicular sites [92], whereas the effects of methylphenidate are dependent on an intact vesicular store of DA [10]. Methylphenidate may actively inhibit the stereotyped behavioral effects of amphetamine in a dose-related manner [91], probably because it inhibits DA uptake in vivo [26,46]. How the pharmacologic differences between methylphenidate and D-amphetamine in rats may be used to better our understanding of hyperactive children is not clear at this time. Pharmacokinetic data for methylphenidate in hyperactive children may or may not be consistent with that of D-amphetamine.

Hungund et al [58] suggested that the low protein binding, resulting in a high percentage of free drug made available for metabolism to pharmacologically inactive metabolites, could explain methylphenidate's brief course of therapeutic action in hyperactive children. Amphetamine also shows low protein binding but has an approximately threefold longer half-life while having a similarly brief duration of therapeutic action. Swanson et al [109,110] reported time-response (cognitive behavior) patterns after single doses of methylphenidate. The maximal behavior effect, favorable or adverse, occurred at 2 to 4 hours, though favorable responders appeared to attain maximal effect earlier than adverse responders. The "behavioral half-life" (time taken for a 50% decline from the maximum effect) was 4 hours. This behavioral half-life more closely approximates the plasma rate of disappearance (half-life) for both methylphenidate and ritalinic acid (methylphenidate's major metabolite) than it does that of D-amphetamine. One might hypothesize that behavioral effect is correlated with the rate of disappearance of methylphenidate and not with the rate of disappearance of D-amphetamine; or, alternatively, maximal clinical effect from both stimulants is related to the absorption phase (oral methylphenidate reaches its peak plasma level at about 2 hours and D-amphetamine at 3 to 4 hours), while the behavioral and pharmacologic half-lives of methylphenidate are coincidental but *not* related. Whether the differences in behavioral variables being measured or the dose levels contribute to an understanding of the mechanism of response for methylphenidate and D-amphetamine is unclear [107]. Pharmacokinetics and dose effects have recently been more thoroughly studied [55,66].

PHARMACOLOGIC, CLINICAL, AND BIOCHEMICAL RESPONSES

Amphetamine and Methodological Considerations

The effects of D-amphetamine and methylphenidate in hyperactive children are well documented and have been studied more intensely than those of any other medications; however, studies earlier than those described in detail above have generally not included accompanying biochemical-dependent variables. A number of other medication trials may be of critical importance in understanding the role that CA may play in the pathophysiology of hyperactive children. Although there have been a number of compounds given to hyperactive children, this section selectively reviews studies which are carefully controlled in terms of ascertaining behavioral effect and which, at the same time, include measurements of accompanying biochemical-dependent variables. Certain other therapeutic trials that lend themselves to a possible understanding of the biochemical changes underlying the behavioral changes are also reviewed.

Of primary importance to the clinician is the understanding that most of the studies cited for review in this chapter were not undertaken in search of an immediate application to the clinical management of hyperactive children, though some studies, such as those on sustained-release preparations and certain drug trials, do have clinical relevance. Absolute values of biochemical levels may be similar from study to study in some cases (i.e., baseline MHPG excretion and blood levels of D-amphetamine at a certain point in time), but, for the most part, absolute levels, because of the many factors that may affect such levels from study to study, are less relevant for understanding than their relative differences within a study.

Piribedil

If the hypothesis of a deficient functioning of DA is correct, one might expect a direct postsynaptic DA agonist to be effective (as opposed to the indirect effects of D-amphetamine and methylphenidate on both NE and DA). One such drug which acts primarily as a postsynaptic DA agonist (with considerably lesser effects as a postsynaptic NE agonist) is piribedil (ET-495). This compound was given in a double-blind, crossover, placebo-controlled trial to eight hyperactive children [15]. There was no significant group effect on behavior or motor activity. Some studies have indicated that low doses of piribedil, apomorphine, and bromocriptine (all direct DA-receptor agonists) have inhibitory presynaptic effects, and high doses of the same compounds may have excitatory postsynaptic effects [24,36,78,82, 94,108,114,115,118] (also see Chapter 13). Both low- and high-dose effects were observed among the hyperactive children, but there were no differences in therapeutic effect at either dose level; side effects were greater at the higher dose. Of particular interest were observations that group MHPG excretion was similar in placebo versus piribedil conditions, though the four children who had a decrease on ABCTRS scores (two significantly so) were also the four who had a decrease in their MHPG excretion; those four children who had an increase in ABCTRS scores also had an increase in MHPG excretion. As expected from studies in adult depression, HVA excretion was decreased in all children when observed after a chronic course of piribedil; this decrease is clear evidence of piribedil's effect on DA metabolism.

Carbidopa

A further assessment of the DA hypothesis is the trial of carbidopa and L-dopa in hyperactive children. Eight hyperactive children were treated with carbidopa and placebo for 3 weeks each in a double-blind, crossover, placebo-controlled trial. Although there was a mild but significant improvement on Factor II of the Conners Teacher Rating Scale (CTRS) without any improvement in motor activity, carbidopa was clearly not as efficacious as D-amphetamine and is not recommended for general use in hyperactivity [68]. Some L-dopa is methylated to 3-O-methyldopa, a metabolite which accumulates in the CNS owing to its half-life. Most dopa is converted to DA, although some is metabolized, in turn, to NE and E. After storage and release from dopaminergic synapses, transformation of DA proceeds rapidly to the principal excretion products: DOPAC and HVA [50]. In human beings, L-dopa therapy results in an increase in CSF HVA [25] and a decrease in 5-HIAA [116] and platelet 5-HT [7]. Autopsy specimens from substantia nigra and striatum in parkinsonian patients treated with L-dopa-carbidopa [89] showed increased DA and HVA without significant changes in NE; 5-HT was not measured. In the study of hyperactive children, plasma NE (both supine and standing) was increased when L-dopa was compared to placebo, but not significantly so; both urinary MHPG and VMA were significantly increased following L-dopa treatment. These findings do indicate an increase in NE metabolism after 2 weeks of L-dopa; however, much of the MHPG and VMA—partially converted from MHPG in the periphery—does not come from the CNS [5,6]. Increased output of plasma NE and the excretion of its metabolites from endogenous L-dopa, however, may not be directly related to the acute plasma NE release seen after a single dose of D-amphetamine. The lack of change in early morning baseline plasma NE in hyperactive children following 2 weeks of D-amphetamine [67] and the decreased excretion of MHPG seen after 2 weeks of D-amphetamine [14,19,99–102] both indicate the importance of taking into account differences in acute effects versus chronic effects.

Mianserin

Another drug of interest which has been used in a pilot trial in hyperactive children is mianserin, a presynaptic, α-adrenergic–receptor blocker [69]. Doses of up to 60 mg/day for 3 weeks in five hyperactive children were not therapeutically effective; side effects of oversedation and postural hypotension, consistent with its major pharmacologic action, resulted in an early termination of the trial. Excretion of MHPG and VMA were not affected. Plasma NE levels increased, possibly reflecting a generalized increase in brain NE, following 3 weeks of mianserin, unlike the lack of plasma baseline NE response following 2 weeks of D-amphetamine [67]. These studies, taken together, may be a further indication that acute release of plasma NE (but not increases in its basal level) may be a critical variable in the therapeutic response observed in hyperactive children.

Tricyclic Antidepressants

Controlled trials indicate that tricyclic antidepressants are generally beneficial to hyperactive children and have generally immediate effects much like D-amphetamine, but the initial response does not seem to be maintained [126]. Imipramine, which the best-controlled studies have used, is primarily a reuptake blocker of both NE and DA. Why there is generally a delayed and lasting response in adult depressives as opposed to the immediate but generally short-term response in hyperactive children is unknown. Childhood enuretics have both a short- and long-term therapeutic response to tricyclics [75,86]. Concomitant biochemical data with tricyclic treatment might elucidate the mechanism of the apparent tolerance that develops.

Effects of some of these drugs and concomitant biochemical effects are shown in Table 10.3. The biochemical changes following the administration of these drugs seem to implicate NE more than DA metabolism as having a role in the pharmacologic therapeutic response in hyperactivity. From the data herein reviewed, one cannot readily hypothesize that hyperactive children can be subdivided into those with disturbed DA metabolism and those with disturbed NE metabolism, a hypothesis that Shekim et al [102] have proposed.

FUTURE DIRECTIONS

More direct studies of hyperactive children versus normal children are important; MAO needs to be studied more thoroughly because it has such an important relationship to compounds (i.e., D-amphetamine) that are effective in treating hyperactive children and because it plays a role in the regulation of the various pathways of phenylalanine metabolism. The COMT findings should be further assessed. The importance of decreased TRM and PHPA excretion and increased PEA excretion following D-amphetamine needs to be further studied as well. Studies of 5-HT metabolism should be carried out to help clarify the currently conflicting data, because an alteration in 5-HT metabolism has been proposed in hyperactive children; also, from animal data, 5-HT is known to be affected by D-amphetamine. The simultaneous study of related metabolites and enzymes in the same child is of particular importance.

Further studies of dose-response relationships to behavioral change and the possibility of receptor supersensitivity and subsensitivity following D-amphetamine treatment would be important. D-amphetamine biotransformation studies have not been done in hyperactive children. Tolerance to D-amphetamine may only relate to some variables in hyperactivity. For example, tolerance may occur with repeated doses at short intervals and not when drug-free intervals exceed the half-life of D-amphetamine.

The carefully controlled prospective studies primarily reviewed in this chapter have contributed substantially to the "data bank" of the biochemical and pharmacologic understanding of hyperactive children, particularly in relationship to CA.

Further drug trials of interest would be controlled studies of MAO inhibitors and new tricyclics with more specific mechanisms of action; drug studies for the evaluation of indoleamine metabolism are also needed. If these drug studies are to pursue explanations for the observations herein reviewed, they must be designed to assess biochemical changes which could relate to clinical responses.

The authors thank Robert D. Hunt, M.D., Edwin J. Mikkelsen, M.D., Dennis L. Langer, M.D., Alan J. Zametkin, M.D., and Marcia D. Minichiello, Research Assistant.

Table 10.3 Behavioral-Biochemical Effects of Different Pharmacologic Compounds on Hyperactive Children

Study	*Drug (dose), Time Course*	*Clinical Effect*	*NE (plasma)*	*MHPG (urine)*	*VMA (urine)*	*HVA (urine)*
Rapoport et al [85] Mikkelsen et al [74]	D-Amphetamine (0.5 mg/kg) single dose	+	↑	NC	—	NC
Brown et al [14] Langer et al [67] Brown et al [19]	D-Amphetamine (0.75 mg/kg/day) 8 days; 2 wk	+	NC	↓	—	NC
Brown et al [15]	Piribedil (40–70 and 80–140 mg/day) 4 wk	NC	—	NC	—	↓
Langer et al [68]	Carbidopa/L-Dopa (50/600 mg/day) 3 wk	+ (minimal)	NC	↑	↑	—
Langer et al [69]	Mianserin (40–60 mg/day)	NC	↑	NC	NC	—

NE = norepinephrine; MHPG = 3-methoxy-4-hydroxyphenylglycol; VMA = vanillylmandelic acid; HVA = homovanillic acid; NC = no change; + = positive response; ↑ = increase; ↓ = decrease.

REFERENCES

1. Arnold LE, Wender PH, McCloskey K, Snyder SH. Levo-amphetamine and dextroamphetamine: comparative efficacy in the hyperkinetic syndrome. Arch Gen Psychiatry 27:816–822, 1972.
2. Bacopoulos NG, Hattos SE, Roth RH. 3,4-Dihydroxyphenylacetic acid and homovanillic acid in rat plasma: possible indicators of central dopaminergic activity. Eur J Pharmacol 56:225–236, 1979.
3. Baldessarini RJ, Harris JE. Effects of amphetamines on the metabolism of catecholamines in the rat brain. J Psychiatr Res 11:41–43, 1974.
4. Bender L, Cottington F. The use of amphetamine sulfate (benzedrine) in child psychiatry. Am J Psychiatry 99:116–121, 1943.
5. Blombery PA, Gordon EK, Kopin IJ, Ebert MH. Metabolism and Turnover of MHPG in the Monkey. In Catecholamines: Basic and Clinical Frontiers, E Usdin, IJ Kopin, and J Barchas (eds), 889–891. New York: Pergamon Press, 1979.
6. Blombery PA, Kopin IJ, Gordon EK, Markey SP, Ebert MH. Conversion of MHPG to vanillylmandelic acid. Arch Gen Psychiatry 37:1095–1098, 1980.
7. Boullin DJ, O'Brien RA. Accumulation of dopamine by blood platelets from normal subjects and parkinsonian patients under treatment with L-dopa. Br J Pharmacol 39:779–788, 1970.
8. Bradley C. The behavior of children receiving benzedrine. Am J Psychiatry 94:577–585, 1937.
9. Bradley C. Benzedrine and dexedrine in the treatment of children's behavior disorders. Pediatrics 5:24–36, 1950.
10. Braestrup C. Biochemical differentiation of amphetamine vs. methylphenidate and Nomifensin in rats. J Pharm Pharmacol 29:463–470, 1977.
11. Brase DA, Loh HH. Possible role of 5-hydroxytryptamine in minimal brain dysfunction. Life Sci 16:1009–1016, 1975.
12. Brown GL, Ebert MH, Hunt RD. Plasma D-amphetamine absorption and elimination in hyperactive children. Psychopharmacol Bull 14:33–35, 1978.
13. Brown GL, Ebert MH, Hunt RD, Bunney WE, Jr. Reliability of behavior and activity responses in hyperactive children following single doses of D-amphetamine. Presented at the Annual Meeting of the American Psychiatric Association, Toronto, 1977.
14. Brown GL, Ebert MH, Hunt RD, Rapoport JL. Urinary 3-methoxy-4-hydroxyphenylglycol and homovanillic acid response to D-amphetamine in hyperactive children. Biol Psychiatry 16:779–787, 1981.
15. Brown GL, Ebert MH, Mikkelsen E, Buchsbaum MS, Bunney WE, Jr. Dopamine agonist piribedil in hyperactive children. Presented at the Annual Meeting of the American Psychiatric Association, Chicago, 1979.
16. Brown GL, Ebert MH, Mikkelsen EJ, Hunt RD. Clinical Pharmacology of D-amphetamine in Hyperactive Children. In Pharmacokinetics of Psychoactive Drugs, LA Gottschalk (ed), 137–153. New York: Spectrum, 1979.
17. Brown GL, Ebert MH, Mikkelsen EJ, Hunt RD. Behavior and motor activity response in hyperactive children and plasma amphetamine levels following a sustained release preparation. J Am Acad Child Psychiatry 19:225–239, 1980.
18. Brown GL, Hunt RD, Ebert MH, Bunney WE, Jr, Kopin IJ. Plasma levels of D-amphetamine in hyperactive children. Psychopharmacology (Berlin) 62:133–140, 1979.

19. Brown GL, Karoum F, Zametkin AJ, Chuang LW, Langer DH, Ebert MH, Rapoport JL, Bunney WE, Jr, Wyatt RJ. Catecholamine excretion in hyperactive boys following D-amphetamine and placebo. Presented at the Annual Meeting of the American Psychiatric Association, Toronto, 1982.
20. Bunney WE, Jr. Neuronal Receptor Function in Psychiatry: Strategy and Theory. In Neuroreceptors—Basic and Clinical Aspects, E Usdin, WE Bunney, Jr, and JJ Davis (eds), 241–255. New York: John Wiley and Sons, Interscience Publication, 1981.
21. Bunney WE, Jr, Murphy DL. Strategies for the Systematic Study of Neurotransmitter Receptor Function in Man. In Pre- and Post-Synaptic Receptors, E Usdin and WE Bunney, Jr. (eds), 283–311. New York: Marcel Dekker, 1975.
22. Burks HF. Effects of amphetamine therapy on hyperkinetic children. Arch Gen Psychiatry 11:604–609, 1974.
23. Carlsson A. Receptor-Mediated Control of Dopamine Metabolism. In Pre- and Post-Synaptic Receptors, E Usdin and WE Bunney, Jr (eds), 49–65. New York: Marcel Dekker, 1975.
24. Carlsson A, Fuxe J, Hamberger B, Lindquist M. Biochemical and histochemical studies on the effects of imipramine-like drugs and (+)-amphetamine on central and peripheral catecholamine neurons. Acta Physiol Scand 67:481–497, 1966.
25. Chase TN. Cerebrospinal fluid monoamine metabolites and peripheral decarboxylase inhibitors in parkinsonism. Neurology (Minneap) 20:36–40, 1970.
26. Chieh CC, Moore KE. Relative potencies of D- and L-amphetamine on the release of dopamine from cat brain in vivo. Res Commun Chem Pathol Pharmacol 7:189–199, 1974.
27. Cohen DJ, Caparulo BK, Shaywitz BA, Bowers MB. Dopamine and serotonin metabolism in neuropsychiatrically disturbed children: cerebrospinal fluid homovanillic acid and 5-hydroxyindoleacetic acid. Arch Gen Psychiatry 34:545–550, 1977.
28. Colburn TR, Smith BA, Guarini JJ, Simmons NJ. An ambulatory activity monitor with solid state memory. ISA Transactions 15:149–154, 1976.
29. Coleman M. Serotonin concentrations in whole blood of hyperactive children. J Pediatr 78:985–990, 1971.
30. Coleman M. Serotonin and central nervous system syndromes of childhood: a review. J Autism Child Schiz 3:27–35, 1973.
31. Conners CK. A teacher rating scale for use in drug studies with children. Am J Psychiatry 126:152–156, 1969.
32. Conners CK. Pharmacotherapy of Psychopathology in Children. In Psychopathological Disorders of Childhood, HC Quay and JS Werry (eds), 316–347. New York: John Wiley and Sons, 1972.
33. Conners CK. Rating scales for use in drug studies with children. Psychopharmacol Bull Special Issue 24–84, 1973.
34. Conners CK, Taylor E, Meo G, Kurtz MA, Fournier M. Magnesium pemoline and dextroamphetamine: a controlled study in children with minimal brain dysfunction. Psychopharmacologia (Berlin) 26:321–336, 1972.
35. Cook JD, Schanberg SM. The effects of methamphetamine on behavior and on the uptake, release, and metabolism of norepinephrine. Biochem Pharmacol 19:1165–1179, 1970.
36. Costall B, Naylor RJ. Dopamine agonist and antagonist activities of piribedil and its metabolites. Naunyn Schmeidebergs Arch Pharmacol 285:71–81, 1974.

37. Coyle JT, Snyder SH. Catecholamine uptake by synaptosomes in homogenates of rat brain: stereospecificity in different areas. J Pharmacol Exp Ther 170:221–231, 1969.
38. Downs DA, Braude MC. Time-action and behavioral effects of amphetamine, ethanol, and acetylmethadol. Pharmacol Biochem Behav 6:671–676, 1977.
39. Ebert MH, van Kammen DP, Murphy DL. Plasma Levels of Amphetamine and Behavioral Response. In Pharmacokinetics of Psychoactive Drugs: Blood Levels and Clinical Response. LA Gottschalk and S Merlis (eds), 157–169. New York: Spectrum-Wiley, 1976.
40. Ebert MH, Kopin IJ. Differential labeling of origins of urinary catecholamine metabolites by dopamine-C^{14}. Trans Assoc Am Physicians 88:256–264, 1975.
41. Ebert MH, Post RM, Goodwin FK. Effect of physical activity on urinary MHPG excretion in depressed patients. Lancet 2:766, 1972.
42. Eisenberg L, Lachman R, Molling PA, Lockner A, Mizelle JD, Conners CK. A psychopharmacologic experiment in a training school for delinquent boys: methods, problems, findings. Am J Orthopsychiatry 33:431–446, 1963.
43. Elchisak MA, Polinsky RJ, Ebert MH, Modlin LT, Kopin IJ. Kinetics of homovanillic acid and determination of its production rate in the rhesus monkey. Life Sci 24:1493–1502, 1979.
44. Elchisak MA, Polinsky RJ, Ebert MH, Powers KJ, Kopin IJ. Contribution of plasma homovanillic acid (HVA) to urine and cerebrospinal fluid HVA in the monkey and its pharmacokinetic disposition. Life Sci 23:2339–2348, 1978.
45. Epstein LC, Lasagna L, Conners CK, Rodriguez A. Correlation of dextroamphetamine excretion and drug response in hyperkinetic children. J Nerv Ment Dis 146:136–146, 1969.
46. Farnebo LO. Effect of D-amphetamine on spontaneous and stimulation-induced release of catecholamines. Acta Physiol Scand [Suppl.] 371:45–52, 1971.
47. Ferguson HB, Pappas BA, Trites RL, Peters DAV, Taub H. Plasma free and total tryptophan, blood serotonin, and the hyperactivity syndrome: no evidence for the serotonin deficiency hypothesis. Biol Psychiatry 16:231–238, 1981.
48. Ferris RM, Tang FLM, Maxwell RA. A comparison of the capacities of isomers of amphetamine, deoxypipradrol and methylphenidate to inhibit the uptake of tritiated catecholamines into rat cerebral cortex, hypothalamus and striatum and into adrenergic nerves of rabbit aorta. J Pharmacol Exp Ther 181:407–416, 1972.
49. Fish B. Drug use in psychiatric disorders of children. Am J Psychiatry 124:31–36, 1968.
50. Goodman Gilman A, Goodman L, Gilman A. Goodman's and Gilman's The Pharmacological Basis of Therapeutics (5th ed). New York: Macmillan, 1980.
51. Greenberg A, Coleman M. Use of blood serotonin levels for the classification and treatment of hyperactive behavior disorders. Neurology (Minneap) 23:428, 1973.
52. Greenberg A, Coleman M. Depressed 5-hydroxyindole levels associated with hyperactive and aggressive behavior: relationship to drug response. Arch Gen Psychiatry 33:331–336, 1976.
53. Greenberg LM, Deem MA, McMahon S. Effect of dextroamphetamine, chlorpromazine, and hydroxyzine on behavior and performance in hyperactive children. Am J Psychiatry 129:532–539, 1972.
54. Greenblatt DJ, Koch-Weser J. Clinical pharmacokinetics. N Engl J Med 293:702–705, 964–970, 1975.
55. Gualtieri CT, Wargin W, Kanoy R, Patrick K, Shen CD, Youngblood W, Mueller

RA, Breese GR. Clinical studies of methylphenidate serum levels in children and adults. J Am Acad Child Psychiatry 21:19–26, 1982.

56. Hauger RL, Skolnick P, Paul SM. Specific [^{3}H] β-phenylethylamine binding sites in rat brain. Eur J Pharmacol 83:147–148, 1982.
57. Huestis RD, Arnold LE, Smeltzer DJ. Caffeine versus methylphenidate and D-amphetamine in minimal brain dysfunction. A double-blind comparison. Am J Psychiatry 132:868–870, 1975.
58. Hungund BL, Perel JM, Hurwic MJ, Sverd J, Winsberg BG. Pharmacokinetics of methylphenidate in hyperactive children. Presented at the Annual Meeting of the Society for Biological Psychiatry, Chicago, 1979.
59. Khan AU, Dekirmenjian H. Urinary excretion of catecholamine metabolites in hyperkinetic child syndrome. Am J Psychiatry 138:108–110, 1981.
60. Knobel M. Psychopharmacology for the hyperkinetic child. Arch Gen Psychiatry 6:198–202, 1962.
61. Kopin IJ. False adrenergic transmitters. Annu Rev Pharmacol 8:377–394, 1968.
62. Kopin IJ. The Influence of False Neurotransmitters on Adrenergic Transmission. In Adrenergic Neurotransmission, GEW Wolstenholme and M O'Connor (eds). 95–104. Boston: Little, Brown and Co., 1968.
63. Kopin IJ. Measuring Turnover of Neurotransmitter in Human Brain. In Psychopharmacology: A Generation of Progress, MA Lipton, A DiMascio, and KF Killam (eds), 933–942. New York: Raven Press, 1978.
64. Kornetsky C. Psychoactive drugs in the immature organism. Psychopharmacologia (Berlin) 17:105–136, 1970.
65. Kuczenski R, Segal DS. Differential effects of D- and L-amphetamine and methylphenidate on rat striatal dopamine biosynthesis. Eur J Pharmacol 30:244–251, 1975.
66. Kupietz SS, Winsberg BG, Sverd J. Learning ability and methylphenidate (Ritalin) plasma concentration in hyperkinetic children: a preliminary investigation. J Am Acad Psychiatry 21:27–30, 1982.
67. Langer DH, Brown GL, Lake CR, Ebert MH. Plasma norepinephrine response to two weeks of D-amphetamine in hyperactive boys. Presented at the Annual Meeting of the American Academy of Child Psychiatry, Washington, DC, 1982.
68. Langer DH, Rapoport JL, Brown GL, Ebert MH, Bunney WE, Jr. Behavioral effects of carbidopa/levodopa in hyperactive boys. J Am Acad Child Psychiatry 21:10–18, 1982.
69. Langer DH, Rapoport JL, Ebert MH, Lake CR, Nee L. Pilot Trial of Mianserin Hydrochloride for Childhood Hyperactivity. In The Psychobiology of Childhood: Profiles of Current Issues, L Greenhill and B Shopsin (eds), 197–210. Jamaica, New York: Spectrum Publications, 1984.
70. Maas JW, Dekirmenjian H, Garver D, Redmond DE, Landis DH. Excretion of catecholamine metabolites following intraventricular injection of 6-hydroxydopamine in the macaca speciosa. Eur J Pharmacol 23:121–130, 1973.
71. Maas JW, Landis DH. In vivo studies of the metabolism of norepinephrine in the central nervous system. J Pharmacol Exp Ther 163:147–162, 1968.
72. Meyerhoff J, Snyder S. Gilles de la Tourette's disease and minimal brain dysfunction: amphetamine isomers reveal catecholamine correlates in an affected patient. Psychopharmacology (Berlin) 29:211–220, 1973.
73. Mikkelsen EJ, Brown GL, Minichiello MD, Millican FK, Rapoport JL. Neurologic status in hyperactive, enuretic, encopretic and normal boys. J Am Acad Child Psychiatry 21:75–81, 1982.

74. Mikkelsen EJ, Lake CR, Brown GL, Ziegler MG, Ebert MH. The hyperactive child syndrome: peripheral sympathetic nervous system function and the effect of D-amphetamine. Psychiatry Res 4:157–169, 1981.
75. Mikkelsen EJ, Rapoport JL, Nee L, Gruenau C, Mendelson W, Gillin JC. Childhood enuresis. I. Sleep patterns and psychopathology. Arch Gen Psychiatry 37:1139–1144, 1980.
76. Millichap JG, Fowler GW. Treatment of minimal brain dysfunction syndromes. Pediatr Clin North Am 14:767–777, 1967.
77. Millichap JG, Johnson FH. Methylphenidate in Hyperkinetic Behavior: Relation of Response to Degree of Activity and Brain Damage. In Clinical Use of Stimulant Drugs in Children, CK Conners (ed), 130–139. Amsterdam: Excerpta Medica, 1975.
78. Morgenroth VH, Walters JR, Roth RH. Dopaminergic neurons: alterations in kinetic properties of tyrosine hydroxylase after cessation of impulse flow. Biochem Pharmacol 25:655–662, 1976.
79. North RB, Harik SI, Snyder SH. Amphetamine isomers: influences on locomotor and stereotyped behavior of cats. Pharmacol Biochem Behav 2:115–118, 1974.
80. Nurnberger JI, Gershon ES, Jimerson DC, Buchsbaum MS, Gold PW, Brown GL, Ebert MH. Pharmacogenetics of D-Amphetamine Response in Man. In Genetic Research Strategies for Psychobiology and Psychiatry, ES Gershon, S Matthysse, XO Breakfield, and RD Ciaranello (eds), 257–268. Pacific Grove, California: Boxwood Press, 1981.
81. Paul SM, Hulihan-Giblin B, Skolnick P. (+)-Amphetamine binding to rat hypothalamus: relation to anorexic potency of phenylethylamines. Science 218:487–490, 1982.
82. Post RM, Gerner RH, Carman JS, Gillin JC, Jimerson DC, Goodwin FK, Bunney WE, Jr. Effects of a dopamine agonist piribedil in depressed patients. Arch Gen Psychiatry 35:609–615, 1978.
83. Powers KG, Ebert MH. Comparison of RIA and GC-MS assays for D-amphetamine. Biomed Mass Spectrom 6:187–190, 1979.
84. Rapoport JL, Lott I, Alexander D, Abramson A. Urinary noradrenaline and playroom behavior in hyperactive boys. Lancet 2:1141, 1970.
85. Rapoport JL, Mikkelsen EJ, Ebert MH, Brown GL, Weise VK, Kopin IJ. Urinary catecholamines and amphetamine excretion in hyperactive and normal boys. J Nerv Ment Dis 166:731, 1978.
86. Rapoport JL, Mikkelsen EJ, Zavadil A, Nee L, Gruenau C, Mendelson W, Gillin JC. Childhood enuresis. II. Psychopathology. Arch Gen Psychiatry 37:1146–1152, 1980.
87. Rapoport JL, Quinn PO, Lamprecht F. Minor physical anomalies and plasma dopamine-beta-hydroxylase activity in hyperactive boys. Am J Psychiatry 131:386–390, 1974.
88. Rapoport JL, Quinn PO, Scribanu N, Murphy DL. Platelet serotonin in hyperactive school age boys. Br J Psychiatry 125:138–140, 1974.
89. Rinne UK, Sonninen MD. Brain catecholamines and their metabolites in parkinsonian patients. Arch Neurol 28:107–110, 1973.
90. Rogeness GA, Hernandez JM, Macedo CA, Mitchell MA. Biochemical differences in children with conduct disorder socialized and undersocialized. Am J Psychiatry 139:307–311, 1982.
91. Ross SB. Antagonism by methylphenidate of the stereotyped behavior produced by (+)-amphetamine in reserpinized rats. Commun J Pharm Pharmacol 30:253–254, 1978.

92. Roth RH, Walters JR, Morgenroth VH. Effects of alterations in impulse flow on transmitter metabolism in central dopaminergic neurons. Adv Biochem Psychopharmacol 12:369–384, 1974.
93. Schanberg SM, Schildkraut JJ, Breese GR, Kopin IJ. Metabolism of normetanephrine-H^3 in rat brain—Identification of conjugated 3-methoxy-4-hydroxyphenylglycol as the major metabolite. Biochem Pharmacol 17:247–254, 1968.
94. Scheel-Kruger J. Comparative studies of various amphetamine analogues demonstrating different interactions with the metabolism of the catecholamines in the brain. Eur J Pharmacol 14:47–59, 1971.
95. Segal DS. Behavioral characterization of D- and L-amphetamine: neurochemical implications. Science 190:475–477, 1975.
96. Shaywitz BA, Cohen DJ, Bowers MB, Jr. CSF amine metabolites in children with minimal brain dysfunction (MBD)—Evidence for alteration of brain dopamine. Pediatr Res 9:385, 1975.
97. Shaywitz BA, Cohen DJ, Bowers MB, Jr. CSF monoamine metabolites in children with minimal brain dysfunction: evidence for alteration of brain dopamine—A preliminary report. J Pediatr 90:67–71, 1977.
98. Shekim WO, Davis LG, Bylund DB, Brunngraber E, Fikes L, Lanham J. Platelet MAO in children with attention deficit disorder and hyperactivity: a pilot study. Am J Psychiatry 139:936–938, 1982.
99. Shekim WO, Dekirmenjian H, Chapel JL. Urinary catecholamine metabolites in hyperkinetic boys treated with D-amphetamine. Am J Psychiatry 134:1276–1279, 1977.
100. Shekim WO, Dekirmenjian H, Chapel JL. Urinary MHPG excretion in minimal brain dysfunction and its modification by D-amphetamine. Am J Psychiatry 136:667–671, 1979.
101. Shekim WO, Dekirmenjian H, Chapel JL, Javaid J, Davis JM. Norepinephrine metabolism and clinical response to dextroamphetamine in hyperactive boys. J Pediatr 95:389–394, 1979.
102. Shekim WO, Javaid J, Dekirmenjian H, Chapel JL, Davis JM. Effects of D-amphetamine on urinary metabolites of dopamine and norepinephrine in hyperactive boys. Am J Psychiatry 139:485–488, 1982.
103. Shetty T, Chase TN. Central monoamines and hyperkinesis of childhood. Neurology (Minneap) 26:1000–1002, 1976.
104. Snyder SH. Stereoselective features of catecholamine disposition and their behavioral implications. J Psychiatr Res 11:31–39, 1974.
105. Snyder SH, Meyerhoff JL. How amphetamine acts in minimal brain dysfunction. Ann NY Acad Sci 205:310–320, 1973.
106. Snyder SH, Taylor KM, Coyle JT, Meyerhoff JL. The role of brain dopamine in behavioral regulation and the actions of psychotropic drugs. Am J Psychiatry 127:199–207, 1970.
107. Sprague RL, Sleator EK. Methylphenidate in hyperkinetic children: differences in dose effects on learning and social behavior. Science 198:1274–1276, 1977.
108. Strombom U. Effects of low doses of catecholamine receptor agonists on exploration in mice. J Neural Transm 37:229–235, 1976.
109. Swanson JM, Kinsbourne J, Roberts W, Zucker MA. Time-response analysis of the effect of stimulant medication on the learning ability of children referred for hyperactivity. Pediatrics 61:21–29, 1978.
110. Swanson JM, Seldin SJ. Serum levels of methylphenidate in hyperactive children: I. Half-life following oral administration: II. The therapeutic range. Workshop on the

Influence of Age on the Pharmacology of Psychoactive Drugs, Washington, DC, 1979.

111. Sweeney DR, Leckman JF, Maas JW, Hattox S, Heninger GR. Plasma-free and conjugated MHPG in psychiatric patients—A pilot study. Arch Gen Psychiatry 37:1100–1102, 1980.
112. Taylor KM, Snyder SH. Differential effects of D- and L-amphetamine on behavior and on catecholamine disposition in dopamine and norepinephrine-containing neurons of rat brain. Brain Res 28:295–309, 1971.
113. Thornburg JE, Moore KE. Dopamine and norepinephrine uptake by rat brain synaptosomes: relative inhibitory potencies of L- and D-amphetamine and amantadine. Res Commun Chem Pathol Pharmacol 5:81–89, 1973.
114. Trabucci M, DiChiara G, Spano PJ. Bromocriptine and the dopaminergic receptors in rat brain. Abstracts of the Collegium Internationale Neuropsychopharmacologicum, Abstract 251. Amsterdam: Elsevier Publishing Co., 1976.
115. Van Voigtlander PF, Moore KE. Involvement of nigro-striatal neurons in the vivo release of dopamine by amphetamine, amantadine and tyramine. J Pharmacol Exp Ther 184:542–552, 1973.
116. Van Woert MH, Bowers MB, Jr. The effect of L-dopa on the monoamine metabolites in Parkinson's disease. Experientia 26:161–163, 1970.
117. Walker HA, Danielson E, Levitt J. Catechol-O-methyltransferase activity in psychotic children. J Autism Child Schiz 6:263–268, 1976.
118. Walters JR, Bunney BS, Roth RH. Piribedil and apomorphine: pre- and postsynaptic effects on dopamine synthesis and neuronal activity. Adv Neurol 9:273–284, 1975.
119. Wehr TA, Muscettola G, Goodwin FK. Urinary 3-methoxy-4-hydroxyphenylglycol circadian rhythm—Early timing (phase-advance) in manic-depressives compared with normal subjects. Arch Gen Psychiatry 37:257–263, 1980.
120. Wender PH. Platelet serotonin levels in children with minimal brain dysfunction. Lancet 2:1012, 1969.
121. Wender PH. Minimal Brain Dysfunction in Children. New York: Wiley-Interscience, 1971.
122. Wender PH. Some speculations concerning a possible biochemical basis of minimal brain dysfunction. Ann NY Acad Sci 205:18–28, 1973.
123. Wender PH, Epstein AS, Kopin IJ, Gordon EK. Urinary monoamine metabolites in children with minimal brain dysfunction. Am J Psychiatry 127:1411–1415, 1971.
124. Zametkin AJ, Brown GL, Karoum F, Rapoport JL, Langer DH, Chuang LW, Wyatt RJ. Urinary phenylethylamine response to D-amphetamine in 12 boys with attention deficit disorder. Am J Psychiatry 141:1055–1058, 1984.
125. Zametkin AJ, Karoum F, Rapoport JL, Brown GL, Wyatt RJ. Phenylethylamine excretion in attention deficit disorder. J Am Acad Child Psychiatry 23:310–314, 1984.
126. Zametkin AJ, Rapoport JL. Tricyclic Antidepressants and Children. In Drugs in Psychiatry. Vol. 1: Antidepressants, G Burrows, TR Norman, and B Davies (eds), 130–147. Amsterdam: Elsevier, 1983.

IV

Affective Disorders and the Catecholamines

11

Norepinephrine in the Affective Disorders: Classic Biochemical Approaches

William Z. Potter
Richard J. Ross
Anthony P. Zavadil III

A unifying theory pursued in basic and clinical research in the affective disorders during the last 15 years is that altered noradrenergic function is central to the pathophysiology of these illnesses—the "catecholamine (CA) hypothesis of affective illness" [14,81,88]. Animal data show that classic antidepressant drugs increase norepinephrine (NE) in the synapse [18,36], and clinical studies report that drugs which deplete NE produce depression in susceptible individuals [19,57,82,97]. Studies on the neuroanatomic distribution of NE-containing neurons and on physiologic function or behaviors influenced by NE are discussed elsewhere in this volume (see Chapters 3 and 5). These investigations show that NE is involved in primary regulatory circuits in brain areas which subserve functions broadly related to appetite, drives, arousal, and "emotions" (including their neuroendocrine and psychophysiologic concomitants). NE serves as well to help integrate these functions with a wide range of other brain components. As reviewed in Chapter 12, at least 50% of patients with affective illness manifest one or more of the following neuroendocrine abnormalities: failure of dexamethasone to suppress cortisol; a blunted thyroid-stimulating hormone (TSH) response to thyrotropin-releasing hormone (TRH); or a blunted growth hormone (GH) response to insulin-induced hypoglycemia or the administration of clonidine, amphetamine, or desipramine (see Chapter 12). Many of these altered neuroendocrine responses may relate to some change of NE function. Moreover, alterations of presynaptic and postsynaptic NE receptors in various tissues generally support the notion of abnormal NE function (see Chapter 12).

This chapter selectively reviews studies which have approached the question of altered noradrenergic function in more classical ways, either by measuring NE or its metabolites in depressed patients or by studying the effects of antidepressant drugs in these individuals. The first section describes the methodologic issues most relevant to investigation of NE function in psychiatric and psychopharmacologic research, our purpose being to highlight the underlying assumptions which are sometimes ignored in the interpretations of data. It is important to realize that rarely do clinical state studies, or those of antidepressant drug action, address whether selected biochemical measures actually reflect noradrenergic function. As we will discuss, these limitations render virtually useless the application of many measures to clinical situations. The second part of the chapter discusses studies preceding the development of assays sensitive enough to measure NE in plasma and cerebrospinal fluid (CSF). The third section includes investigations which focus on NE itself.

METHODOLOGIC ISSUES

With the advent of sensitive, specific assays for NE and its abundant metabolites, the concentrations of all these substances can be accurately measured in plasma and other samples. The interpretation of such data is generally based on the implicit assumption that observed differences in plasma concentrations are due to differences in the rates of entry of the measured substances into the plasma pool [56]. Plasma concentrations of NE metabolites are assumed to reflect the activity of NE neurons [98]. However, factors other than the rate of entry into the pool may influence the concentration of NE (or metabolites) in the plasma, a problem discussed in more depth in Chapter 1. We highlight those considerations which are most relevant to the interpretation of studies with psychiatric patients and ignore the possible problem of arterial-venous differences [42]. Particularly in the case of NE metabolites (Figure 11.1), a factor that should be considered in collecting and interpreting data is the constancy of the fraction of NE that is converted to the metabolite. In other words, the rate of entry of the metabolite into the plasma pool could be increased by increased amounts of NE entering the metabolic pathway (production rate) or by an increased fractional conversion of a constant amount of precursor to a particular metabolite (metabolic rate). Because both the rate of production and the rate of metabolism are altered by drugs and perhaps disease processes, a detailed exposition of this phenomenon is necessary to understand available clinical data.

Consider the simplest model for NE kinetics in which the concentration of NE in the plasma at any time is a function of three variables: the rate in (R_i); the volume of distribution (V_d); and the rate out (R_o) (Figure 11.2). R_i is probably a composite of NE escaping into the circulation following release at nerve endings and at the adrenal medulla as well as nonspecific "leakage" from axons. R_o is probably a composite of uptake of NE by nerve endings or extraneuronal sites, metabolism, and excretion in the urine. In real-life situations, because the half-life of NE in the plasma is relatively short [33], an interval of 10 minutes should be adequate to change from one steady-state condition to another. By definition, in the steady-state situation the rate of NE entry into the pool is equal to the rate of exit (i.e., $R_i = R_o$). Furthermore, $R_i = R_o = V_d \times C \times K_e$, where C is

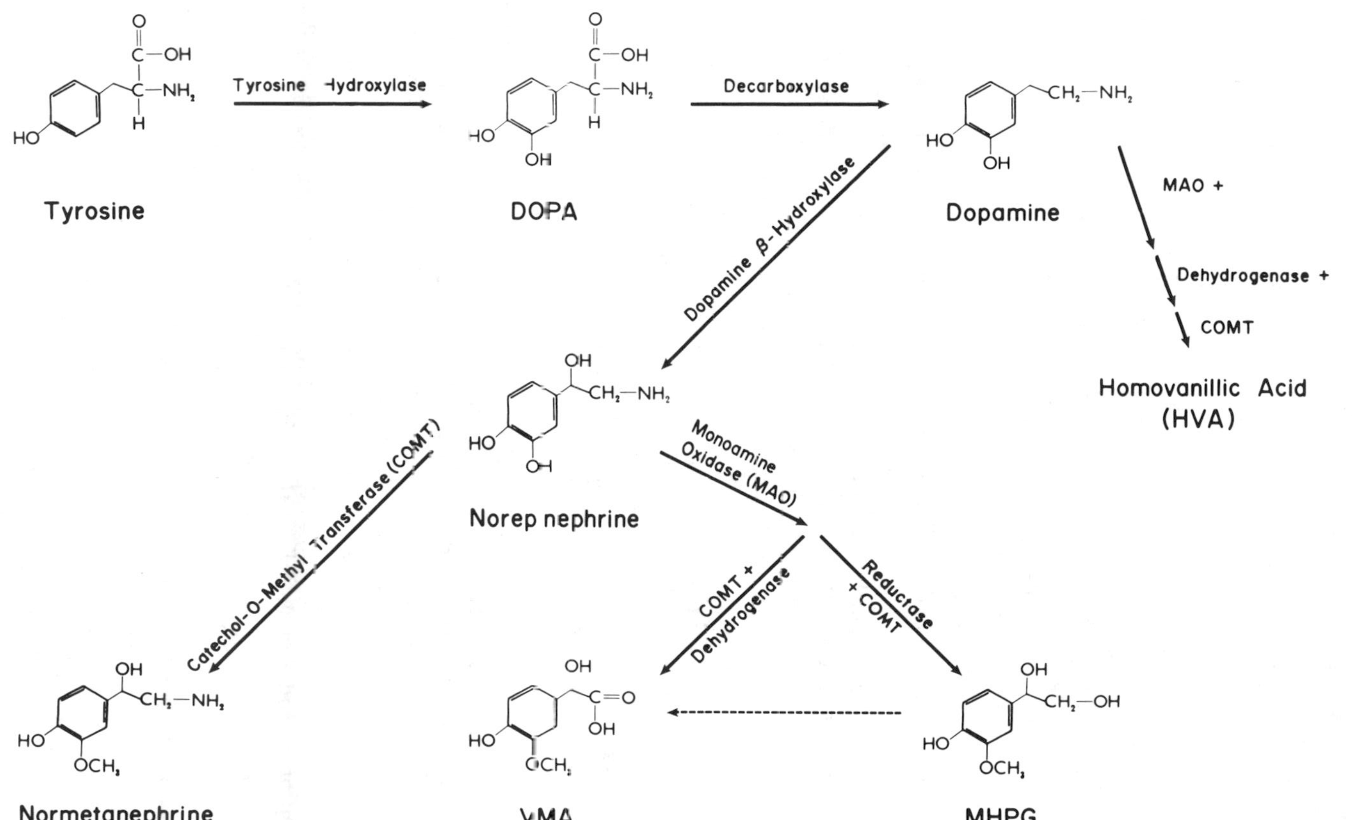

Figure 11.1 Pathways of norepinephrine synthesis and metabolism in human beings. The primary deamination of norepinephrine is believed to occur intraneuronally. Released norepinephrine can be metabolized directly to normetanephrine, which can be converted to 3-methoxy-4-hydroxyphenylglycol (MHPG) and vanillylmandelic acid (VMA) extraneuronally (pathways not shown).

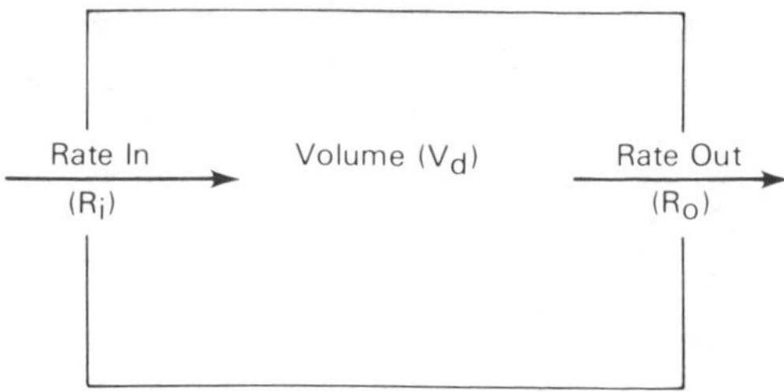

Figure 11.2 One compartment kinetic model of three variables controlling the concentration of norepinephrine in plasma: rate in (R_i); volume of distribution (V_d); and rate out (R_o).

the concentration of NE and K_e is the elimination rate constant (the fraction of the pool that is cleared of NE in a unit of time). Rearranging this equation ($C = R_i/V_d \times K_e$) shows that the measured variable, C, is a function of V_d and K_e as well as R_i. Thus, concentrations of NE in the plasma can be increased or decreased in the absence of any change in R_i (production rate) if V_d, K_e, or both change. Because these factors are rarely measured in clinical NE studies, the magnitude of their interindividual variations is not well characterized in groups of different age, physical condition, etc. Fitzgerald et al [33] showed that the clearance (Clearance = $V_d \times K_e$) of infused NE varied by 360% in five normotensive men aged 32.4 ± 1.9 years. These subjects were matched for posture, age, race, gender, salt intake, cigarette use, caffeine intake, and the time of sampling—factors known to influence plasma NE concentrations. This clearance difference would result in plasma NE concentrations of 100 and 360 pg/ml in individuals with identical input rates. Thus, plasma NE would be a very poor measure of the effective NE concentration in the synapse acting on the receptors.

There may be strategies for dealing with this problem which would apply to NE metabolites as well. An approach being applied by a few investigators which allows for correction of differences in NE clearance is to infuse NE at a constant rate for 10 to 20 minutes, measure the plasma level, and calculate the clearance rate. A shortcoming of this approach is that one must make an assumption about the contribution of endogenous NE to the measured plasma level. When infused NE has no effect on blood pressure or pulse, it can be assumed that the infused NE has no effect on the rate of release of endogenous NE. However, this assumption is probably incorrect when NE is infused rapidly enough to reduce the pulse rate. (See Chapter 1 for details on the effects of infused NE.) A recent study using high specific activity radiolabeled NE seems to have avoided some of these difficulties in attempting to distinguish altered NE clearance ($V_d \times K_e$) from altered release (R_i). Essler et al [30a] found that in a small group of depressed patients both release of NE ("spillover rate" in their terminology) and the elimination rate (K_e) of the first component of a bioexponential NE disappearance curve were increased although overall clearance was unaltered. They interpreted this as evidence of increased neuronal uptake in the depressed patients [30a] which would increase the V_d term in the model above.

The possible consequences of not accounting for these kinetic variables is seen in an investigation in which the infusion methodology was used [107]. These investigators showed that the difference in plasma NE between young and old persons in the standing position cannot be explained by differences in the disappearance rate of NE from the circulation. However, their calculations of the half-time for NE were based on average data for the groups at each time point rather than averaging the $t_{1/2}$ calculated for each subject. Furthermore, they assumed that the endogenous NE made no contribution to the plasma concentration of NE during the infusion. If this is the case, however, it is difficult to explain why the plasma NE did not drop to subbaseline levels when the infusion was stopped, unless compensatory reflexes were involved.

In summary, investigations comparing the plasma concentrations of NE in different groups should control posture, age, race, gender, salt intake, cigarette use, caffeine intake, time of sampling, and prandial condition. Because it is likely that most NE measured in the periphery is released in the periphery, the measurement may yield little information about the state of noradrenergic systems in the brain [51]. It is known that plasma and CSF concentrations of NE are significantly, but not highly, correlated ($r = 0.59$) in certain patient groups [108]; extrapolation of this relationship to all groups may not be warranted.

There are additional methodologic considerations influencing interpretations based on metabolite measurements. First, concentrations of NE metabolites in plasma are determined by the same factors as are concentrations of NE. With metabolites, however, the R_i is determined by two variables: the R_i for the precursor, NE, and the fractional conversion of the precursor of the product. Interpreting metabolite data, therefore, is even more complex than interpreting NE data. The discovery of 3-methoxy-4-hydroxyphenylglycol (MHPG) as the major metabolite of centrally administered NE in mammals [87] and the demonstration that it is the major CSF metabolite of NE [65] suggest that the measurement of MHPG excretion in the urine might reflect its rate of production in the brain. The work of Maas et al [64] showed that in human beings there is a change in the concentration of unconjugated MHPG between the radial artery and the internal jugular vein. The average difference in six normal volunteers and four patients was 0.7 ± 0.1 ng/ml. In subjects whose radial artery/internal jugular vein difference and urinary excretion of MHPG were measured concurrently, MHPG produced in the brain could account for more than 60% of the MHPG found in the urine if MHPG derived from the brain was excreted unchanged in the urine. However, the assumption that MHPG is not metabolized in the periphery is contradicted by studies of peripherally administered MHPG in humans [9,66], which indicate that most MHPG is excreted in the urine as vanillylmandelic acid (VMA). These results suggest that a variable fraction of the MHPG derived from the brain is excreted in the urine as free or conjugated MHPG. Thus, it is unlikely that observed differences in the excretion rates of MHPG in the urine are primarily the result of altered excretion rates of MHPG formed in the brain.

It appears equally unlikely that the concentration of any other metabolite of NE in any single tissue can be used as a reliable measure of NE activity in the brain. Nevertheless, as discussed in the following section, studies of NE metabolites may prove to be of more than heuristic value.

CLINICAL STUDIES ANTEDATING MEASURES OF NOREPINEPHRINE

Early studies of noradrenergic function in affective illness focused on normetanephrine (NM), which was thought to best reflect NE released into the synapse [4,52]. In an intraindividual comparison of patients with bipolar illness, urinary levels of NM (measured spectrophotometrically) were found to be relatively low during depression and relatively high during hypomania [90]. In subsequent comparisons across individuals of diagnostic subgroups, no statistically significant differences in urinary NM levels were found [62,93]. This was interpreted to mean that NM would primarily reflect the activity of the peripheral sympathetic nervous system (SNS) and hence be of no direct relevance for affective illness [92]. As discussed in the following paragraphs, this interpretation may be too simplistic. On the other hand, NM by itself remains unlikely to provide useful information about affective illness.

Findings that most NE in the central nervous system (CNS) ultimately metabolizes to MHPG (see the previous discussion, Methodologic Issues) and that comparisons of urinary MHPG excretion across diagnostic groups and patients yield significant differences [26,37,63,91] spurred study of urinary MHPG. Regardless of uncertainty as to its source, urinary MHPG has been found to be relatively low both in subjects with affective illness and in specific mood states (Tables 11.1 through 11.3). Table 11.1 summarizes most of the literature during the last decade that studied the excretion of MHPG in patients with affective illness, normal volunteers, or both. Patients with affective illness have an overall lower urinary MHPG excretion rate than normal volunteers, if weighted means are compared. Inspection of the actual values in each study, however, reveals widely different absolute values for both patients and volunteers, with a range of almost 300%. There is no evidence that these differences can be accounted for by factors such as age, gender, diet, activity, time of year, anxiety or other psychological factors, medical illnesses, or drugs—all of which have been reported to influence urinary MHPG under certain circumstances (for review see reference 78). Because the gas chromatography method used to quantitate MHPG involves an elaborate calculation of recovery following extraction and enzymatic hydrolysis, there may be systematic interlaboratory differences [10,25]; this was recently confirmed in a comparison of results from gas chromatography assays using electron capture detection versus mass spectrometric detection [70]. These factors limit the comparison of laboratory groups to patterns of MHPG differences and not to absolute values. Thus, what constitutes "low" or "high" levels of MHPG in patients is dependent as much on geography as on the values themselves.

Nonetheless some overall consistent findings have emerged. Table 11.2 demon-

Table 11.1 MHPG Excretion in All Studies, Not Taking Gender into Account

	*Major or Primary Depression**			
Source	*All Types*	*Unipolar*	*Bipolar*	*Normal*
Maas et al [63]	1059 (16)			1517 (11)
Fawcett et al [32]	998 (11)			
Shaw et al [96]	1401 (22)	1401 (22)		
Schildkraut et al [91]		1800 (6)	1240 (5)	
Maas et al [62]	1228 (68)			1502 (40)
Bond and Howlett [10]				2006 (13)
DeLeon-Jones et al [26]	1032 (21)	1069 (16)	911 (5)	1348 (21)
Joseph et al [49]				2740 (13)
Sachetti et al [86]	845 (5)	845 (5)		
Beckmann and Goodwin [5]	1540 (24)			
Sharpless [95]	1688 (20)			1884 (11)
Garfinkel et al [34]	1320 (8)		1320 (8)	1600 (10)
Schildkraut et al [93]		1950 (16)	1209 (12)	
Hollister et al [46]				1888 (17)
Sweeney et al [101]	902 (24)			
Taube et al [103]	791 (14)			
Cobbin et al [21]	1333 (35)	1046 (28)	2485 (7)	
Coppen et al [22]	1580 (23)			1680 (27)
Hollister et al [45]	2016 (17)			
Beckmann and Goodwin [6]	1544 (41)	1820 (21)	1090 (11)	1328 (15)
Tang et al [102]				1349 (6)
Potter et al [79]	1650 (70)	1790 (28)	1460 (19)	1850 (27)
Weighted means	1380 (419)	1491 (142)	1387 (67)	1701 (211)

MHPG = 3-methoxy-4-hydroxyphenylglycol.

* Values are means of micrograms of MHPG per 24-hour urine either taken directly from tables in articles or calculated from raw data. Numbers in parentheses indicate number of subjects.

strates that urinary MHPG values are consistently higher in men than in women. Comparisons within a laboratory should therefore be sex-matched. Table 11.3 presents intrastudy comparisons of unipolar and bipolar depressed patients without specifying the gender of the subject. Those that do allow for analysis by gender are indicated in Table 11.2. Because women tend to predominate among unipolars

Table 11.2 MHPG Excretion in Studies Specifying Values by Gender

Source	*Major or Primary Depression*			Normal
	All Types	*Unipolar*	*Bipolar*	*Normal*
Maas et al [63]	M(7) = 1337 F(9) = 892			
Fawcett et al [32]	M(5) = 1080 F(6) = 930			
Maas et al [62]	M(20) = 1390 F(48) = 1160			M(19) = 1670 F(21) = 1350
DeLeon-Jones et al [26]	F(21) = 1032	F(16) = 1069	F(5) = 911	F(21) = 1348
Beckmann and Goodwin [5]	M(8) = 1671 F(16) = 1474			
Joseph et al [49]				M(13) = 2740
Sachetti et al [86]	M(5) = 845	M(5) = 845		
Sharpless [95]	M(10) = 2019 F(10) = 1357			M(6) = 2105 F(5) = 1618
Hollister et al [46]				M(11) = 2071 F(6) = 1551
Sweeney et al [101]	F(24) = 902			
Taube et al [103]	F(14) = 791	F(14) = 791		F(10) = 1029
Cobbin et al [21]		M(9) = 1899 F(19) = 949	M(2) = 2335 F(5) = 2544	
Coppen et al [22]	M(10) = 1730 F(13) = 1480			M(10) = 2190 F(17) = 1370
Hollister et al [45]	M(11) = 2249 F(6) = 1590			
Beckmann and Goodwin [6]	M(10) = 1680 F(31) = 1500	M(6) = 2040 F(15) = 1430	M(2) = 1070 F(9) = 1090	M(7) = 1440 F(8) = 1230
Potter et al [79]	M(30) = 1810 F(40) = 1530	M(15) = 1890 F(13) = 1670	M(8) = 1600 F(11) = 1370	M(9) = 1890 F(18) = 1830
Weighted means	M(116) = 1668 F(238) = 1249	M(35) = 1769 F(77) = 1161	M(12) = 1634 F(30) = 1405	M(75) = 2023 F(106) = 1419

MHPG = 3-methoxy-4-hydroxyphenylglycol; M = male; F = female.

* Values are means of micrograms of MHPG per 24-hour urine either taken directly from tables in articles or calculated from raw data. Numbers in parentheses indicate number of subjects.

and excrete less MHPG than men, there is a bias to lowering the mean unipolar values. Even with this bias and including the study by Cobbin et al [21], a small difference in the urinary excretion of MHPG between unipolar and bipolar depressed patients is seen. Excluding Cobbin's results yields a more striking difference and emphasizes the agreement among the remaining three separate groups, both in their original and replication studies, that bipolars excrete less MHPG than unipolars. Because Cobbin et al [21] found mean values for MHPG excretion in bipolars

Table 11.3 MHPG in Studies Which Compare Unipolar and Bipolar Depressions

Source	*Unipolar*	*Bipolar*
Schildkraut et al [91]	1800 (6)	1240 (5)
DeLeon-Jones et al [26]	1069 (16)	911 (5)
Schildkraut et al [93]	1950 (16)	1209 (12)
Cobbin et al [21]	1046 (28)	2485 (7)
Beckmann and Goodwin [6]	1820 (21)	1090 (11)
Potter et al [79]	1790 (28)	1460 (19)
Weighted means	1537 (115)	1396 (59)
Weighted means without Cobbin	1695 (87)	1250 (52)

MHPG = 3-methoxy-4-hydroxyphenylglycol.

to be almost two times those reported by any other group, (see Table 11.1), selective exclusion of this study may be justified.

The predominant evidence, therefore, points to a true reduction of urinary MHPG excretion in bipolar depression. This would be consistent with an interpretation that total NE synthesis, release, and metabolism (turnover) is decreased during bipolar depression. Supporting this interpretation, Linnoila et al [59] found that within a group of depressed patients there is an approximate 0.90 correlation between the urinary excretion of NE and each of its three major metabolites—MHPG, NM, and VMA. As discussed in the preceding section, it is currently not possible to determine whether the primary site of abnormality is centrally or peripherally located. Furthermore, it may be an inappropriate distinction, because altered MHPG and presumably altered NE, NM, and VMA excretion can be a reflection of events that originate centrally, peripherally, or both [39].

Changes in the urinary excretion of MHPG during different clinical states also suggest alterations of NE turnover. Longitudinal studies in a small number of patients, followed by studies of different groups, show that urinary MHPG excretion is low during bipolar depression and elevated during hypomania (or mania) [11,40,48,73,91,105]. Moreover, probable drug-induced hypomania in amphetamine abusers is also associated with elevated MHPG [94]. Drugs which can produce stimulation of noradrenergic receptors can precipitate mania or hypomania [39], although altered urinary excretion of MHPG or other biochemical changes have not been documented in most cases. Thus, two lines of evidence support a view that mania involves a hyperadrenergic state: (1) urinary excretion of MHPG, a major NE metabolite, is increased in mania and hypomania; and (2) compounds which at least acutely increase stimulation of NE receptors can precipitate mania or hypomania. Recent investigations agree that plasma MHPG is increased during hypomania or mania in nonmedicated [47] as well as in medicated patients [41]. Despite the apparent agreement of studies using either urinary excretion or plasma concentrations of MHPG, when both are obtained from the same group of patients, no significant correlation between these measures has been found [100]. Moreover, plasma and urinary MHPG do not appear to correlate in the same patient studied longitudinally [47]. These failures to demonstrate such a relationship emphasize the difficulties in interpreting either urinary or plasma MHPG values in isolation and presumably reflect independent variance of the factors contributing to absolute levels of MHPG (see Methodologic Issues).

The status of CSF MHPG in affective illness has also been investigated although there are numerous problems in the interpretation of the measurements [38]. Whatever the interpretation, neither baseline nor post probenecid values of CSF MHPG are clearly altered in depression or its subtypes; CSF baseline MHPG values also do not differ between depressed patients and healthy controls [1].

Concentrations of MHPG in urine and CSF of depressed patients have been measured before and after treatment with antidepressant drugs. Whether changes are simply a function of drug treatment cannot be definitively ascertained in such patient studies, because clinical states tend to change during the time between measurements (3 to 4 weeks). There is little data to suggest, however, that changes parallel clinical improvement or deterioration. Thus, CSF MHPG has no known potential as a clinical tool.

Despite some animal studies which report increased MHPG following long-term (2-week) treatment with relatively high doses of tricyclic antidepressants [84], most clinical investigations show a decrease. For instance, treatment with nortriptyline, imipramine, desipramine, or chlorimipramine reduces MHPG in the CSF [2,3,69,76]. In some instances, the extent of reduction is significantly correlated with tricyclic concentration, which would be expected if the change were drug induced [77]. The few studies which include measurements of urinary MHPG change in patients treated with tricyclic antidepressants usually find a reduction, although the data are more variable [5,21,71]. Because all tricyclics or their active metabolites found in vivo are potent inhibitors of NE uptake, a drug-induced reduction of MHPG could be explained in at least two ways: (1) decreased uptake would decrease intraneuronal metabolism of NE to MHPG and increase extraneuronal metabolism to such metabolites as NM (see Figure 11.1); and (2) increased intrasynaptic NE secondary to decreased reuptake could produce a feedback inhibition of total NE turnover.

A recent investigation focused on the urinary excretion of NE and its three major metabolites (MHPG, NM, and VMA) in depressed patients before and after treatment with desmethylimipramine (DMI). The study showed that both of the previously discussed mechanisms can contribute to MHPG reduction—the NM/MHPG ratio is increased in all patients indicating altered metabolism away from MHPG and the total turnover (combined total production and metabolism) of NE (NE + MHPG + NM + VMA) is decreased [59].

Treatment with monoamine oxidase inhibitors (MAO-I) only decreases MHPG if the MAO-I blocks the enzyme responsible for the deamination of NE. Consistent with this expectation, CSF MHPG is reduced in patients treated with both mixed inhibitors and a specific inhibitor of MAO-A but not by a specific inhibitor of MAO-B [68]. Urinary excretion of MHPG as well as VMA is also extensively reduced (by more than 80%) by treatment with the MAO-A inhibitor, clorgyline [68]. Of greater interest is that total excretion of NE and its major metabolites is reduced by more than 50% in depressed patients [60]. As in the case of the tricyclic antidepressants, the reduction shows that there may be some feedback inhibition of NE synthesis, release, or both [59].

Thus, pharmacologic studies indicate that the major classes of drugs used in the treatment of depression influence the major metabolites of NE in a way consistent with some compensatory decrease of total turnover. The simplest interpretation is that effective intrasynaptic NE is increased by the treatments. In Chapter 12, Siever et al present a review of much more basic data consistent with this suggestion.

CLINICAL STUDIES OF NOREPINEPHRINE

The CA hypothesis of affective illness has also been tested by measuring NE itself. In general, these investigations have compared either NE concentrations in depressed patients with those in control subjects or NE concentrations in animals or human beings before and after antidepressant drug treatment. NE has been assayed in plasma, CSF, and urine, as well as in the brain. The methodologic issues involved in the collection of samples for assaying NE and the interpretation of NE concentrations are reviewed previously in this chapter in Methodologic Issues and elsewhere in this volume (see Chapter 1).

Most animal studies have measured levels of NE in the brain, omitting CSF which is often studied in human beings. Direct comparison might be possible with the few human studies using postmortem brains. In the hypothesis relating the etiology of depression to noradrenergic function, it is generally assumed that the neurotransmitter deficit must occur at synapses within the CNS. Because the blood-brain barrier is relatively impermeable to NE [108], but relatively permeable to MHPG, measures of NE in the CSF may better reflect brain noradrenergic activity. Even if NE in the CSF turns out to reflect brain noradrenergic activity, it is unlikely that NE concentrations per se will prove to be a marker of psychiatric illness because major physiologic processes are linked to NE. This point is elaborated in the following discussion.

Analogously, levels of plasma NE have been seen as indicators of SNS activity [56]. However, as already mentioned, central and peripheral noradrenergic function seem to be anatomically and physiologically related [39]. For example, there are noradrenergic inputs onto brainstem nuclei which influence sympathetic outflow, and the local application of CA in these regions can markedly influence blood pressure [30]. This may help explain the finding that in human beings there is a stronger correlation between blood pressure and CSF NE than between blood pressure and plasma NE [53]. Conversely, levels of plasma NE may provide important insights into aspects of central noradrenergic activity.

NE levels have been measured in a number of nonpsychiatric illnesses (most of these data are reported and discussed in this volume). Studies have also been designed to establish whether levels of NE in patients with affective disorders are abnormal. Using a radioenzymatic assay for NE and epinephrine (E), the combined resting plasma CA level in a heterogeneous group of depressed patients was significantly greater than that in a control population [106]. Separate determinations of the levels of NE and E in the patient group showed that each was elevated over the mean value found in the control subjects. The total plasma CA level correlated positively with the degree of anxiety, and it tended to parallel clinical improvement. The finding of elevated plasma NE in patients with a range of depressive diagnoses was confirmed in a subsequent study [55]. There is much scatter in the data, however, and a direct relationship to depression has not been demonstrated.

In a study of CSF NE in patients with affective illnesses, a higher level of NE existed in both depressed and manic patients compared with a control group with a neurologic disorder [27]. Post et al [74] observed a higher mean NE level in patients during mania than during depression. However, they found no significant difference between the level of CSF NE in the depressed state and that in the control condition. Christensen et al [20], also using a radioenzymatic assay, confirmed that a group of patients with unipolar or bipolar depression had normal CSF NE levels. In the same patients, however, they observed a reduced concentration of CSF E, which increased with clinical improvement. It is difficult to interpret these observations.

CSF studies in which fluid samples are obtained by standard lumbar puncture are not as well standardized as studies of plasma NE; for example, the subjects may not have had the same degree of habituation to the stress of needle insertion, and a fixed period of time may not have elapsed between the insertion of the needle and the collection of the sample. Depending on the magnitude and the latency of the response of the CSF NE level to the lumbar puncture procedure itself, measurements made in various clinical states might reflect differential responsiveness to a stressor rather than physiologic processes fundamental to particular affective states. Furthermore, the gradient that exists for CSF NE with later samples showing higher NE levels than initial samples provides an additional source of variance [109]. Given all of these factors and the either modest or inconsistent abnormalities of NE, it appears very unlikely that CSF measures of this neurotransmitter will have clinical utility in the near future.

There have also been reports of integrated urinary measures of CA in patients with affective disorders. An early study showed that patients with neurotic depressive reactions had normal urinary levels of NE and E [28]. Subsequently, the concentrations of both NE and E were reported to be higher in a group with psychotic depressive reactions than in a group with neurotic depressive reactions [15]. There have been several attempts to sequentially monitor urinary CA in patients cycling between depression and mania; there is evidence that the level of urinary NE rises before the switch into mania and remains elevated in the manic state (see Figure 12.1 in Chapter 12) [16,75].

As previously noted, another paradigm which has been used in studying the importance of NE levels in affective illness has been the measurement of CA levels in brain tissue, plasma, or CSF before and after short- or long-term antidepressant drug treatment and electroconvulsive therapy (ECT). Rats given a single dose of imipramine, protriptyline, or DMI showed no change in the level of brain NE, whereas rats treated with any of these drugs for a period of 3 weeks had a significantly lower level of brain NE compared to controls [89]. A subsequent study indicated that the level of NE in rat brain declined after 1 week of treatment with DMI [67]. Monkeys receiving imipramine over a long period of time had increased CSF NE within 24 hours of the beginning of drug administration, and again during the period of drug withdrawal [58]. There has been particular interest in documenting the biochemical changes which occur after the long-term administration of the antidepressant drugs, because the therapeutic effect in humans is typically not manifested until the second or third week of treatment.

If the antidepressant drugs have a common mode of action involving the alteration of the level of an endogenous CA, it might be expected that the effects of MAO-I, lithium, or ECT would parallel those of the tricyclic compounds. The administration of pargyline to rabbits, however, led to a rise in brain NE after a single dose and to a further rise after repeated doses [99]. Phenelzine, tranylcypromine, and clorgyline, administered over a long period of time to rats, produced initial elevations of brain NE and a subsequent decline toward baseline [17]. Animal studies do not, of course, necessarily predict what will happen in human beings.

The effects of the antidepressant drugs on CA levels have been investigated in human beings, mainly following tricyclic compounds. An increment in plasma NE has been demonstrated in eneuretic boys treated for 13 days with imipramine (see Chapter 9). There is evidence, though, that the tricyclic drugs can produce different physiologic effects in children than in adults. In particular, there seems to be an elevation of diastolic blood pressure in children rather than the systolic hypotension often described in older depressed patients [35,54]. Because NE released during activation of the SNS is significantly involved in blood pressure regulation, and because the plasma NE level reflects the degree of sympathetic activity, the question arises as to whether a comparable effect of the tricyclic drugs on the plasma NE level can be observed in the older population, which generally tends to receive these compounds. Nonetheless, young adults also show elevated NE and diastolic blood pressure after another tricyclic antidepressant, desipramine [85], and middle-aged depressed adults treated with imipramine, doxepin, or amitriptyline had elevated NE without significant changes in blood pressure [104]. It might also be speculated that there is a differential response among diagnostic subgroups. Conceivably this could explain the findings of unchanged plasma NE in depressed outpatients treated with amitriptyline [83].

There have been several studies on the effects of MAO-I on CA levels in human beings. Postmortem brain specimens from elderly, terminally ill patients treated over a long period of time with various MAO-I showed elevated hypothalamic NE concentrations [7]. Depressed patients treated for at least 4 weeks with the relatively specific MAO-A inhibitors, pargyline and clorgyline, had a decrement in the mean plasma NE level with no change in the mean CSF level [68]. Depressed patients treated with the less specific drug, phenelzine, also had a decrease in the mean plasma NE concentration [83]. It should be noted that effective antidepressants can either elevate (tricyclics) or lower (MAO-I) plasma NE; obviously this variable cannot be used as an index of therapeutic effect.

Lithium, administered either over a long or short period of time to rats, had little or no effect on NE levels in the brain [8,23,44,73]. Few studies involving ECT administration to animals have included determinations of CA levels. There are several reports of an increase in brain NE or presumed NE release following a single shock [29,31]. There are also studies describing an increase in brain NE following long-term treatment with ECT [29,50]. A decrease, or no significant change, in brain NE has also been noted [12,43]. One study of patients receiving ECT demonstrated increases in plasma NE and E within minutes of the procedures [72]. As mentioned in the discussion, Clinical Studies Antedating Measures of Norepinephrine, human studies measuring the effect of drugs on a biochemical variable must consider the confounding effect of altered clinical state. Even without this problem, it does not appear likely that measures of NE alone in any tissue will yield valuable information on the effects of lithium or ECT.

To conclude this section, we return to the evidence that at least some groups of patients within the range of major depressive disorders have elevated plasma NE under the probably stressful conditions of study. Under conditions of rest, depressed patients may not show elevated NE [104]. Possibly because of confounding sources of variance, comparable studies done on CSF have not yielded consistent results. Assuming that no difference exists between depressed patients and normal controls in the rate of clearance of NE from the plasma (through either neuronal or extraneuronal uptake) the increased concentration of circulating NE in depressed patients probably reflects an increased spillover of NE from the sympathetic neuroeffector junction to the plasma compartment. If the NE concentration gradient from the neuroeffector region to the plasma remains constant, changes in the concentration of circulating NE could reflect changes in the actual intrajunctional concentration of NE. The general validity of this assumption has been questioned [13], but not in relationship to variables which are likely to pertain to dysthymic states. Thus, depression may be characterized by peripheral adrenergic hyperactivity in response to normal stressors. Support for this hypothesis is provided by the observation that patients with affective disorders may display a marked tachycardia [55].

The relevance of biochemical and physiologic observations made in the periphery to central noradrenergic function, which presumably relates more directly to the pathophysiology of depression, remains to be elucidated. Possibly noradrenergic synapses in the CNS of depressed patients contain an increased concentration of intrasynaptic NE. This would not be predicted by the CA hypothesis of affective illness previously mentioned. If there is general hyperactivity of noradrenergic function in depression, the ability of MAO-I antidepressants to lower plasma NE might be seen as consistent. However, as previously noted, the administration of two tricyclic antidepressants has been associated with either a rise in the plasma NE level or no significant change. The interpretation of these direct measures of circulatory NE remains open. It is hoped that a more functional measure such as the release of NE in response to stress will better distinguish subgroups of patients or patients from controls or both. Such a possibility is currently under investigation.

CONCLUSIONS

It should be apparent that no general statement concerning the role of altered noradrenergic function in affective illness is possible on the basis of existing data. Direct measures of NE discussed in Clinical Studies Antedating Measures of Norepinephrine do not provide any evidence of a deficit; if anything, they point to a hyperactivity of noradrenergic function in at least some forms of depressive illness. In contrast, measurement of metabolites of NE, especially MHPG, indicate that, at least in bipolar patients, noradrenergic function is decreased in depression and increased in mania. The pharmacologic evidence is confusing because antidepressants, depending on their type and on the subject population, are reported to both increase and decrease NE, its metabolites, or both. It may ultimately be found that most antidepressants decrease total NE turnover, presumably because they increase functional intrasynaptic NE with feedback inhibition of synthesis [59]. Future studies must account for multiple sources of variance, with special emphasis on age, gender, and diagnosis, and must be designed to assess whether alterations in NE or its metabolites reflect changes in intrasynaptic NE, total turnover, clearance, or metabolism. With such data, it will be possible to answer whether overall noradrenergic function is increased or decreased and in what subgroups of affective illness. Knowing this will not sufficiently clarify whether altered noradrenergic function plays a causal role in affective illness but it may permit specification of clinical experiments which would provide a real test of the "CA hypothesis."

We continue to view the applications of all of these measures as appropriate to clinical experiments and *not* to clinical practice. The use of such biochemical measures as urinary MHPG in the diagnosis and treatment of affective illness would appear premature. Despite dramatic success in such areas as differentiating types of "idiopathic" hypotension with NE measures, we must realize that our ability to biochemically subtype the major chronic, variable, and recurrent syndromes of hypertension and depression is rudimentary. There is no question that NE is somehow involved but at what level remains an object of active research.

REFERENCES

1. Asberg M, Bertilsson L, Thoren P, Traskman L. CSF Monoamine Metabolites in Depressive Illness. In Depressive Disorders, S Garattini (ed), 293–335. FK Schattaner Verlag Stuttgait, 1978.
2. Asberg M, Bertilsson L, Tuck D, Cronholm B, Sjoquist F. Indoleamine metabolites in the cerebrospinal fluid of depressed patients before and during treatment with nortriptyline. Clin Pharmacol Ther 14:277–286, 1973.

3. Asberg M, Ringberger VA, Sjoquist F, Thoren P, Traskman L, Tuck RJ. Monoamine metabolites in cerebrospinal fluid and serotonin uptake inhibition during treatment with chlorimipramine. Clin Pharmacol Ther 21:201–207, 1977.
4. Axelrod J. Noradrenaline: fate and control of its biosynthesis. Science 173:598–606, 1971.
5. Beckmann H, Goodwin, FK. Antidepressant response to tricyclics and urinary MHPG in unipolar patients. Arch Gen Psychiatry 32:17–22, 1975.
6. Beckmann H, Goodwin FK. Urinary MHPG in subgroups of depressed patients and normal controls. Neuropsychobiology 6:91–100, 1980.
7. Bevan Jones AB, Pare CMB, Nicholson WJ, Price K, Stacey RS. Brain amine concentrations after monoamine oxidase inhibitor administration. Br Med J 1:17–19, 1972.
8. Bliss EL, Ailion J. The effect of lithium upon brain neuroamines. Brain Res 24:305–310, 1970.
9. Blombery PA, Kopin IJ, Gordon EK, Markey SP, Ebert MH. Conversion of MHPG to vanillylmandelic acid. Arch Gen Psychiatry 37:1095–1098, 1980.
10. Bond PA, Howlett DK. Measurement of the two conjugates of 3-methoxy-4-hydroxyphenylglycol in urine. Biochem Med 10:219–228, 1974.
11. Bond PA, Jenner JA, Sampson DA. Daily variation of the urine content of 3-methoxy-4-hydroxyphenylglycol in two manic-depressive patients. Psychol Med 2:81–85, 1972.
12. Breitner C, Picchioni A, Chin L. Neurohormone levels in brain after CNS stimulation including electrotherapy. J Neuropsychiatry 5:153–158, 1964.
13. Brown MJ, Lhoste FJM, Zamboulis C, Ind PW, Jenner DA, Dollery CT. Estimation of sympathetic activity in essential hypertension. Clin Pharmacol Ther 31:16–22, 1982.
14. Bunney WE, Jr., Davis JM. Norepinephrine in depressive reactions: A review. Arch Gen Psychiatry 13:483–494, 1965.
15. Bunney WE, Jr., Davis JM, Weil-Malherbe H, Smith ERB. Biochemical changes in psychotic depression. Arch Gen Psychiatry 16:448–460, 1967.
16. Bunney WE, Jr., Goodwin FK, Murphy DL, House KM, Gordon EK. The "switch process" in manic-depressive illness. II. Relationship of catecholamines, REM sleep, and drugs. Arch Gen Psychiatry 27:304–309, 1972.
17. Campbell IC, Murphy DL, Gallager DW, Tallman JF, Marshall EF. Neurotransmitter-Related Adaptation in the Central Nervous System Following Chronic Monoamine Oxidase Inhibition. In Monoamine Oxidase: Structure, Function, and Altered Functions, TP Singer RW Von Korff, Murphy DL (eds), 517–530. New York: Academic Press, 1979.
18. Carlsson A, Corrodi H, Fuxe K, Hokfelt T. Effect of some antidepressant drugs on the depletion of intraneural brain catecholamine stores caused by 4-alpha-dimethyl-meta-tyramine. Eur J Pharmacol 5:367–373, 1969.
19. Carlsson A, Rosengren E, Bertler A, Nilsson J. Effect of Reserpine on the Metabolism of Catecholamines. In Psychotropic Drugs, S Garrattini and V Ghetti (eds), 363–372. Amsterdam: Elsevier, 1957.
20. Christensen NJ, Vestersaard P, Sirensen T, Rafaelsen OJ. Cerebrospinal fluid adrenaline and noradrenaline in depressed patients. Acta Psychiatr Scand 61:178–182, 1980.
21. Cobbin DM, Requin-Blow B, Williams LR, Williams WO. Urinary MHPG levels and tricyclic antidepressant drug selection. Arch Gen Psychiatry 36:1111–1115, 1979.
22. Coppen A, Roma Roo VA, Ruthuen CRJ, Goodwin BL, Sandler M. Urinary 4-hydroxy-3-methoxyphenylglycol is not a predictor for clinical response to amitriptyline in depressive illness. Psychopharmacology (Berlin) 64:95–97, 1979.

23. Corrodi H, Fuxe K, Hokfelt T, Schou M. The effect of lithium on cerebral monoamine neurons. Psychopharmacologia (Berlin) 11:345–353, 1967.
24. Corrodi H, Fuxe K, Schou M. The effect of prolonged lithium administration on cerebral monoamine neurons in the rat. Life Sci 8:643–651, 1969.
25. Dekirmenjian H, Maas JW. An improved procedure of 3-methoxy-4-hydroxy-phenylethylene glycol determination by gas liquid chromatography. Anal Biochem 35:113–122, 1970.
26. DeLeon-Jones FD, Maas JW, Dekirmenjian H, Sanchez J. Diagnostic subgroups of affective disorders and their urinary excretion of catecholamine metabolites. Am J Psychiatry 132:1141–1148, 1975.
27. Dencker SJ, Haggendal J, Malm U. Noradrenaline content of cerebrospinal fluid in mental diseases. Lancet 2:754, 1966.
28. Drujan BD, Sourkes TL, Layne DS, Murphy GF. The differential determination of catecholamines in urine. Can J Biochem Physiol 37:1153–1159, 1959.
29. Ebert MH, Baldessarini RJ, Lipinski JF, Beru K. Effects of electroconvulsive seizures on amine metabolism in the brain. Arch Gen Psychiatry 29:397–401, 1973.
30. Elliott JM. The central noradrenergic control of blood pressure and heart rate. Clin Exp Pharmacol Physiol 6:569–579, 1979.
30a. Essler M, Turbott J, Schwarz R, Leonard P, Bobik A, Skews H, Jackson G. The peripheral kinetics of norepinephrine in depressive illness. Arch Gen Psychiatry 39:295–300, 1982.
31. Essman WB. Neurochemical changes in ECS and ECT. Semin Psychiatry 4:55–65, 1972.
32. Fawcett J, Maas JW, Dekirmenjian H. Depression and MHPG excretion. Arch Gen Psychiatry 26:246–251, 1972.
33. FitzGerald GA, Hossman V, Hamilton C, Davies D, Reid J, Dollery CT. Interindividual variation in the kinetics of infused norepinephrine. Clin Pharmacol Ther 26:669–675, 1979.
34. Garfinkel PE, Warsh JJ, Stancer HC, Goelse DD. CNS monoamine metabolism in bipolar affective disorder. Arch Gen Psychiatry 34:735–739, 1977.
35. Glassman AH, Bigger JT, Giardina EV, Kantor SJ, Perel JM, Davies M. Clinical characteristics of imipramine-induced orthostatic hypotension. Lancet 1:468–472, 1979.
36. Glowinski J, Axelrod J. Inhibition of uptake of tritiated noradrenaline in the intact rat brain by imipramine and structurally related compounds. Nature 204:1318–1319, 1964.
37. Goodwin FK, Beckmann H. Urinary MHPG in unipolar and bipolar affective disorders. Sci Proc Am Psychiatr Assoc 128:96–97, 1975.
38. Goodwin FK, Post RM. Studies of Amine Metabolites in Affective Illness and in Schizophrenia: A Comparative Analysis. In Biology of the Major Psychoses, DX Freedman (ed), vol. 54, 299–332. New York: Raven Press, 1975.
39. Goodwin FK, Potter WZ. Noradrenergic Function in Affective Illness. In Neuro-Psychopharmacology, B Saletu (ed), 127–137. Proceedings of the 11th Collegium Internationale Neuro-Psychopharmacologium (CINP) Congress. New York: Pergamon Press, 1979.
40. Gordon EK, Greenspan K, Schildkraut JJ, Baer L, Aronoff MS, Durell J. Catecholamine metabolism in affective disorders: III. MHPG and other catecholamine metabolites in patients treated with lithium carbonate. J Psychiatry Res 7:171–183, 1970.

41. Halaris AE. Plasma 3-methoxy-4-hydroxyphenylglycol in manic psychosis. Am J Psychiatry 135:493–494, 1978.
42. Halter JB, Pflug AE, Tolas AG. Arterial-venous difference of plasma catecholamines in man. Metabolism 29:9–12, 1980.
43. Hinesley RK, Norton JA, Aprison MH. Serotonin, norepinephrine and 3,4-dihydroxyphenylethylamine in rat brain parts following electroconvulsive shock. J Psychiatry Res 6:143–152, 1968.
44. Ho AKS, Loh HH, Craves F, Hitzemann RJ, Gershon S. The effect of prolonged lithium treatment on the synthesis rate and turnover of monoamines in brain regions of rats. Eur J Pharmacol 10:72–78, 1970.
45. Hollister LE, Davis KL, Berger PA. Subtypes of depression based on excretion of MHPG and response to nortriptyline. Arch Gen Psychiatry 37:1107–1110, 1980.
46. Hollister LE, Davis KL, Overall JE, Anderson T. Excretion of MHPG in normal subjects. Arch Gen Psychiatry 35:1410–1415, 1978.
47. Jimerson DC, Nurnberger JI, Post RM, Gershon ES, Kopin IJ. Plasma MHPG in rapid-cyclers and healthy twins. Arch Gen Psychiatry 38:1287–1290, 1981.
48. Jones FD, Maas FJ, Dekirmenjian M, Fawcett JA. Urinary catecholamine metabolites during behavioral changes in a patient with manic-depressive cycles. Science 179:300–302, 1973.
49. Joseph MH, Baker HF, Johnstone EL, Crow TJ. Determination of 3-methoxy-4-hydroxyphenylglycol conjugates in urine. Application to the study of central noradrenaline metabolism in unmedicated chronic schizophrenic patients. Psychopharmacology (Berlin) 51:47–51, 1976.
50. Kety SS, Javoy F, Thierry A, Julou L, Glowinski J. A sustained effect of electroconvulsive shock on the turnover of norepinephrine in the central nervous system of the rat. Proc Natl Acad Sci USA 58:1249–1254, 1967.
51. Kopin IJ. Assessing Norepinephrine Metabolism in Human Brain: Past, Present and Future. In Psychiatry and the Biology of the Human Brain: A Symposium Dedicated to Seymour S Kety, S Matthysse (ed), 89–101. Amsterdam: Elsevier North Holland, 1981.
52. Kopin IJ, Gordon EK. Metabolism of administered and drug-released norepinephrine 7-H3 in rat. J Pharmacol Exp Ther 140: 207–219, 1963.
53. Lake CR, Gullner H-G, Polinsky RJ, Ebert MH, Ziegler MG, Bartter FC. Essential hypertension: Central and peripheral norepinephrine. Science 211:955–957, 1981.
54. Lake CR, Mikkelsen EJ, Rapoport JL, Zavadil AP, Kopin IJ. Effect of imipramine on norepinephrine and blood pressure in enuretic boys. Clin Pharmacol Ther 26:647–653, 1979.
55. Lake CR, Pickar D, Ziegler MG, Lipper S, Slater S, Murphy DL. High plasma norepinephrine levels in patients with major affective disorders. Am J Psychiatry 139:1315–1318, 1982.
56. Lake CR, Ziegler MG, Kopin IJ. Use of plasma norepinephrine for evaluation of sympathetic neuronal function in man. Life Sci 18:1315–1326, 1976.
57. Lemieux G, Dangnon A, Genest J. Depressive states during Rauwolfia therapy for arterial hypertension: a report of 30 cases. Can Med Assoc J 74:522–526, 1956.
58. Lerner P, Major LF, Ziegler M, Dendel PS, Ebert MH. Central noradrenergic adaptation to long-term treatment with imipramine in rhesus monkeys. Brain Res 200:220–224, 1980.
59. Linnoila M, Karoum F, Calil HM, Kopin IJ, Potter WZ. Alteration of norepinephrine

metabolism with desipramine and zimelidine in depressed patients. Arch Gen Psychiatry 39:1025–1028, 1982.

60. Linnoila M, Karoum F, Potter WZ. Effect of low-dose clorgyline on 24-hour urinary monoamine excretion in patients with rapidly cycling bipolar affective disorder. Arch Gen Psychiatry 39:513–516, 1982.
61. Linnoila M, Karoum F, Potter WZ. High correlation of norepinephrine and its major metabolite excretion rates. Arch Gen Psychiatry 39:521–523, 1982.
62. Maas JW, Dekirmenjian H, Jones F. The Identification of Depressed Patients Who Have a Disorder of NE Metabolism and/or Disposition. In Frontiers in Catecholamine Research, E Usdin and S Synder (eds), 1091–1096. New York: Pergamon Press, 1973.
63. Maas JW, Fawcett JA, Dekirmenjian H. 3-Methoxy-4-hydroxyphenylglycol (MHPG) excretion in depressive states: A pilot study. Arch Gen Psychiatry 19:129–134, 1968.
64. Maas JW, Hattox SE, Greene NM, Landis DH. 3-Methoxy-4-hydroxyphenylglycol production by human brain in vivo. Science 205:1025–1029, 1979.
65. Maas JW, Landis H, Dekirmenjian H. The occurrence of free versus conjugated MHPG in non-human and human primate brain. Psychopharmacol Commun 2:403–410, 1976.
66. Mardh G, Sjoquist B, Anggard E. Norepinephrine metabolism in man using deuterium labelling: The conversion of 4-hydroxy-3-methoxyphenylglycol to 4-hydroxy-3-methoxy mandelic acid. J Neurochem 36:1181–1185, 1981.
67. McMillen BA, Warnack W, German DC, Shore PA. Effects of chronic desipramine treatment on rat brain noradrenergic responses to α-adrenergic drugs. Eur J Pharmacol 61:239–246, 1980.
68. Murphy DL, Pickar D, Jimerson D, Cohen RM, Garrick NA, Karoum F, and Wyatt RJ. Biochemical Indices of the Effect of the Selective MAO Inhibitors, Clorgyline, Pargyline and Deprenyl in Man. In Clinical Pharmacology in Psychiatry, E Usdin, SG Dahl, LF Gram, and O Lingjaerde (eds), 307–316. London: Macmillan, 1981.
69. Muscettola G, Goodwin FK, Potter WZ, Claeys MM, Markey SP. Imipramine and desipramine in plasma and spinal fluid. Relationship to clinical response and serotonin metabolism. Arch Gen Psychiatry 35:621–625, 1978.
70. Muscettola G, Potter WZ, Gordon EK, Goodwin FK. Methodological issues in the measurement of urinary MHPG. Psychiatry Res 4:267–276, 1981.
71. Perry GF, Fitzsimmons B, Shapiro L, Irwin P. Clinical study of mianserin, imipramine, and placebo in depression. Br J Clin Pharmacol 5:355–415, 1978.
72. Pina-Cabral JM, Rodrigues C. Blood catecholamine levels, factor VIII and fibrinolysis after therapeutic electroshock. Br J Haematol 28:371–380, 1974.
73. Poitou P, Bohuon C. Catecholamine metabolism in the rat brain after short- and long-term lithium administration. J Neurochem 25:535–537, 1975.
74. Post RM, Lake CR, Jimerson DC, Bunney WE, Wood JH, Ziegler MG, Goodwin FK. Cerebrospinal fluid norepinephrine in affective illness. Am J Psychiatry 135:907–912, 1978.
75. Post RM, Stoddard FJ, Gillin JC, Buchsbaum MS, Runkle DC, Black KE, Bunney WE. Alterations in motor activity, sleep, and biochemistry in a cycling manic-depressive patient. Arch Gen Psychiatry 34:470–477, 1977.
76. Potter WZ, Calil HM, Extein I, Gold PW, Wehr TA, Goodwin FK. Specific norepinephrine and serontonin uptake inhibitors in man: a cross-over study with pharmacokinetic, biochemical, neuroendocrine and behavioral parameters. Acta Psychiatr Scand 63[Suppl 290]: 152–165, 1981.

77. Potter WZ, Calil HM, Zavadil AP, Jusko WJ, Sutfin T, Rapoport JL, Goodwin FK. Steady-state concentrations of hydroxylated metabolites of tricyclic antidepressants in patients: relationship to clinical effect. Psychopharmacol Bull 16:32–34, 1980.
78. Potter WZ, Muscettola G, Goodwin FK. Sources of Variance in Clinical Studies of MHPG. In MHPG: Basic Mechanisms and Psychopathology, JW Maas (ed), 145–165. New York: Academic Press, 1983.
79. Potter WZ, Muscettola G, Pickar D, Goodwin FK. Unpublished data, 1983.
80. Powis G. The binding of catecholamines to human serum proteins. Biochem Pharmacol 24:707–712, 1975.
81. Prange AJ, Jr. The pharmacology and biochemistry of depression. Dis Nerv Syst 25:217–221, 1964.
82. Quetsch RM, Achor RWP, Litin EM, Fawcett RL. Depressive reactions in hypertensive patients: a comparison of those treated with Rauwolfia and those receiving no specific antihypertensive treatment. Circulation 19:366–375, 1959.
83. Robinson DS, Johnson GA, Corcella J, Nies A, Howard D, Cooper TB. Plasma 3,4-dihydroxyphenylglycol, catecholamines, and antidepressant drug levels during treatment of depression. Clin Pharmacol Ther 29:277, 1981.
84. Roffman M, Kling MA, Cassens G, Orsulak PJ, Reigle TG, Schildkraut JJ. The effects of acute and chronic administration of tricyclic antidepressants of MHPG-SO_4 in rat brain. Psychopharmacol Commun 1:195–206, 1977.
85. Ross RJ, Zavadil AP, III, Calil HM, Linnoila M, Kitanaka I, Blombery P, Kopin IJ, Potter WZ. Effects of desmethylimipramine on plasma norepinephrine, pulse and blood pressure. Clin Pharmacol Ther 33:429–437, 1983.
86. Sachetti E, Smeraldi E, Cagnasso M, Biondi PA, Bellodi L. MHPG, amitriptyline and affective disorders: a longitudinal study. Int Pharmacopsychiatry 11:157–162, 1976.
87. Schanberg SM, Schildkraut JJ, Breese GR, Kopin IJ. Metabolism of norepinephrine-H^3 in rat brain. Identification of conjugated 3-methoxy-4-hydroxyphenylglycol as the major metabolite. Biochem Pharmacol 17:247–254, 1968.
88. Schildkraut JJ. The catecholamine hypothesis of affective disorders: a review of supporting evidence. Am J Psychiatry 122:509–522, 1965.
89. Schildkraut JJ. Norepinephrine Metabolism after Short- and Long-Term Administration of Tricyclic Antidepressant Drugs and Electroconvulsive Shock. In Neurobiological Mechanisms of Adaptation and Behavior, AJ Mandell (ed), 137–153. New York: Raven Press, 1975.
90. Schildkraut JJ, Green R, Gordon EK, Darrell J. Normetanephrine excretion and affective state in depressed patients treated with imipramine. Am J Psychiatry 123:690–700, 1966.
91. Schildkraut JJ, Keeler BA, Grob EL, Kantrowich J, Kartmann E. MHPG excretion and clinical classification in depressive disorders. Lancet 1:1251–1252, 1973.
92. Schildkraut JJ, Orsulak PJ, Gudeman JG, Schatzberg AF, Rohde WA, LaBrie RA, Cahill JF, Cole JO, Frazier SA. Norepinephrine Metabolism in Depressive Disorders: Implications for a Biochemical Classification of Depressives. In Depression, Biology, Psychodynamics and Treatment, JO Cole, AF Schatzberg, and SA Frazier (eds), 75–101. New York: Plenum Press, 1978.
93. Schildkraut JJ, Orsulak PJ, Schatzberg AF, Gudeman JE, Cole JO, Rohde WA, LaBrie RA. Toward a biochemical classification of depressive disorders. Arch Gen Psychiatry 35:1427–1433, 1978.
94. Schildkraut JJ, Watson R, Draskoczy PR, Hartmann E. Amphetamine withdrawal: depression and MHPG excretion. Lancet 2:485–486, 1971.

95. Sharpless NS. Determination of 3-methoxy-4-hydroxyphenylglycol in urine and the effect of diet on its excretion. Res Commun Chem Pathol Pharmacol 18:257–273, 1977.
96. Shaw DM, O'Keefe R, MacSweeney DA, Brooksbank BWL, Noguera R, Coppen A. 3-Methoxy-4-hydroxyphenylglycol in depression. Psychol Med 3:333–336, 1973.
97. Shore PA, Brodie BB. Influence of Various Drugs on Serotonin and Norepinephrine in the Brain. In Psychotropic Drugs, S Garattini and V Ghetti (eds), 423–427. Amsterdam: Elsevier, 1957.
98. Silverberg AB, Skah SD, Haymond MW, Cryer PS. Norepinephrine: hormone and neurotransmitter in man. Am J Physiol 234:252–256, 1978.
99. Spector S, Hirsch CW, Brodie BB. Association of behavioral effects of pargyline, a non-hydrazide MAO inhibitor with increase in brain norepinephrine. Int J Neuropharmacol 2:81–93, 1963.
100. Sweeney DR, Leckman JF, Maas JW, Hattox S, Heninger GR. Plasma free and conjugated MHPG in psychiatric patients. A pilot study. Arch Gen Psychiatry 37:1100–1103, 1980.
101. Sweeney DR, Maas JW, Heninger GR. State anxiety, physical activity, and urinary 3-methoxy-4-hydroxyphenethyleneglycol excretion. Arch Gen Psychiatry 35:1418–1423, 1978.
102. Tang SW, Stancer HC, Takahashi S, Shephard RJ, Warsh JJ. Controlled exercise elevates plasma but not urinary MHPG and VMA. Psychiatry Res 4:12–20, 1981.
103. Taube SL, Kirstein LS, Sweeney DR, Heninger GR, Maas JW. Urinary 3-methoxy-4-hydroxyphenlyglycol and psychiatric diagnosis. Am J Psychiatry 135:78–82, 1978.
104. Veith RC, Raskind MA, Barnes RF, Gunbrecht G, Ritchie JL, Halter JB. Tricyclic antidepressants and supine, standing, and exercise plasma norepinephrine levels. Clin Pharmacol Ther 33:763–769, 1983.
105. Wehr TA. Phase and biorhythm studies in affective illness. In WE Bunney, Jr. (moderator), The switch process in manic-depressive psychosis. Ann Intern Med 87:319–335, 1977.
106. Wyatt RJ, Portnoy B, Kupfer DJ, Snyder F, Engelman K. Resting plasma catecholamine concentrations in patients with depression and anxiety. Arch Gen Psychiatry 24:65–70, 1971.
107. Young JB, Rowe JW, Pallotta JA, Sparrow D, Landsberg L. Enhanced plasma norepinephrine response to upright posture and oral glucose administration in elderly human subjects. Metabolism 29:532–539, 1980.
108. Ziegler MG, Lake CR, Wood JH, Brooks BR, Ebert MH. Relationship between norepinephrine in blood and cerebrospinal fluid in the presence of a blood-cerebrospinal fluid barrier for norepinephrine. J Neurochem 28:677–679, 1977.
109. Ziegler MG, Wood JH, Lake CR, Kopin IJ. Norepinephrine and 3-methoxy-4-hydroxyphenylglycol gradients in human cerebrospinal fluid. Am J Psychiatry 134:565–568, 1977.

12

Norepinephrine in the Affective Disorders: Receptor Assessment Strategies

Larry J. Siever
Thomas W. Uhde
William Z. Potter
Dennis L. Murphy

Classic pharmacologic approaches have provided an extensive but controversial body of evidence indicating alterations in monoamine availability in affective disorders [134, Chapter 11]. However, investigation during the last decade has been increasingly devoted to evaluation of monoamine receptor alterations in the net functional activity of neurotransmitter systems in the affective disorders and their treatments. Changes in receptor responsiveness are hypothesized to play a role in the etiology of depression [7,13,25,30,141,142,144] and mania [13], as well as in the mechanisms of action of antidepressant medications [21,142,149,166].

We review the evidence for hypotheses implicating noradrenergic receptor dysfunction in the affective disorders, with particular attention to clinical studies which shed light on this relatively new area (Table 12.1).

METHODOLOGIES

There are many techniques with which to evaluate receptor function in preclinical studies including receptor-binding assays, single-cell recordings, and measurement of the production of receptor "second messenger" substances such as cyclic adenosine 3',5'-monophosphate (cAMP).

The first approach consists of a direct determination of receptor number and affinity in specific tissues obtained by measuring the degree to which receptor agonists or antagonists compete with radiolabeled ligands for receptor-binding sites [155]. In the second approach, alterations in the firing rates of well-defined neuronal populations in response to local application of exogenous pharmacologic agents may provide information about the responsiveness of the receptors on which these

Table 12.1 Approaches to the Study of Receptor Responsiveness in Psychiatric Patients

I. Peripheral Receptors
  A. Tissue-Binding Studies
    1. Platelet
    2. Leukocyte
    3. Lymphocyte
    4. Adipocyte
    5. Fibroblast
  B. Pharmacologic Challenge
    1. Tyramine
    2. Norepinephrine
    3. Phenylephrine
II. Central Receptors
  A. Tissue-Binding Studies: Postmortem Studies
  B. Pharmacologic Challenge
    1. Amphetamine
    2. L-Dopa
    3. Insulin-induced Hypoglycemia
    4. Desmethylimipramine
    5. Clonidine

agents act [1]. In the third approach, the production of chemical messengers such as cAMP in response to pharmacologic agents may be measured in vitro or in vivo. As the generation of such substances is coupled to receptor activation [61], inferences may be made regarding the responsiveness of the mediating receptor. Such approaches lend themselves to preclinical studies of pharmacologically induced alterations in receptor responsiveness.

The clinical application of such methodologies is more problematic, particularly if an assessment of central receptors is desired (see Table 12.1). Central nervous system (CNS) tissue is not available for such techniques except in postmortem brain studies, which are restricted by considerations of availability and deterioration secondary to storage. Furthermore, in the case of the affective disorders, such studies would be further complicated by difficulties with diagnosis and effects of prior medication. For these reasons, postmortem studies focusing on receptors have not been reported in depressed patients. Peripheral tissues such as platelets [74], lymphocytes [189], leukocytes [52], fibroblasts [93], and adipose tissue [171] also have receptors similar in character to those observed centrally. Thus, both binding and cAMP generation can be measured in vitro from samples of these human tissues.

Another approach that has been successful in exploring receptor function in the affective disorders is the pharmacologic challenge strategy [125,144]. In this method, a pharmacologic agent that directly or indirectly stimulates neurotransmitter receptors is administered to patients, and specific neuroendocrine, biochemical, physiologic, or behavioral responses to the challenge are evaluated. These responses may provide an indirect index of receptor responsiveness in patients with affective disorders and may be used to evaluate possible effects of antidepressant medications on the relevant receptors. Evidence from these lines of investigation are reviewed in the following discussion.

TISSUE RECEPTOR STUDIES

Platelets

The platelet has attracted particular interest as a model of receptor function because of the common characteristics of biogenic amine uptake and storage it shares with CNS neurons [106]. α-adrenergic receptors, which have pharmacologic similarities to central α-adrenergic receptors [176], have been identified on human platelets [74]. Direct ligand-binding studies [36,37,54,74,75,176] can determine α-adrenergic receptor density on the platelet membrane, and the degree of inhibition of the prostaglandin E_1 ((PGE_1)-stimulated cAMP response by norepinephrine (NE) [74,75,107,183] may provide an index of the physiologic responsiveness of these α-adrenergic receptors.

A variety of ligands are used in receptor-binding studies, including radiolabeled dihydroergocryptine (^{3}H-DHE); ^{3}H-yohimbine, an α_2-adrenergic antagonist; and ^{3}H-clonidine, an α_2-adrenergic agonist. α_2-adrenoreceptor binding may encompass both high-affinity and low-affinity sites, with ^{3}H-yohimbine labeling both sites and ^{3}H-clonidine labeling the majority of the high-affinity sites [37,176]. ^{3}H-DHE measures all high- and low-affinity sites and perhaps other sites as well [37,176]. One study demonstrated increased clonidine binding in patients with major depressive disorders compared with normal controls [54], and another preliminary study reported increased ^{3}H-DHE binding in the platelets of affective disorder patients compared with controls [75]. However, a third preliminary study using yohimbine as a ligand has failed, as yet, to confirm these findings [36,176]. Differences in developing methodologies and in the patient populations may account for these discrepancies, but this potential finding seems worthy of further investigation.

The interpretation of these findings, however, is complicated by the fact that platelet α_2-adrenoreceptors, although similar, may not be identical to central α_2-adrenoreceptors. Perhaps more pertinent, receptor numbers may be regulated in equilibrium with circulating plasma catecholamine (CA) levels, which presumably differ from the intrasynaptic NE levels to which central α-adrenergic receptors are exposed. Interestingly, plasma NE levels appear to be higher in depressed patients than in controls [81,87,145,191], so that if peripheral receptor alterations were secondary consequences of the increased circulating NE, one might expect α_2-adrenergic receptors to decrease rather than increase in depressed patients. We are currently measuring plasma NE levels concurrently with receptor binding in affectively disordered patients.

There is emerging evidence for an alteration of physiologic responsiveness in the platelets of depressed patients. Although three groups have failed to find differences between depressed patients and controls in the cAMP response to PGE_1

or NE [75,107,184], recent data suggest that NE inhibition (at submaximal NE concentrations) of PGE_1-stimulated cAMP may be decreased in depressed patients [144a]. Increases in binding might thus be compensatory to decreased postreceptor efficiency. Such a decreased responsiveness parallels decreased α_2-adrenergic receptor–mediated responses to central noradrenergic challenges. Further studies are required of the physiologic responsiveness of the platelet α_2-adrenergic receptor and the catalytic proteins that mediate its interaction with adenyl cyclase. At present, these methodologies do not have clinical predictive value, although it is conceivable that evaluation of platelet α_2-adrenergic receptor responsiveness may help diagnose a depressive subgroup in the future.

Leukocytes

β-adrenergic receptors located on leukocytes [52] mediate the cAMP response to isoproterenol, NE, and epinephrine (E) [114,115]. One study suggested that cAMP production in response to NE and isoproterenol is decreased in depressed patients as compared with either normal subjects or schizophrenics [114]. This finding does not appear to be specific to depressed patients, however, as it is observed in manic patients as well [47]. These results raise the possibility that β-adrenergic sensitivity may be decreased in depressed patients. One possible explanation for this finding, however, is that β-adrenergic receptors are downregulated by increased levels of circulating plasma NE in both depressed and manic patients. This possibility seems more plausible when one considers the studies which suggest that adrenergic-receptor responsiveness in peripheral tissue may have an inverse relationship with circulating plasma CA levels [69,79,91,145,150]. This finding must also be evaluated with caution, though it too deserves further exploration.

CHALLENGE STRATEGIES

Peripheral Challenges

Administration of peripherally acting pharmacologic agents permits an indirect evaluation of peripheral noradrenergic receptors. Physiologic indices such as blood pressure, pupil size, or pulse depend in part on the mediation of peripheral adrenergic receptors. Changes in these variables in response to agents with noradrenergic activity may thus reflect the activity of peripheral adrenergic receptors.

Pupillary Response

Pupillometry allows the measurement of pupillary responses to locally applied pharmacologic agents which act on cholinergic or adrenergic receptors in the pupil. Increased constriction in response to cholinergic challenges in depressed patients compared with controls has been reported, but as of yet no differences have been reported for the pupillary dilatation response to adrenergic agents such as phenylephrine [150a].

Pressor Response

The pressor response to exogenous administration of adrenergic agents is mediated by peripheral α-adrenergic receptors. The magnitude of the pressor response to these agents may therefore reflect responsiveness of the autonomic nervous system and perhaps of peripheral α-adrenergic receptors. Because it appears that generalized abnormalities of noradrenergic function might be detectable peripherally, this approach has been applied in the comparison of depressed patients and controls.

NE itself was one of the first challenges to be studied in depressed patients. Its effects are primarily peripheral, as it does not seem to penetrate the blood-brain barrier [193]. Prange et al [120] demonstrated that a group of depressed patients in remission showed a greater response to NE than they did in the depressed state. However, Prange et al did not study a distinct control population. Because studies have indicated that plasma NE may be elevated in depressed patients [81, 87,145,191], a refractory response to exogenous NE might be expected in the depressive state, with an increase on remission, in conjunction with a normalization of autonomic activity.

Other studies have shown an enhanced pressor response to tyramine (TRM) in depressed patients compared with controls [33,51,57]. The same augmented pressor response in depressed patients is observed in response to the direct noradrenergic agonist, phenylephrine, and to NE in these same studies [31,51]. Another study (D. Pickar, personal communication, 1982), however, showed no increase in the blood pressure response to TRM in depressed patients compared with controls. In this study, depressed patients had a greater variance in their response to TRM than did age-matched controls, and an older group of depressed patients showed a trend toward a decreased pressor response in comparison to the two matched younger groups. These results raise the possibility of heterogeneity in the depressed population on this measure, as may also exist with plasma NE levels [81]. This study also suggested an inverse relationship between the pressor response to TRM and plasma NE levels across patients and controls. One possible explanation for these results is that depressed patients differ in the degree of sympathetic arousal, reflected in differences in plasma NE levels and responsiveness to pressor agents. Older patients with high sympathetic activity as indicated by elevated plasma NE levels may have less sensitive receptors than younger depressed patients (D Pickar, personal communication, 1982). It is also of interest to note that changes in pressor response to TRM accompanied changes in clinical state in one cycling bipolar patient [119], suggesting that these peripheral changes may accompany centrally mediated alterations in mood.

Central Challenges

Drugs that alter noradrenergic activity in the CNS may affect subjective state, behavior, physiologic indices, amine metabolites, and levels of circulating hormones. These responses provide a basis for evaluating the responsiveness of the noradrenergic system centrally and, in some cases, may permit preliminary inferences as to the degree of responsiveness of central adrenergic receptors.

Behavioral Responses

Amphetamine was the first and most widely used pharmacologic agent found to affect central noradrenergic neurons. The interpretation of NE system responses to amphetamine is somewhat problematic because it appears to affect the dopaminergic [104], serotonergic [70], and cholinergic systems [39] as well as the noradrenergic system.

A variety of behavioral and subjective responses, ranging from euphoria and activation to retardation and fatigue, have been reported after amphetamine administration [22,144]. The activation, excitation, or euphoriant response is the most commonly reported and appears to have the greatest association with other biologic or behavioral measures in depressed patients. For example, Fawcett and Siomopoulus [48] reported that mood elevation in response to amphetamine significantly predicts a positive therapeutic response to long-term administration of tricyclic antidepressants. Furthermore, patients with low baseline excretion of urinary 3-methoxy-4-hydroxyphenylglycol (MHPG) tend to respond positively to both short-term amphetamine and later long-term tricyclic administration [90]. Another study [179] supported an association in depressed patients between the activation, euphoriant, or antidepressant response to amphetamine and the antidepressant efficacy of a 4-week trial of imipramine. A later study [6] also supported the hypothesis that patients with lower baseline urinary excretion of MHPG experience increased euphoria and activation in response to amphetamine. Most recently, Nurnberger et al [111] reported that remitted bipolar patients with low baseline plasma MHPG have increased excitation responses to amphetamine as compared to those with high baseline plasma MHPG. Among their normal subjects, those with high baseline plasma MHPG have the greater excitation response.

Clonidine, which acts directly on α_2-adrenergic autoreceptors that inhibit noradrenergic firing and NE release, causes sedation in human subjects, but the degree of sedation does not differ between depressed patients and controls [25]. Clonidine appears to be effective in the treatment of opiate withdrawal [59].

These studies do not permit any specific inferences about the responsiveness of noradrenergic receptors because amphetamine has effects on multiple neurotransmitter systems and, even within the noradrenergic system, enhances activity by increasing presynaptic availability of NE. However, it is interesting to note that in all studies examining affective disorder patients, those with low urinary or plasma MHPG, which, perhaps, reflects decreased noradrenergic activity, show an increased behavioral response to amphetamine. One might expect the converse, which is seen in normals, i.e., subjects with evidence of increased presynaptic noradrenergic availability, as may be reflected by increased baseline plasma MHPG, would respond more to the releasing properties of amphetamine. These results may be explained by intervening compensatory alterations in receptor responsiveness in the affective disorder patients. If the receptor responsiveness of depressed patients is greater in those with lowered noradrenergic metabolite levels and less in those with increased noradrenergic metabolite levels, these results may become more comprehensible. This possibility is considered further in relation to neuroendocrine responses to noradrenergic challenges.

Neuroendocrine Responses

Growth Hormone

Growth hormone (GH) is regularly increased by agents which enhance noradrenergic activity. In animals, spontaneous GH release appears to be mediated by α-adrenergic receptors and blocked by phentolamine [173]. The receptors are likely to be of the α_2-adrenergic type, because the selective α_2-adrenergic agonist clonidine stimulates GH in rodents [170], primates [17], and human beings [82]. This stimulation is blocked by the α_2-adrenergic antagonists piperoxane and yohimbine, but only weakly by the α_1-adrenergic antagonist prazosin in primates [100]. It appears that at least some of the relevant receptors are in the hypothalamic area; NE, locally applied to the hypothalamus, will elicit a GH response in animal studies [172]. Stimulation of these receptors appears to lead to the release of GH-releasing factor, for the GH response to clonidine in rats occurs in the presence of antibodies to somatostatin [42]. Electrical stimulation of limbic structures, including the locus coeruleus (LC), will also initiate GH release in animals [96]. On the basis of this evidence, the assumption is made that subcortical noradrenergic structures, also hypothesized to be important in the regulation of mood, stimulate hypothalamic postsynaptic α-adrenergic receptors to elevate GH.

Long-term administration of reserpine, which increases adrenergic receptor binding [177], also increases the magnitude of the GH response to clonidine in animals compared with the clonidine-induced GH response observed prior to or during short-term reserpine administration [46]. Preliminary results have also suggested that 6-hydroxydopamine (6-OHDA) treatment, which increases postsynaptic α-adrenoreceptor binding [175], also enhances the GH response to clonidine in rats (L Siever, C Tamminga, and A Pert, unpublished data, 1981). This preliminary evidence supports the possibility that the magnitude of the GH response to clonidine may, in some instances, provide an index of the responsiveness of central postsynaptic α-adrenergic receptors, although the methodology is at best indirect, and contributions of other neuromodulators to the response are difficult to exclude.

Numerous studies have indicated that endogenously depressed patients have a relatively diminished GH response to psychopharmacologic challenges presumed to increase noradrenergic activity (Table 12.2). Langer et al [84] reported that endogenously depressed patients have a lesser response to amphetamine, which increases noradrenergic release [104], than do normal controls, whereas reactively depressed patients have a greater response. Controls were not age- and sex-matched in this study. Furthermore, Checkley and Crammer [23,24] found no difference between the GH response to methamphetamine in depressed patients compared with psychiatric controls or those same patients in remission. A third study reported that the GH response to amphetamine is blunted in most endogenously depressed patients, although this response does not appear to be specific to this patient group [49]. Another recent study, however, showed no appreciable decrease in the GH response to amphetamine in depressed patients [64]. Because some patients with blunted GH responses to the selective α_2-adrenergic agonist, clonidine, have shown adequate GH response to amphetamine, it seems likely that amphetamine effects

Table 12.2 Neuroendocrine Responses to Agents Altering Noradrenergic Activity in the Affective Disorders

Challenge	*Neuro-endocrine Response*	*Blocked by Noradrenergic Antagonists*	*Response in Unipolar Depression*	*Response in Bipolar Depression*	*Response in Mania*
Insulin-induced hypoglycemia	GH	+	↓	? ↑	↓
L-Dopa	GH	+	? ↓	? ↑	↓
Amphetamine or derivatives	GH;	+	↓	?	?
	cortisol		↓	?	?
Desmethyl-imipramine	GH		↓	?	?
Clonidine	GH	+	↓	? ↑	?

GH = growth hormone; ↓ = decreased; ↑ = increased.

subsensitivity (L Siever, T Insel, and J Hamilton, unpublished data, 1982).

Desmethylimipramine (DMI), which blocks reuptake of NE in the synapse, can induce a GH response. This response, which is blocked in many endogenously depressed patients but not in reactive depressive patients, does not occur when the patients are in remission [80]. Studies from the National Institute of Mental Health have supported this finding (W Potter, personal communication, 1982). This response is also blocked by yohimbine but not by methysergide or propranalol (G Laakman, personal communication, 1981).

The insulin tolerance test also results in a GH elevation secondary to the induced hypoglycemia. This elevation seems to be contingent on α-adrenergic receptor stimulation, as α-adrenergic antagonists will block the response [10]. Again, the magnitude of this response may depend on the sensitivity of α-adrenergic receptors, although the degree to which hypoglycemia is induced may influence the GH response. Studies from several groups have indicated that the depressive subjects' GH response to the insulin tolerance test is deficient [43,132,133,144]. Even normal, postmenopausal subjects, who tend to have a blunted response to the insulin tolerance test, had higher GH response than depressive, postmenopausal subjects [62]. One study [56] showed a significant correlation between the peak GH response to hypoglycemia and elevation of 24-hour urinary MHPG excretion above the norm for each sex, as determined prior to the test. The regression line for this correlation is shifted more to the right in manic patients than in depressed patients. The positive correlation observed in all patients suggests that the GH response may depend on noradrenergic availability, reflected in the urinary MHPG excretion. The decreased responsiveness observed in manic patients, however, raises the possibility that these patients may have less sensitive postsynaptic α-adrenergic receptors. Another study [16] found evidence for a reduced GH response to the insulin tolerance test in manic as well as in depressed patients. An enhanced GH response to the test in some bipolar depressed patients has been observed [133], although the number of bipolar subjects in this study was too small to permit a definite conclusion.

L-dihydroxyphenylalanine (L-dopa) also stimulates GH release. In animals, this stimulation is blocked by phentolamine, an α-adrenergic antagonist [76], but not by pimozide, a dopaminergic antagonist [97]. L-dopa may thus achieve this effect as a precursor for NE rather than for dopamine (DA). A diminished GH response to L-dopa is reported in primarily unipolar depressed patients as compared with controls [133]. However, there is no marked difference between menopausal depressed subjects and menopausal controls, suggesting that earlier results may have been due to the large number of postmenopausal women in the depressed sample [130]. In this study as well, the greatest elevations in GH are generally observed among the bipolar depressed subjects, although again the bipolar sample was small. Another study [60] noted that bipolar depressed patients manifest an enhanced GH response to L-dopa compared with unipolar depressed patients or controls, although these results have not been replicated [88].

The interpretation of all these studies suffers from the lack of specificity of the challenges. Most have effects on the dopaminergic and, in some cases, the serotonergic system as well as the noradrenergic system. Furthermore, interpreting responses of adrenergic receptors is complicated because most of the challenges act by enhancing presynaptic noradrenergic availability, which may depend on factors such as rate of synthesis, readiness for release, and rate of inactivation of NE.

Use of the selective noradrenergic agonist, clonidine, allows for a somewhat cleaner dissection of the role of the noradrenergic receptors themselves in this response. Clonidine acts directly on α_2-adrenergic receptors without enhancing release or blocking reuptake of NE. Effects on the histamine system, however, have been reported in animals [50], but not consistently in humans [184]. Although clonidine may decrease NE release centrally, it is unlikely to affect baseline levels of GH which are already depressed. Therefore, the response should reflect its postsynaptic effects. Clonidine stimulates GH release in normal subjects [82], but several studies have indicated that this response is blunted in depressed patients [20,25,98,150] even with age- and sex-matched controls and when controlling for postmenopausal status [150]. These studies provide the clearest evidence that postsynaptic α_2-adrenergic responsiveness is decreased in depressed patients.

Further examination of the mechanism and cause of the blunted GH response in depression is required. These findings may reflect a depletion of GH or GH-releasing factor or an excessive inhibition by somatostatin. These possibilities seem less likely, though, because the GH response to apomorphine has been found to be similar in depressed patients and normal subjects [88], and spontaneous GH secretory bursts of normal magnitude can be observed in depressed patients [49]. It remains to be ascertained if this finding is a state-dependent marker or represents a vulnerability factor in the onset of depression. The GH response to DMI appears to normalize after remission in depressed patients [80], but this response may depend in part on presynaptic noradrenergic availability, which may also increase after remission. Preliminary studies from our group suggest that at least some depressed patients off medications and in remission may continue to have blunted GH response to clonidine [147]. Matussek et al [98] suggested that decreased postsynaptic sensitivity may represent a broader vulnerability marker for depression, as it is observed in heavy drinkers who have abstained from alcohol for several weeks and who may have a predisposition to affective disorders. Postmenopausal women also tend to have blunted GH responses to clonidine [98,150] and may also have a higher risk for affective disorders [77]. We have also observed blunted GH responses to clonidine in many patients with obsessive-compulsive disorders [143], which may have biologic mechanisms in common with the affective disorders [71]. Thus, although it is clear that this finding cannot be considered specific for the depressive state, it remains to be determined whether the blunted GH response to clonidine in nondepressed subjects is compatible with such a vulnerability hypothesis and if it will be observed in depressed patients in remission as suggested in the preliminary studies [147]. We have speculated that α-adrenergic receptors may become subsensitive if exposed over a prolonged period to excesses of NE in a relatively dysregulated noradrenergic system [142a,145,147,150]. Extreme elevations of plasma NE in some patients may be associated with decreased blood pressure response to TRM, mediated by peripheral α-adrenergic receptors, as well as a blunted GH response to clonidine [145]. This lead requires further exploration because the relationship between noradrenergic availability and receptor responsiveness in humans is not well understood.

The data from these accumulated studies indicate the possibility of relatively enhanced α-adrenergic sensitivity in a subgroup of bipolar patients. Other studies demonstrate that these patients have lower excretion of urinary MHPG, possibly reflecting decreases in total body intraneuronal metabolism of NE (see Chapter 11). If this decreased turnover is paralleled by decreased intrasynaptic availability of NE, one might expect an enhanced α-adrenergic responsiveness in relation to such decreased NE levels. In one study [150], we did observe the most robust GH responses to clonidine in patients with low plasma MHPG. In our study [150] and in the study of Matussek et al [98], augmented GH responses to clonidine were observed in several young bipolar patients. It is conceivable that enhanced α-adrenergic responsiveness in some bipolar depressed patients enhances susceptibility to a manic switch triggered by increases in intrasynaptic NE concentrations [13,144]. During prolonged periods of increased intrasynaptic noradrenergic concentration, as is sometimes observed later in the manic phase, α-adrenergic sensitivity may be downregulated (Figure 12.1). This model is consistent with the reduced GH responses to the insulin tolerance test [16] and to L-dopa challenge [60] observed in manic patients.

With techniques now available to more accurately assay the concentration of NE and its metabolites in body fluids (see Chapters 1, 2, and 11), and pharmacologic challenges and receptor-binding approaches developed to assess receptor function, simultaneous assessment of presynaptic and postsynaptic components of noradrenergic activity may allow a better understanding of these possible relationships.

In the future, the GH response to clonidine may have clinical utility. The

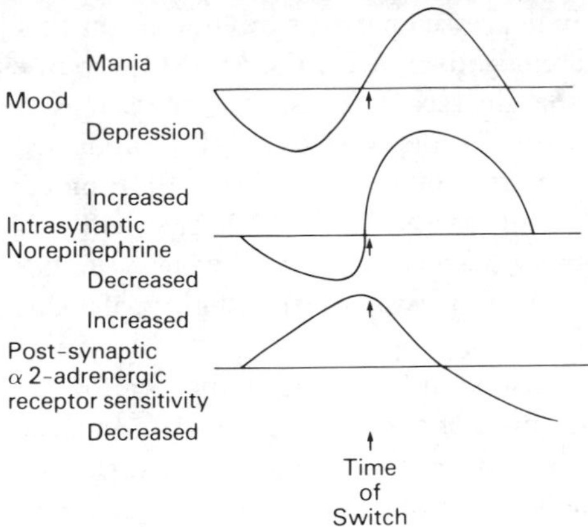

Figure 12.1 The switch to mania, according to this model, occurs when increases in intrasynaptic norepinephrine stimulate supersensitive postsynaptic receptors. The increased postsynaptic receptor sensitivity reflects upregulation secondary to the previously decreased intrasynaptic norepinephrine.

replicability of the finding suggests that it may be an important biologic marker for depression. In a small preliminary sample of men and premenopausal women, a blunted GH response distinguished depressed patients from controls with a sensitivity of 73% and a specificity of 7% (L Siever, T Uhde, and D Murphy, unpublished data, 1982). However, because of the pervasiveness of blunted GH response in postmenopausal women and the frequent baseline GH elevations that may occur unless there is a long acclimatization period (1–2 hours) prior to the procedure, there may be restrictions to its diagnostic utility. Another possibility that requires exploration is that the GH response to clonidine may predict treatment response with patients with blunted GH responses requiring higher doses of antidepressants because of the lesser responsiveness of noradrenergic receptors.

Cortisol

Cortisol plasma levels increase in response to both amphetamine and methylamphetamine in human beings [9,23,24,131]. This effect also seems to be noradrenergically mediated; apomorphine does not change cortisol levels [83], and thymoxamine, a selective α-adrenergic antagonist, blocks the cortisol response to amphetamine [122]. Propranolol enhances the peak cortisol response to methylamphetamine, suggesting an inhibitory influence of β-adrenergic receptors on this response [122]. Checkley and Crammer [23,24] found a relatively decreased cortisol response to amphetamine in depressed patients compared with other psychiatric patients and with depressed patients' responses when in remission. Sachar et al [132] reported that cortisol levels of depressed patients actually decrease in response to amphetamine, contrary to the increase observed in normal subjects. Cortisol decreases in response to clonidine in depressed patients but not in controls [147]. Plasma cortisol concentrations correlate negatively with the MHPG response to clonidine, suggesting decreased α_2-adrenergic receptor responsiveness may be associated with the hypercortisolemia observed in depression [147]. Diminished receptor-receptor responsiveness may decrease the inhibitory effects of NE on cortisol, which clonidine may restore [147]. Overall, these studies are consistent with other studies showing decreased α-adrenergic receptor responsiveness in depressed patients compared with controls and even raise the possibility of an enhanced β-adrenergic inhibitory influence.

The cortisol response could serve as a marker for noradrenergic receptors, although further clarification of the relative roles of α-adrenergic and β-adrenergic receptors is needed. More specific information on this question may be available from studying responses to amphetamine concomitant with the use of selective α-adrenergic or β-adrenergic blockers.

Other Hormones

There is little evidence that prolactin release is appreciably modulated by noradrenergic activity. Changes in prolactin after amphetamine administration [153] are likely to reflect serotonergic or dopaminergic influences rather than noradrenergic influences, and DMI [80] and clonidine [82] have no effect on plasma prolactin.

Plasma β-endorphin levels increase in response to intravenous [29], but not oral, administration of amphetamine. β-endorphin does not, however, appear to increase in response to clonidine in humans [174], making this an unlikely function of α-adrenergic stimulation.

In summary, these neuroendocrine responses cannot presently be interpreted to reflect activity of specific noradrenergic receptors.

Biochemical Responses

Changes in plasma or CSF NE or its metabolites in response to drugs that alter noradrenergic activity may provide an index of noradrenergic receptor responsiveness. Clonidine decreases both plasma NE [98,147] and plasma MHPG [20,147] by decreasing sympathetic outflow from the CNS [78]. These decreases may reflect clonidine's actions on presynaptic α_2-adrenergic autoreceptors which inhibit noradrenergic release [85]; they function as part of a feedback inhibitory system by which NE modulates its own release. Increased release of NE thus appears to dampen further release, "buffering" the release pattern of NE. The decrement in plasma NE and plasma MHPG may provide a potential index of α_2-adrenergic autoreceptor sensitivity. Preliminary studies have shown no notable differences between the decrement in plasma NE or MHPG to clonidine in depressed patients compared with controls [98,151]. Recent data from a larger series of patients, however, show a significantly decreased plasma MHPG response to clonidine in depressed patients compared with age- and sex-matched controls [147].

In an early study [90], individuals with low baseline urinary MHPG, who have a behavioral response of activation to amphetamine, showed an increase in urinary MHPG after amphetamine administration; those with higher baseline urinary MHPG generally did not have as great an activation response to amphetamine and showed a slight decrease in MHPG. These results may indicate that amphetamine increases NE release, thus decreasing intraneuronal NE metabolism as may, for example, be observed with DMI administration (see Chapter 11). Increased MHPG in subjects with low MHPG may reflect the behavioral activation observed in these subjects. Nurnberger et al [110,111] also observed decreases in plasma MHPG with amphetamine administration. However, as these effects are partly mediated by presynaptic mechanisms, interpretation regarding receptor responsiveness is problematic.

Physiologic Responses

Changes in blood pressure response to central noradrenergic challenges may partially reflect noradrenergic receptor sensitivity, as the noradrenergic system plays an important role in the central regulation of blood pressure. The increase in blood pressure observed with amphetamine does not appear to differ between depressed patients and controls [84]. Clonidine decreases blood pressure by acting on central α_2-adrenergic receptors, perhaps partially mediated by autoreceptors in the LC [193]. There appear to be no differences in this decrement between depressed patients and controls [20,147].

Body temperature also decreases as a result of clonidine administration. As temperature increases with noradrenergic enhancement [169], the decrement observed with clonidine may also reflect α_2-adrenergic autoreceptor responsiveness.

Rapid eye movement (REM) sleep is suppressed by both amphetamine [58] and clonidine [3] and may provide another avenue for assessing possible differences in receptor responsiveness in depressed patients compared with controls.

Most of these physiologic responses have not been systematically compared in depressed patients and controls; because of the complex physiologic regulation of these functions, interpretation of changes may be difficult.

IMPLICATIONS OF RECEPTOR STUDIES FOR MODELS OF NORADRENERGIC REGULATION IN THE AFFECTIVE DISORDERS

The studies cited in this and the previous chapter present an inconsistent and even paradoxical picture of noradrenergic function in the affective disorders. NE metabolites may be greater than, less than, or the same as control values depending on the study (see Chapter 11). The blunted GH response to clonidine suggests decreased responsiveness of central postsynaptic α-adrenergic receptors [18,25, 98,150] and possibly decreased central presynaptic α_2-adrenergic receptor responsiveness [147]. α_2-adrenergic binding in platelets is increased in some [54,75] but not all subjects [36] and may be less than or no different than control values [75,107, 144a,183] in functional responsiveness. These inconsistencies may reflect methodologic differences between the studies and thus may be artifactual. Alternatively, apparent inconsistencies may partially reflect assumptions about the functioning of the noradrenergic system that are too simplistic for use in interpreting the actual complexity of noradrenergic regulation in these disorders. For example, it has been assumed that net noradrenergic activity is either increased or decreased in depression, and studies have attempted to confirm or refute this hypothesis. A different set of assumptions might permit a different, although speculative, model of the alterations of noradrenergic activity in the affective disorders and may be more consistent with evidence to date.

Most of the studies discussed in this and the previous chapter measure biologic values at one or two time points and do not permit an integrated picture of changes in these values over time. Studies have demonstrated daily and seasonal rhythms of noradrenergic activity [186] as well as more transient oscillations in NE release as measured by plasma MHPG [63]. Furthermore, it is quite possible that noradrenergic receptor responsiveness and intrasynaptic concentrations of NE may change during a single affective episode [13]. A more dynamic perspective may be required to understand the possible alteration in the noradrenergic system of affective disorder patients.

Animal studies have suggested that CA receptors are regulated relative to ambient concentrations of antagonists and agonists including the CA neurotransmitters themselves [139,157,175]. Excessive levels of amines may downregulate amine receptors, and relative deficits may upregulate these receptors. Alterations in levels of NE may thus cause secondary adaptive changes in NE receptors. Receptors with the same pharmacologic profile of responsiveness may not be regulated identically because anatomically different receptor populations may be exposed to different neurotransmitter concentrations. Differences may also exist in the regulation of different subpopulations of receptors depending in part on the sensitivity of contiguous receptor populations on the same membrane. For example, changes in β-adrenergic density may alter α_2-adrenergic binding in animal tissues [92]. Perhaps the disparity between the blunted GH response to clonidine and the normal hypotensive response to clonidine in some studies of depressed patients [20,147,150] may reflect differences in the regulation of different populations of α_2-adrenergic receptors.

Finally, depressed patients are likely to represent a biologically heterogeneous syndrome. One possible subdivision is between unipolar and bipolar patients, although there may be further heterogeneity within these subgroups. The next section of this chapter briefly elaborates on possible models of noradrenergic dysfunction that may apply to the unipolar and bipolar depressed subgroups.

Unipolar Depression

Cumulatively, a number of studies of a large subgroup of depressed patients, particularly of the unipolar type, have suggested that postsynaptic α-adrenergic receptors may have blunted responsiveness. If the decreased neuroendocrine responsiveness does represent subsensitivity of postsynaptic α_2-adrenergic receptors, such a subsensitivity could reflect a primary receptor defect or a downregulation secondary to increased noradrenergic activity. Downregulation of postsynaptic α_2-adrenergic receptors by repeated exposure to increased levels of NE is a possibility that is compatible with evidence for a dysregulation of noradrenergic transmission in depressed patients.

Observations of elevated plasma NE [81] and 24-hour urinary MHPG excretion in a subgroup of depressed, especially unipolar, patients [see Chapter 11; 135,136], may reflect such a dysregulation with periodic excessive release of NE superimposed on a relatively low baseline NE activity [142a] (Figure 12.2). Integrated measures of NE metabolites over time may reflect these possible increases resulting in a net increase in metabolite excretion or, in some cases, a relative decrease if these peaks are not prominent. Daily patterns of plasma MHPG also suggest a more dysregulated, oscillatory pattern in depressed patients [63]. Depressed patients have increased sensitivity to alterations of the noradrenergic system in response to changes in diet and exercise [108,186], and an altered circadian pattern of urinary MHPG excretion and plasma MHPG as compared with controls [63,186]. These responses are consistent with a model that suggests that the noradrenergic system may not be well buffered in depressed patients. Decreased responsiveness of presynaptic inhibitory α_2-adrenergic receptors in depressed patients, as suggested by a recent study [147], may result in less sensitively regulated release of NE with "overshoots" of release and subsequent decreased concentrations in the synapse [142a]. Animal studies have suggested increases of noradrenergic release with acute stress and an ensuing depletion of noradrenergic stores after chronic stress [30,159]. A depressive episode triggered by stress may be reflected biologically by an increased dysregulation of noradrenergic release, with excessive release acutely. During longer periods, however, the sustained adequate levels of NE in the synapse which are required to maintain optimal noradrenergic functioning are lacking. The subjective concomitants of these noradrenergic changes might be anergia during troughs of noradrenergic activity punctuated with episodes of anxiety or agitation during the peaks, in contrast to specific activation of the noradrenergic system that is required to sustain optimal arousal and goal-directed activity.

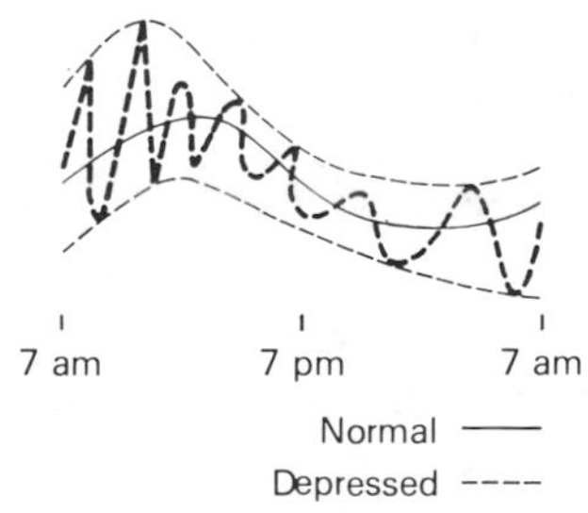

Figure 12.2 Model of noradrenergic activity in depression.

Estrogens increase α_2-adrenergic receptor sensitivity in some tissues [188], hence their withdrawal on menopause might contribute to α_2-adrenergic subsensitivity. A decrease in target organ receptor responsiveness in the periphery (e.g., cardiac adrenergic receptors) may be accompanied by increases in presynaptic NE availability, a process which may have parallels in the CNS. Such a model would predict that depression, associated with increased noradrenergic activity and postsynaptic α-adrenergic subsensitivity, would occur most frequently in older individuals, particularly postmenopausal women [145,150].

Bipolar Depression

Metabolite studies suggest that a relative deficiency of presynaptic noradrenergic activity characterizes the bipolar depressed patients (see Chapter 11). It is interesting to note that although bipolar depressed patients may show blunted neuroendocrine responses, increased responses to pharmacologic challenge have also been observed in this patient subgroup [60,133]. We wonder if these increased responses may represent supersensitization of postsynaptic receptors secondary to decreased levels of intrasynaptic NE [156]. Studies with α-methyl-*p*-tyrosine (AMPT) support such a model. The withdrawal of AMPT in patients may be accompanied by elation and decreased sleep suggesting a postsynaptic noradrenergic receptor supersensitivity, which is blocked by lithium [12]. Thus, postsynaptic supersensitivity owing to decreases in intrasynaptic NE may trigger elation and perhaps, in susceptible individuals, mania [13] (see Figure 12.1).

In patients with sustained decreases in noradrenergic activity, presynaptic α_2-adrenergic receptor sensitivity might also be expected to increase, tending to set the equilibrium set-point of noradrenergic activity at a lower than optimal level. Increases in postsynaptic responsiveness would therefore be offset and might only sensitize the system to transient shifts from equilibrium. There is preliminary evidence peripherally for increased presynaptic α-adrenergic responsiveness to phenylephrine in bipolar depressed patients [150a]; the most relevant studies have been done primarily with unipolar patients [20,147]. It has been suggested that increased α-adrenergic binders in the platelets of some depressed patients [54,75] reflect increased presynaptic α-adrenergic receptor sensitivity.

A shift in the set-point of presynaptic noradrenergic activity would be required to elicit mania. This switch might be initiated by a stimulus overriding feedback inhibition. Such a stimulus might be an external stressor or an internal state change, such as a shift in sleep stages. Such a shift may also involve other neurotransmitter or receptor systems. Could excitatory presynaptic β-adrenergic receptors, which may stimulate noradrenergic release peripherally [158], be stimulated centrally by an acute increase in peripheral CA overriding the feedback inhibition? Withdrawal of propranolol facilitates the switch to mania in rapidly cycling patients, suggesting that β-adrenergic receptors may play a role in the switch process (A Lewy, personal communication, 1982). Later in mania, increases in noradrenergic activity might desensitize postsynaptic receptors and account for the blunted neuroendocrine responses observed in manic patients [16,60]. It follows that interlocking cyclic oscillations of receptors and presynaptic neurotransmitter activity may parallel the alternating mood swings observed in the cycling bipolar patient [13].

In summary, many unipolar depressed patients may manifest a dysregulation of noradrenergic activity with episodic elevations in intrasynaptic NE associated with postsynaptic noradrenergic receptor subsensitivity. In some bipolar depressed patients, increased receptor responsiveness might permit a tonic inhibition of noradrenergic activity but also confer a vulnerability to a switch to mania. The noradrenergic system may be a regulator which finely tunes the organism's attention and responsiveness to meaningful environmental stimuli [142a]. Therefore, it is possible that a dysregulation of this system may have maladaptive consequences in terms of mood and arousal. Although the models previously discussed are rather speculative, they may form a heuristic framework for more sophisticated testing of the hypothesis that noradrenergic function is altered in depressed patients.

NORADRENERGIC RECEPTOR CHANGES ACCOMPANYING ANTIDEPRESSANT TREATMENT

Animal Studies

A number of noradrenergic receptor changes consistently accompany antidepressant treatment in animals [21], some of which are summarized briefly (Table 12.3). The most consistent effect observed in animal studies is the reduction of NE or isoproterenol-stimulated cAMP production in rat brain after long-term antidepressant treatment [162,163,180,181]. In the case of NE-stimulated cAMP accumulation, the effect is only partially mediated by β adrenergic receptors [11]. β-adrenergic receptor binding is reduced with antidepressant treatment [4,8,28,117]. In some cases, single unit recordings in the cingulate cortex or the cerebellum,

Table 12.3 Evidence Supporting Changes in Noradrenergic Receptor Sensitivity Associated with Long-term Antidepressant Treatment

β-Adrenergic receptor changes
↓ cAMP production
↓ Electrophysiologic responsiveness
↓ Binding of β-adrenergic antagonists
α_1-Adrenergic receptor changes
↑ Electrophysiologic responsiveness
↑ or no change in binding of α_1-adrenergic antagonists
α_2-Adrenergic receptor changes
↓ Electrophysiologic, biochemical responsiveness
↓, ↑, or no change in binding of α_2-adrenergic agonists or antagonists

cAMP = cyclic adenosine 3′,5′-monophosphate; ↓ = decreased; ↑ = increased.

where NE responsiveness is probably mediated by β-adrenergic receptors, indicate decreased responsiveness to NE after long-term tricyclic or monoamine oxidase inhibitor (MAO-I) treatment [113,138]. β-adrenergic receptors are also assumed to be responsible for the lack of change in NE responsiveness in the hippocampus [40,53], although baseline firing in the hippocampus decreases after long-term treatment [67]. Although exceptions may be noted in several of the paradigms, these studies consistently suggest decreases in β-adrenergic binding and responsiveness after long-term antidepressant treatment and the possibility of additional diminution in responsiveness distal to the β-adrenergic recognition site.

α-adrenergic binding, using the radioligand WB-4101 (an α_1 antagonist), reportedly increased after long-term amitriptyline administration in one study [123], but no changes in binding have been observed after long-term tricyclic administration in other studies [66,117,128]. Electrophysiologic studies have suggested increases in responsiveness to NE in the facial nucleus and lateral geniculate nucleus [101], where these responses appear to be mediated by α_1-adrenergic receptors, and in the amygdala [182], where noradrenergic receptors do not have clear α- or β-adrenergic pharmacologic profiles. Animal behavioral studies have also suggested enhanced α_1-adrenergic responsiveness after long-term antidepressant treatment and electroconvulsive therapy (ECT) [38,94,95,103]. As α agonists may inhibit the cAMP response to NE [102], it is conceivable that enhanced α_1-adrenergic receptor activation may contribute to the decreased cAMP production observed after chronic antidepressant treatment. Although binding studies are controversial, perhaps because of the existence of multiple binding sites with different affinities [123] and the variety of antidepressants tested, several studies have suggested increased responsiveness of α_1-adrenergic receptors after antidepressant treatment.

Variable changes in α_2-adrenergic receptors, as measured by the binding of either ^{3}H-clonidine or ^{3}H-*p*-aminoclonidine are reported after antidepressant drug administration [160]. Three to 4 days of desipramine or iprindole administration causes α_2 receptors to increase [73,124], whereas no change or a decrease in α_2 receptors occurs with long-term administration of amitriptyline [118,154], and a decrease occurs with long-term clorgyline administration [31,32]. Electrophysiologic studies show decreases in LC responsiveness after treatment with some of the tricyclic antidepressants and clorgyline [165,167]. Studies in the cardiovascular system also have indicated decreased responsiveness of α_2-adrenergic receptors after long-term tricyclic administration [34,35]. CNS studies have indicated decreased biochemical responses to the α_2-adrenergic agonist, clonidine, after long-term treatment with some of the tricyclic antidepressants [161,167,168]. These studies are somewhat discrepant, perhaps because the radioligands employed in the binding studies label predominantly postsynaptic α_2-adrenergic receptors in rat brain. The physiologic studies may, on the other hand, selectively assess the responsiveness of presynaptic "autoreceptors" which inhibit noradrenergic release [85]. Furthermore, duration of antidepressant administration varies, with the increases observed only after short-term antidepressant treatment [73,124,187], and time course considerations play an important role in α_2-adrenergic desensitization [36]. The cumulative evidence suggests that presynaptic α_2-adrenergic desensitization occurs after long-term administration of many of the typical antidepressants.

It is problematic to base explanations of clinical phenomena in humans on the results of rodent studies. Moreover, inconsistencies among animal studies, particularly discrepancies between binding and physiologic studies, need further investigation before assuming that these reported receptor changes are important in the mechanism of action of the antidepressants. Differences in methodologies, specific antidepressants employed, anatomic regions examined, and duration or dose of antidepressant treatment may account for many of the differences among studies. Antidepressants may also vary in their specific effects on different noradrenergic receptor subtypes, but these receptor changes, in conjunction with other presynaptic antidepressant actions, may alter the net functioning of the noradrenergic system similarly. According to such a model, the sequence and relationship of these receptor changes for individual antidepressants may be useful in understanding net effects.

For example, antidepressants may enhance the "efficiency" of noradrenergic transmission in response to specific stimulation while attenuating nonspecific activity in the unstimulated state. The baseline firing rate of the LC is decreased by long-term DMI and imipramine administration [5,99,164] and by long-term administration of the MAO-I clorgyline (15). This decrease in firing rate may be mediated by α-adrenergic receptors, as the decrease is blocked by the α-adrenergic antagonists, phenoxybenzamine [5] or dibozane [99]. Increased intrasynaptic NE, secondary to reuptake blockade or MAO inhibition, may decrease noradrenergic firing and release through its action on inhibitory presynaptic α_2-adrenergic receptors. The firing rate is more depressed in short-term than in long-term treatment [99] compatible with desensitization of α_2-adrenergic autoreceptors, presumably owing to downregulation by long term increases in ambient NE concentrations.

Levels of NE and its metabolites decrease initially after tricyclic antidepressant treatment [5,99,109,126,137] and return to normal [5,92] or higher-than-normal levels after longer-term treatment in animals [99,127,137]. The return to normal levels does not necessarily occur in humans (see Chapter 11). Because firing rates decline after long-term treatment, the effective intrasynaptic NE concentration per nerve impulse may be increased after long-term antidepressant administration [99]. DMI acutely decreases baseline firing and MHPG accumulation [99], but it does not acutely alter the increase in MHPG induced in the cortex-hippocampus by LC stimulation [5]. Chronic antidepressant treatment may thus increase the "signal-to-noise" ratio, that is, the ratio of intrasynaptic NE concentrations during periods of enhanced noradrenergic impulse flow compared with the concentrations observed during the unstimulated state.

Studies of the hippocampus have supported this model of antidepressant action [67,68]. Hippocampal neurons, inhibited by NE via β-adrenergic receptors, increase their firing in animals treated over the long term with DMI compared with untreated controls [67]. However, no difference in hippocampal firing is observed between the DMI-treated animals and untreated controls when both groups of animals are electrically stimulated at the LC [67]. Because β-adrenergic receptors become subsensitive after long-term DMI administration, presynaptic noradrenergic activity under stimulated conditions would have to be enhanced after long-term DMI administration to offset the decreased β-adrenergic receptor responsiveness. The level of presynaptic activity, however, is apparently insufficient to do so under unstimulated conditions.

Postsynaptic receptor changes may alter the stimulated noradrenergic activity depending on the receptor subtype. Increases in α_1-adrenergic responsiveness may amplify noradrenergic activity. As α-adrenergic receptors have been implicated in reward behavior [65,157], these effects may enhance the positive reinforcing effects of noradrenergic activity. The β-adrenergic system has been implicated in alarm and arousal functions in primates [121], and, in this receptor system, subsensitivity may dampen the internal overarousal often observed in depressed patients.

Whether these postsynaptic changes are functions of the presynaptic changes previously discussed is not clear. For example, β-adrenergic desensitization appears to depend on the integrity of presynaptic noradrenergic neurons because 6-OHDA prevents this effect [140,190]. A net cancellation of the opposing effects of the two treatments, however, cannot be excluded. Decreases in α_2-adrenergic binding precede β-adrenergic subsensitization during clorgyline administration [31]. Phenoxybenzamine and yohimbine, which block inhibiting presynaptic α_2-adrenergic receptors, accelerate the onset of β-adrenergic subsensitivity when concurrently administered with antidepressants [116,187]. These results also suggest that β-adrenergic receptor changes may be secondary to increased noradrenergic availability. However, direct effects on β-adrenergic receptor binding and/or effects distal to the recognition site may occur. The changes on α_1-adrenergic receptors may be secondary consequences of α_1-adrenergic blockade because, in binding studies, increases are most clearly observed after administration of the more potent α_1-adrenergic antagonist, amitriptyline [123]. If so, this effect would not be apparent during treatment when the α_1-adrenergic antagonist effects predominate. However, iprindole, which does not have α_1-adrenergic blocking activity [45], also results in physiologic, postsynaptic, α_1-adrenergic sensitization [101].

Although the sequence and character of these changes may vary with antidepressants, they result in a common end-point of enhanced noradrenergic efficiency. For example, mianserin, a potent α_2-adrenergic antagonist [44], would *not* be expected to downregulate α_2-adrenergic receptors, and long-term treatment with mianserin does not in fact dampen rodent brain responsiveness to clonidine [161]. Its acute blocking effects, however, may also enhance noradrenergic release by dampening feedback inhibition when noradrenergic impulse flow is increased. These considerations may apply to amitriptyline at higher doses as well, as amitriptyline also has α_2-adrenergic blocking activity [45]. Zimelidine, which specifically affects serotonergic uptake and cell firing [41], also changes noradrenergic metabolite concentrations in the same manner as DMI, suggesting that it may have at least indirect effects on the noradrenergic system [86]. Iprindole, although not a noradrenergic reuptake blocker, may act to enhance noradrenergic efficiency by altering release mechanisms [190]. Cocaine and amphetamine, which both increase the release and block reuptake of CA [14], may be less effective antidepressants, as their effects are too short-lived to result in the secondary receptor adaptive changes previously discussed. Whereas these considerations are speculative, they illustrate that common effects on the noradrenergic system could plausibly be achieved by different underlying mechanisms of action. It is of interest that DA autoreceptors may become subsensitive with long-term antidepressant treatment [27], suggesting that similar mechanisms may also apply to other aminergic systems.

These models serve to indicate the ways in which antidepressant treatment may help reverse the dysequilibria of the noradrenergic system suspected in the affective disorders. Based on antidepressant drugs' actions on noradrenergic receptors, the possibility of altered presynaptic α_2-adrenergic receptor responsivity, decreased postsynaptic α-adrenergic receptor responsivity, and increased β-adrenergic responsivity in the depressive disorders should be explored. These are, in fact, alterations suggested by studies of depressed patients discussed earlier, although evidence is still preliminary in clinical studies.

Clinical Studies

Few clinical studies to date have used the previously described strategies to assess receptor responsiveness during antidepressant treatment. Binding studies of the platelet, however, have suggested that the density of α_2-adrenergic receptors decreases after long-term tricyclic antidepressant treatment, consistent with animal studies demonstrating decreased responsiveness of these autoreceptors [55]. A decreased platelet cAMP response to short-term administration of salbutamol, a β_2-adrenergic agonist, has followed long-term treatment with this antidepressant [7].

In some studies, neuroendocrine challenges have been used as indirect measurements of central receptor responsiveness in patients before and after antidepressant treatment, as discussed previously. Enhancement of the GH response to clonidine has been reported after chronic DMI treatment in one study (S Checkley, personal communication, 1982) but not in another. This response to clonidine is not altered in patients over a long period of time with clorgyline [148]. Because the GH response to clonidine appears to be mediated by α_2-adrenergic receptors, the possibility that antidepressant treatment enhances postsynaptic α_2-adrenergic activity is not supported by the studies to date.

Finally, the hypotensive effect of clonidine is blunted in patients receiving DMI [19,26] and long-term clorgyline [142,149]. This effect appears to require long- rather than short-term administration, at least with the MAO-I, clorgyline [149]. The MHPG response to clonidine is also decreased by chronic DMI treatment [19]. As both the MHPG and hypotensive responses may partially reflect α_2-adrenergic autoreceptor activity, these results support the possibility that α_2-adrenergic autoreceptors are subsensitized by long-term antidepressant treatment in the clinical setting. Downregulation of autoreceptors would alter the feedback inhibition of intrasynaptic NE on noradrenergic release, presumably allowing increased concentrations of NE in the synapse and perhaps accounting for the delayed onset of therapeutic efficacy of the antidepressants. Although this phenomenon may not apply to some of the atypical antidepressants, which have not yet been tested in this paradigm in clinical studies, autoreceptor desensitization may be of heuristic value in understanding the sequence of events leading to increased noradrenergic availability for some of the more typical noradrenergic antidepressants.

Preliminary evidence from clinical studies, therefore, suggests that α_2-adrenergic autoreceptors are downregulated with some antidepressant treatments; their effects on postsynaptic α-adrenergic receptors are less clear. Evidence for β-adrenergic subsensitization and increased responsiveness of α_1 receptors after antidepressant treatments has not been as adequately investigated in the clinical setting as in animal studies. Further exploration of the effects of antidepressants on both α-adrenergic receptors and β-adrenergic receptors is indicated.

CONCLUSIONS

Accumulating evidence suggests that noradrenergic receptor responsiveness may be abnormal in the affective disorders and may be altered by long-term antidepressant treatment. We have emphasized the possibility of dysfunctional noradrenergic states that may differ between patient subgroups. In particular, we suggest that a subgroup of unipolar patients may be characterized by α-adrenergic postsynaptic subsensitivity accompanied by episodic elevations of central presynaptic noradrenergic availability. Other unipolar and bipolar patients may be marked by low central noradrenergic turnover coupled with presynaptic and postsynaptic α_2-adrenergic supersensitivity. Mania may be accompanied by increases in NE turnover and gradual development of postsynaptic noradrenergic subsensitivity. The possibility of increased central β-adrenergic responsivity in the affective disorders should also be explored.

Such alterations are compatible with disorders of other neurotransmitter systems. For example, decreased serotonergic activity may be a characteristic of many patients with affective disorder, [105] and has been suggested as the biologic basis of depression in patients who have no evidence of decreased noradrenergic activity [89]. Because serotonin (5-hydroxytryptamine; 5-HT), may have an inhibitory influence on noradrenergic systems, a relative deficit of 5-HT may account for the increased noradrenergic turnover postulated in the "low sensitivity" unipolar patients. Cholinergic supersensitivity may play an etiologic role in depression [151, 152]. A cholinergic-noradrenergic imbalance, with a predominance of cholinergic tone, might account for a noradrenergic deficit in some depressed patients because cholinergic systems inhibit noradrenergic activity [72]. We have evidence that, of eight subjects, all those with a blunted GH response to clonidine (suggesting a noradrenergic receptor subsensitivity), showed enhanced depressive responses to cholinergic challenge, suggesting a cholinergic receptor supersensitivity [146]. Nurnberger et al [111] reported a negative correlation between the activation response to amphetamine and the decrease in REM latency induced by arecoline. Although speculative, these possibilities are reminders that these neurotransmitter systems do not exist in isolation and their interaction, particularly in patients with affective disorders, requires further study.

Testing such models requires careful attention to clinical characteristics of patient populations, including dimensions such as unipolar-bipolar or agitated-retarded, and to the clinical state and phase of the patient (e.g., early depression or late mania).

Scrutiny of data for possible biologic subgroups and characterization of such subgroups may aid in the clinical understanding of these heterogeneous disorders. Multiple measurements over time in the same individuals may allow for better comparisons of state variables, particularly in bipolar patients. Simultaneous determination of indices of presynaptic noradrenergic turnover, of postsynaptic receptor responsivity, and examination of the relationship between these variables may lead to a better understanding of the integrated functioning of the noradrenergic system.

Responses to psychologic stress or pharmacologic challenge may be particularly important in evaluating a dysregulation of noradrenergic systems that may not appear in baseline measurements. By analogy, the malfunction of a home heating system with a faulty thermostat may not be apparent on a spring day but will manifest itself under winter conditions. Because the furnace and heating capacities are intact, only by changing the thermostat can the underlying problem be rectified.

In bipolar depression, the "thermostat" of the noradrenergic system may be locked into dysfunctionally decreased levels of activity by excessive presynaptic inhibition, and in some forms of unipolar depression, a marked dysregulation may lead to variable noradrenergic activity with deficient postsynaptic receptor responsiveness.

Antidepressants may stabilize the noradrenergic system by decreasing baseline firing (or "noise") and enhancing the response to stimulation (or the "signal") through the release of increased amounts of NE per nerve impulse [142a,149]. Subsensitization of presynaptic α_2-adrenergic receptors may release noradrenergic neurons from excessive inhibition. Increased postsynaptic α_2-adrenergic receptor responsivity may increase noradrenergically mediated reinforced behavior in response to stimulation, and β-adrenergic subsensitivity may decrease excessive arousal or anxiety in these patients in response to vicissitudes of baseline firing or trivial environmental stimulation. These models, although speculative, underscore the importance of conceptualizing neurotransmitter-receptor interactions in dynamic terms and attempting to formulate approaches that might provide information as to how these dynamics may be altered in depression.

REFERENCES

1. Aghajanian GK. Tricyclic Antidepressants and Single Cell Responses to Serotonin and Norepinephrine: A Review of Chronic Studies. In Neuroreceptors: Basic and Clinical Aspects, E Usdin, WE Bunney Jr, and JM Davis (eds), 27–35. New York: John Wiley & Sons, 1981.

2. Ashcroft GW, Eccleston D, Murray LG, Glen AIM, Crawford TBB, Pullar IA, Shields PJ, Walter DS, Blackburn IM, Connechan J, Loren M. Modified amine hypothesis for the aetiology of affective illness. Lancet 2:573–577, 1972.
3. Autret A, Minz M, Beillevaire T, Cathala H-P, Schmitt H. Effects of clonidine on sleep patterns in man. Eur J Clin Pharmacol 12:319–322, 1977.
4. Benerjee SP, Kung LS, Riggi SJ, Chanda SK. Development of β-adrenergic receptor subsensitivity by antidepressants. Nature 268:455–456, 1977.
5. Bareggi SR, Markey K, Genovese K. Effects of single and multiple doses of desipramine (DMI) on endogenous levels of 3-methoxy-4-hydroxyphenylglycol-sulfate (MOPEG-SO) in rat brain. Eur J Pharmacol 50:301–306, 1978.
6. Beckman H, van Kammen DP, Goodwin FK, Murphy DL. Urinary excretion of 3-methoxy-4-hydroxyphenylglycol in depressed patients: modifications by amphetamine and lithium. Biol Psychiatry 11:377–387, 1976.
7. Belmaker RH. Receptors, adenylate cyclase, depression, and lithium. Biol Psychiatry 16:333–350, 1981.
8. Bergstrom DA, Kellar KJ. Adrenergic and serotonergic receptor binding in rat brain after chronic desmethylimipramine treatment. J Pharmacol Exp Ther 209:256–261, 1979.
9. Besser GM, Butler PWP, Landon J, Rees L. Influence of amphetamines on plasma corticosteroid and growth hormone levels in man. Br Med J 4:528–530, 1969.
10. Blackard WG, Heidingsfelder SA. Adrenergic receptor control mechanism for growth hormone secretion. J Clin Invest 47:1407–1414, 1968.
11. Blumberg JB, Vetulani J, Stawarz RJ, Sulser F. The noradrenergic cyclic AMP generating system in the limbic forebrain: Pharmacological characterization in vitro and possible role of limbic noradrenergic mechanisms in the mode of action of antipsychotics. Eur J Pharmacol 37:357–366, 1976.
12. Bunney WE, Jr, Kopanda RT, Murphy DL. Sleep and behavioral changes possibly reflecting central receptor hypersensitivity following catecholamine synthesis inhibition in man. Acta Psychiatr Scand 56:189–203, 1977.
13. Bunney WE, Jr, Post RM, Anderson AE, Kopanda RT. A neuronal receptor sensitivity mechanism in affective illness (a review of evidence). Commun Psychopharmacol 1:393–405, 1977.
14. Caldwell J, Sever PS. The biochemical pharmacology of abused drugs. I. Amphetamines, cocaine, and LSD. Clin Pharmacol Ther 16:625–638, 1974.
15. Campbell IC, Murphy DL, Gallager DW, Tallman JF, Marshall EF. Neurotransmitter-Related Adaptation in the Central Nervous System Following Chronic Monoamine Oxidase Inhibition. In Monoamine Oxidase: Structure, Function and Altered Functions, TP Singer, RW Von Korff, and DL Murphy (eds), 517–530. New York: Academic Press, 1979.
16. Casper RC, Davis JM, Pandey GN, Garver DL, Dekirmenjian H. Neuroendocrine and amine studies in affective illness. Psychoneuroendocrinology 2:105–113, 1977.
17. Chambers JW, Brown GM. Neurotransmitter regulation of growth hormone and ACTH in the rhesus monkey: effects of biogenic amines. Endocrinology 98:420–428, 1976.
18. Charney DS, Heninger GR, Sternberg DE. Failure of chronic antidepressant treatment to alter growth hormone response to clonidine. Psychiatry Res 7:135–138, 1982.
19. Charney DS, Heninger GR, Sternberg DE, Redmond DE, Leckman JF, Maas JW, Roth RH. Presynaptic adrenergic receptor sensitivity in depression. Arch Gen Psychiatry 38:1334–1340, 1981.

20. Charney DS, Heninger GR, Sternberg DE, Redmond DE, Leckman JF, Maas JW, Roth RH. Adrenergic receptor sensitivity in depression. Effects of clonidine in depressed patients and healthy patients. Arch Gen Psychiatry, 39:290–294, 1982.
21. Charney DS, Menkes DB, Heninger GR. Receptor sensitivity and the mechanism of action of antidepressant treatment. Arch Gen Psychiatry 38:1160–1180, 1981.
22. Checkley SA. A new distinction between the euphoric and the antidepressant effects of methylamphetamine. Br J Psychiatry 133:417–423, 1978.
23. Checkley SA. Corticosteroid and growth hormone responses to methylamphetamine in depressive illness. Psychol Med 9:107–116, 1979.
24. Checkley SA, Crammer JL. Hormonal responses to methylamphetamine in depression: a new approach to the noradrenaline depletion hypothesis. Br J Psychiatry 131:582–586, 1977.
25. Checkley SA, Slade AP, Shur E. Growth hormone and other responses to clonidine in patients with endogenous depression. Br J Psychiatry 138:51–55, 1981.
26. Checkley SA, Slade AP, Shur E, Dowling S. A pilot study of the mechanism of action of desipramine. Br J Psychiatry 138:248–251, 1981.
27. Chiodo LA, Antelman SM. Repeated tricyclics induce a progressive dopamine autoreceptor subsensitivity independent of daily drug treatment. Nature 287:451–454, 1980.
28. Clements-Jewery S. The development of cortical β-adrenoceptor subsensitivity in the rat by chronic treatment with trazodone, doxepin, and mianserin. Neuropharmacology 17:779–781, 1978.
29. Cohen MR, Nurnberger JI, Pickar D, Gershon E, Bunney WE, Jr. Dextroamphetamine infusions in normals result in correlated increases of plasma β-endorphin and cortisol immunoreactivity. Life Sci 29:1243–1247, 1981.
30. Cohen RM, Campbell IC, Cohen MR, Torda T, Pickar D, Siever LJ, Murphy DL. Presynaptic noradrenergic regulation during depression and antidepressant treatment. Psychiatr Res 3:93–105, 1980.
31. Cohen RM, Campbell IC, Dauphin M, Tallman JF, Murphy DL. Changes in alpha- and beta-receptor densities in rat brain as a result of treatment with monoamine oxidase inhibiting (MAO-I) antidepressants. Neuropharmacology, 21:293–298, 1982.
32. Cohen RM, Ebstein RP, Daly JW, Murphy DL. Chronic effects of a monoamine oxidase-inhibiting antidepressant: Decreases in functional alpha-adrenergic autoreceptors precede the decrease in norepinephrine-stimulated cyclic AMP systems in rat brain. J Neurosci 2:1588–1595, 1982.
33. Coppen A, Ghose K. Peripheral alpha-adrenoreceptor and central dopamine receptor activity in depressive patients. Psychopharmacologia (Berlin) 59:171–177, 1978.
34. Crews FT, Smith CB. Presynaptic alpha-receptor subsensitivity after long-term antidepressant treatment. Science 202:322–324, 1978.
35. Crews FT, Smith CB. Potentiation of responses to adrenergic nerve stimulation in isolated rat atria during chronic tricyclic administration. J Pharm Exp Ther 215:143–149, 1980.
36. Daiguji M, Meltzer HY, Tong C, U'Prichard DC, Young M, Kravitz H. α_2-Adrenergic receptors in platelet membranes of depressed patients: no change in number of ^{3}H-yohimbine affinity. Life Sci 29:2059–2064, 1981.
37. Daiguji M, Meltzer HY, U'Prichard DC. Human platelet α_2-adrenergic receptors: labeling with $_3$H-yohimbine, a selective antagonist ligand. Life Sci 28:2705–2707, 1981.
38. David M. Agonist indexed changes in behavior as a measure of functional changes in receptor sensitivity following chronic administration of antidepressant drugs. Ab-

stracts of the Annual Meeting of the American College of Neuropsychopharmacology, p. 41, 1981.

39. Deffenu G, Bartolini A, Pepeu G. Effects of Amphetamine on Cholinergic Systems of the Cerebral Cortex of the Cat. In Amphetamines and Related Compounds, E Costa and S Garattini (eds), 357–368. New York: Raven Press, 1970.

40. DeMontigny C, Aghajanian GK. Tricyclic antidepressants: long-term treatment increases responsivity of rat forebrain neurons to serotonin. Science 202:1303–1306, 1978.

41. DeMontigny C, Blier P, Caillé C, Kouassl E. Pre- and post-synaptic effects of zimelidine and norzimelidine on the serotoninergic system: single cell studies in the rat. Acta Psychiatr Scand 63 [Suppl 290]:79–90, 1981.

42 Eden S, Eriksson E, Martin JB, Modigh K. Evidence for a growth hormone–releasing factor mediating alpha-adrenergic influence on growth hormone secretion in the rat. Neuroendocrinology 33:24–27, 1981.

43. Endo M, Endo J, Nishikubo M, Yamaguchi T, Hatotani N. Endocrine Studies in Depression. In Psychoneuroendocrinology Workshop Conference of the International Society for Psychoneuroendocrinology, N Hatotani and S Karger (eds), 22–31. Basel: Karger, 1974.

44. Engberg G, Syensson TH. Mianserin: direct activation of brain norepinephrine neurons by blocking α_2-receptors. Commun Psychopharmacol 4:233–239, 1980.

45. Enna SJ, Kendall DA. Interaction of antidepressants with brain neurotransmitter receptors. J Clin Psychopharmacol 1:125–165, 1981.

46. Eriksson E, Eden S, and Modigh K. Up- and down-regulation of central postsynaptic α_2 receptors reflected in the growth hormone response to clonidine in reserpine-pretreated rats. Psychopharmacology 77:327–331, 1982.

47. Extein I, Tallman J, Smith CC, Goodwin FK. Changes in lymphocyte beta-adrenergic receptors in depression and mania. Psychiatry Res 1:191–197, 1979.

48. Fawcett J, Siomopoulos V. Dextroamphetamine response as a possible predictor of improvement with tricyclic therapy in depression. Arch Gen Psychiatry 25:247–255, 1971.

49. Feinberg M, Greden JF, Carroll BJ. The effect of amphetamine on plasma cortisol in patients with endogenous and non-endogenous depression. Psychoneuroendocrinology 6:355–357, 1981.

50. Finch L, Harvey CA, Hicks PE, Owens DA. Clonidine-induced hypotension: further evidence for a central interaction with histamine H_2-receptor antagonists in the rat. Neuropharmacology 17:307–313, 1978.

51. Friedman M. Does receptor supersensitivity accompany depressive illness? Am J Psychiatry 135:107, 1978.

52. Galant SP, Duriseti L, Underwood S, Insel PA. Leukocyte β-adrenergic receptor assay in normals and asthmatics. N Engl J Med 299:933–936, 1978.

53. Gallager DW, Bunney WE, Jr. Failure of chronic lithium treatment to block tricyclic antidepressant–induced 5-HT supersensitivity. Naunyn Schmiedebergs Arch Pharmacol 307:129–133, 1979.

54. Garcia-Sevilla JA, Zis AP, Hollingsworth PJ, Greden JF, Smith CB. Platelet α_2-adrenergic receptors in major depressive disorder. Arch Gen Psychiatry 38:1327–1333, 1981.

55. Garcia-Sevilla JA, Zis AP, Zelnic TC, Smith CB. Tricyclic antidepressant drug treatment decreases α_2 adrenoreceptors on human platelet membranes. Eur J Pharmacol 69:121–123, 1981.

56. Garver DL, Pandey GN, Dekirmenjian H, DeLeon-Jones F. Growth hormone and catecholamines in affective disease. Am J Psychiatry 132:1149–1154, 1975.
57. Ghose K, Turner P, Coppen A. Intravenous tyramine pressor response in depression. Lancet 1:1317–1318, 1975.
58. Gillin JC, Mendelson WB, Sitaram N, Wyatt RJ. The neuropharmacology of sleep and wakefulness. Annu Rev Pharmacol Toxicol 18:563–579, 1978.
59. Gold MS, Redmond DE, Jr, Kleber HD. Clonidine blocks acute opiate withdrawal symptoms. Lancet 2:599–602, 1978.
60. Gold PW, Goodwin FK, Wehr T, Rebar R, Sack R. Growth hormone and prolactin response to levodopa in affective illness. Lancet 2:1308–1309, 1976.
61. Greengard P. Possible role for cyclic nucleotides and phosphorylated membrane proteins in postsynaptic actions of neurotransmitters. Nature 260:101–108, 1976.
62. Gruen PH, Sachar EJ, Altman N, Sassin J. Growth hormone responses to hypoglycemia in postmenopausal depressed women. Arch Gen Psychiatry 32:31–33, 1975.
63. Gwirtsman HE, Halaris AE, DeMet EM, Decker PI, Rino RM. Abnormal diurnal norepinephrine metabolism in depression. New Research Abstracts of the 135th Annual Meeting of the American Psychiatric Association, No. 20, 1982.
64. Halbreich U, Sachar EJ, Asnis GM, Quitkin F, Nathan RS, Halpern FS, Klein DF. Growth hormone response to dextroamphetamine in depressed patients and normal subjects. Arch Gen Psychiatry 39:189–192, 1982.
65. Herberg LJ, Stephens DN, Franklin KBJ. Catecholamines and self-stimulation: Evidence suggests a reinforcing role for noradrenaline and motivational role for dopamine. Pharmacol Biochem Behav 4:575–582, 1976.
66. Hu HY, Davis TM, Pandey GN. Characterization of alpha-adrenergic receptors in guinea pig cerebral cortex: effect of chronic antidepressant treatment. Psychopharmacology (Berlin) 74:201–203, 1981.
67. Huang YH. Chronic desipramine treatment increases activity of noradrenergic postsynaptic cells. Life Sci 25:709–716, 1979.
68. Huang YH, Maas JW, Hu G. The time course of noradrenergic pre- and post-synaptic activity during chronic desipramine treatment. Eur J Pharmacol 68:41–47, 1980
69. Hui KKP, Conolly ME. Increased numbers of beta-receptors in orthostatic hypotension due to autonomic dysfunction. N Engl J Med 304:1473–1476, 1981.
70. Innes IR. Action of dexamphetamine on 5-hydroxytryptamine receptors. Br J Pharmacol 21:427–435, 1963.
71. Insel TR, Kahn NH, Guttmacher LP, Cohen RM, Murphy DL. The dexamethasone suppression test in patients with primary obsessive-compulsive disorders. Psychiatry Res 6:153–160, 1982.
72. Janowsky DS, El-Yousef MK, Davis JM, Sekerke HJA. Cholinergic-adrenergic hypothesis of mania and depression. Lancet 2:632–638, 1972.
73. Johnson RW, Reisine T, Spotnitz S, Wiech N, Ursillo R, Yamamura HI. Effects of desipramine and yohimbine on α_2- and β-adrenoreceptor sensitivity. Eur J Pharmacol 67:123–127, 1980.
74. Kafka MS, Tallman FJ, Smith CC. Alpha-adrenergic receptors on human platelets. Life Sci 21:1429–1438, 1977.
75. Kafka MS, van Kammen DP, Kleinman JE, Nurnberger JI, Siever LJ, Uhde TWE, Polinsky RJ. Alpha-adrenergic receptor function in schizophrenia, affective disorder and some neurological diseases. Commun Psychopharmacol 4:477–486, 1981.
76. Kansal PC, Buse J, Talbert OR, Buse MG. The effect of L-dopa on plasma growth hormone, insulin and thyroxine. J Clin Endocrinol Metab 38:253–256, 1977.

77. Kielholz P. Diagnosis and therapy of the depressive states. Doc Geigy Acta Psychosom (N Am) 1:37, 1959.
78. Kobinger W, Pichler L. Centrally induced reduction in sympathetic tone—a postsynaptic α-adrenoceptor stimulating action of imidazolines. Eur J Pharmacol 40:311–320, 1976.
79. Krall JF, Connelly M, Weisbart R, Tuck ML. Age-related elevation of plasma catecholamine concentration and reduced responsiveness of lymphocyte adenylate cyclase. J Clin Endocrinol Metab 52:863–867, 1981.
80. Laakman von G, Benkert O, Neulinger E, Werger KV, Erhardt F. Beeinflussing der Hypophysen-Vorderlappen-hormon-Sekretion nach akuter und chronischer Gabe von Desipramin. Arzneimittelforsch 28:1292–1294, 1978.
81. Lake CR, Pickar D, Ziegler MG, Lipper S, Slater S, Murphy DL. High plasma norepinephrine levels in patients with major affective disorders. Am J Psychiatry, 139:1315–1318, 1982.
82. Lal S, Tolis G, Martin JB, Brown GM, Guyda H. Effect of clonidine on growth hormone, prolactin, luteinizing hormone, follicle-stimulating hormone and thyroid-stimulating hormone in the serum of normal men. J Clin Endocrinol Metab 41:827–832, 1975.
83. Lal S, de la Vega CE, Sourkes TL, Friesen HG. Effect of apomorphine on growth hormone, prolactin, luteinizing hormone and follicle stimulating hormone levels in human serum. J Clin Endocrinol Metab 37:719–724, 1973.
84. Langer G, Heinze G, Reim B, Matussek N. Reduced growth hormone responses to amphetamine in "endogenous" depressive patients: studies in normal, "reactive" and "endogenous" depressive, schizophrenic, and chronic alcoholic subjects. Arch Gen Psychiatry 33:1471–1475, 1976.
85. Langer SZ. Modern Concepts of Adrenergic Transmission. In Neurotransmitter Systems and Their Clinical Disorders, N Legg (ed), 29–51. London: Academic Press, 1980.
86. Linnoila M, Karoom F, Calil HM, Kopin IJ, Potter WZ. Alterations of norepinephrine metabolism in the desipramine and zimelidine in depressed patients. Arch Gen Psychiatry 39:1025–1028.
87. Louis WJ, Doyle AE, Anavekar SN. Plasma noradrenaline concentration and blood pressure in essential hypertension, phaeochromocytoma and depression. Clin Sci Mol Med 48:2395–2425, 1975.
88. Maany I, Mendals J, Frazer A, Brunswick D. A study of growth hormone release in depression. Neuropsychobiology 5:282–289, 1979.
89. Maas JW. Biogenic amines and depression: biochemical and pharmacological separation of two types of depression. Arch Gen Psychiatry 32:1357–1361, 1975.
90. Maas JW, Fawcett JA, Dekirmanjian H. Depression and MHPG excretion. Arch Gen Psychiatry 26:252–262, 1972.
91. MacKenzie TB, Popkin MK, Sheppard TR, Stillner V, Davis CM, Fenimore DC. Changes in beta-adrenergic receptor sensitivity associated with stress. Lancet 1:322, 1980.
92. Maggi A, U'Prichard DC, Enna SJ. β-adrenergic regulation of α_2-adrenergic receptors in the central nervous system. Science 207:645–647, 1980.
93. Maguire ME, Wiklund RA, Anderson HJ, Gilman AG. Binding of [^{125}I] Iodohydroxybenzylpindolol to putative β-adrenergic receptors of rat glioma cells and other cell clones. J Biol Chem 251:1221–1231, 1976.
94. Maj J, Mogilnicka E, Kordecka A. Chronic treatment with antidepressant drugs:

potentiation of apomorphine-induced aggressive behavior in rats. Neurosci Lett 13:337–341, 1979.

95. Maj J, Mogilnicka E, Kordecka-Magiera A. Effects of chronic administration of antidepressant drugs on aggressive behavior induced by clonidine in mice. Pharmacol Biochem Behav 13:153–154, 1979.

96. Martin JB, Kontor J, Mead P. Plasma GH responses to hypothalamic, hippocampal and amygdaloid electrical stimulation: Effects of variation in stimulus parameters and treatment with α-methyl-p-tyrosine (α-MT). Endocrinology 92:1354–1361, 1973.

97. Massala A, Delitala G, Alagna S, Devilla L. Effects of pimozide on levodopa-induced growth hormone release in man. Clin Endocrinol 7:253–256, 1977.

98. Matussek N, Ackenheil M, Hippius H, Muller F, Schröder H-Th, Schuttes H, Wasilewski B. Effect of clonidine on growth hormone release in psychiatric patients and controls. Psychiatr Res 2:25–36, 1980.

99. McMillen BA, Warnack W, German DC, Shore PA. Effects of chronic desipramine treatment on rat brain noradrenergic responses to α-adrenergic drugs. Eur J Pharmacol 61:239–246, 1980.

100. McWilliam JR, Meldrom BS. Noradrenergic regulation of growth hormone secretion in the baboon. Endocrinology 112:254–259, 1983.

101. Menkes DB, Aghajanian GK, McCall RB. Chronic antidepressant treatment enhances α-adrenergic and serotonergic responses in the facial nucleus. Life Sci 27:45–55, 1980.

102. Mobley PL, Sulser F. Norepinephrine-stimulated cyclic AMP accumulation in rat limbic forebrain slices: partial mediation by a subpopulation of receptors with neither α nor β characteristics. Eur J Pharmacol 60:221–227, 1979.

103. Modigh K. Electroconvulsive shock and postsynaptic catecholamine effects: increased psychomotor stimulant action of apomorphine and clonidine in reserpine pretreated mice by repeated ECS. J Neural Transm 36:19–32, 1975.

104. Moore KE. The actions of amphetamines on neurotransmitters: a brief review. Biol Psychiatry 12:451–462, 1977.

105. Murphy DL, Campbell FC, Costa JL. The brain serotonergic system in the affective disorders. Prog Neuropsychopharmacol 2:1–31, 1978.

106. Murphy DL, Costa JL. Utilization of Cellular Studies of Neurotransmitter-Related Enzymes and Transport Processes in Man for the Investigation of Biological Factors in Behavioral Disorders. In The Psychobiology of Depression, J Mendels (ed), 27–46. New York: Spectrum Publications, 1975.

107. Murphy DL, Donelly C, Moskowitz J. Catecholamine receptor function in depressed patients. Am J Psychiatry 131:1389–1391, 1974.

108. Muscettola G, Wehr T, Goodwin FK. Effects of diet in urinary MHPG excretion in depressed patients and normal control subjects. Am J Psychiatry 134:914–916, 1977.

109. Nielsen M, Braestrup C. Chronic treatment with desipramine caused a sustained decrease of 3,4-dihydroxyphenylglycolsulphate and total 3-methoxy-4-hydroxyphenylglycol in the rat brain. Naunyn Schmiedebergs Arch Pharmacol 300:87–92, 1977.

110. Nurnberger JI, Gershon ES. Genetic Considerations in the Epidemiology of Psychoactive Drug Use. In Epidemiological Impact of Psychotropic Drugs, G Tognoni, C Bellantuono, and M Lader (eds), 19–31. Amsterdam: Elsevier North Holland Biomedical Press, 1981.

111. Nurnberger JI, Jr, Gershon ES, Sitaram H, Gillin JC, Brown G, Ebert M, Gold P, Jimerson D, Kessler L. Dextroamphetamine and arecoline as pharmacogenetic probes in normals and remitted bipolar patients. Psychopharmacol Bull 17:80–82, 1981.

112. Olpe HR. Differential effects of chlorimipramine and clorgyline on the sensitivity of cortical neurons to serotonin: effects of chronic treatment. Eur J Pharmacol 69:375–377, 1981.
113. Olpe HR, Schellenberg A. Reduced sensitivity of neurons to noradrenaline after chronic treatment with antidepressant drugs. Eur J Pharmacol 63:7–13, 1980.
114. Pandey GN, Dysken MW, Garver DL, Davis JM. Beta-adrenergic receptor function in affective illness. Am J Psychiatry 136:675–678, 1979.
115. Parker CW, Smith JW. Alterations in cyclic AMP production in human bronchial asthma. I. Leukocyte responsiveness to β-adrenergic agents. J Clin Invest 52:48–59, 1973.
116. Paul SM, Crews FT. Rapid desensitization of cerebral cortical β-adrenergic receptors induced by desmethylimipramine and phenoxybenzamine. Eur J Pharmacol 62:349–350, 1980.
117. Peroutka SJ, Snyder SH. Chronic antidepressant treatment decreases spiroperidol-labeled serotonin receptor binding. Science 210:88–90, 1980.
118. Peroutka SJ, Snyder SH. Regulation of serotonin (5-HT_2) receptors labeled with ^{3}H-spiroperidol by chronic treatment with the antidepressant amitriptyline. J Pharmacol Exp Ther 215:582–587, 1980.
119. Pickar D, Cohen RM, Murphy DL, Fried D. Tyramine infusions in bipolar illness: behavioral effects and longitudinal changes in pressor sensitivity. Am J Psychiatry 136:1460–1463, 1979.
120. Prange AJ, McCurdy RL, Cochrane CM. The systolic blood pressure response of depressed patients to infused norepinephrine. J Psychiatr Res 5:1–13, 1967.
121. Redmond DE. Alterations in the Function of the Nucleus Locus Coeruleus: A Possible Model for Studies of Anxiety. In Animal Models in Psychiatry and Neurology, I Hanin and E Usdin (eds), 293–304. New York: Pergamon Press, 1977.
122. Rees L, Butler PWP, Gosling C, Besser GM. Adrenergic blockade and the corticosteroid and growth hormone responses to methylamphetamine. Nature 228:565–566, 1970.
123. Rehavi M, Ramot O, Yavetz B, Sokolovsky M. Amitriptyline: long-term treatment elevates α-adrenergic and muscarinic receptor binding in mouse brain. Brain Res 194:443–453, 1980.
124. Reisine TD, U'Prichard DC, Wiech NL, Ursillo RC, Yamamura HI. Effects of combined administration of amphetamine and iprindole on brain adrenergic receptors. Brain Res 188:587–592, 1980.
125. Risch SC, Kalin NH, Murphy DL. Pharmacological challenge strategies: implications for neurochemical mechanisms in affective disorders and treatment approaches. J Clin Psychopharmacol 1:238–243, 1981.
126. Roffler-Tarlov S, Schildkraut JJ, Draskoczy PR. Effects of acute and chronic administration of desipramine on the content of norepinephrine and other monoamines in the rat brain. Biochem Pharmacol 22:2923–2926, 1973.
127. Roffman M, Kling MA, Cassens G, Orsulak PJ, Reigle TG, Schildkraut JJ. The effects of acute and chronic administration of tricyclic antidepressants on MHPG-SO_4 in rat brain. Psychopharmacol Commun 1:195–206, 1977.
128. Rosenblatt JE, Pert CB, Tallman JF, Pert A, Bunney WE, Jr. The effect of imipramine and lithium on α- and β-receptor binding in rat brain. Brain Res 160:186–191, 1979.
129. Rosloff BN, Davis JM. Decrease in brain NE turnover after chronic DMI treatment: No effect with iprindole. Psychopharmacology (Berlin) 56:335–341, 1978.

130. Sachar EJ, Altman N, Gruen PH, Glassman A, Halpern FS, Sassin J. Human growth hormone response to L-dopa in relation to menopause, depression and plasma level of L-dopa. Arch Gen Psychiatry 32:502–503, 1975.
131. Sachar EJ, Asnis G, Nathan RS, Halbreich U, Tabrizi MA, Halpern FS. Dextroamphetamine and cortisol on depression. Arch Gen Psychiatry 37:755–757, 1980.
132. Sachar EJ, Finkelstein J, Hellman L. Growth hormone responses in depressive illness. I. Responses to insulin tolerance test. Arch Gen Psychiatry 25:263–269, 1971.
133. Sachar EJ, Frantz AB, Altman N, Sassin J. Growth hormone and prolactin in unipolar and bipolar depressed patients. Responses to hypoglycemia and L-dopa. Am J Psychiatry 130:1362–1367, 1973.
134. Schildkraut JJ. The catecholamine hypothesis of affective disorders: a review of supporting evidence. Am J Psychiatry 122:509–522, 1965.
135. Schildkraut JJ, Orsulak PJ, LaBrie RA, Schatzberg AF, Gudeman JE, Cole JO, Rhode WE. Toward a biochemical classification of depressive disorders: II. Application of multivariate discriminant function to analysis of data on urinary catecholamines and metabolites. Arch Gen Psychiatry 35:1436–1439, 1978.
136. Schildkraut JJ, Orsulak PJ, Schatzberg AF, Gudeman JE, Cole JO, Rhode WE, LaBrie RA. Toward a biochemical classification of depressive disorders: I. Differences in urinary excretion of MHPG and other catecholamine metabolites on clinically defined subtypes of depression. Arch Gen Psychiatry 35:1427–1433, 1978.
137. Schildkraut JJ, Roffman M, Orsulak PJ, Schatzberg AF, Kling MA, Reigle TG. Effects of short- and long-term administration of tricyclic antidepressants and lithium on norepinephrine turnover in brain. Pharmakopsychiatr Neuropsychopharmakol 9:193–202, 1976.
138. Schultz JR, Siggins GR, Schocker FW, Turck M, Bloom FE. Effects of prolonged treatment with lithium and tricyclic antidepressants on discharge frequency, norepinephrine responses and beta-receptor binding in rat cerebellum: electrophysiological and biochemical comparison. J Pharmacol Exp Ther 216:28–38, 1981.
139. Schwartz JC, Costentin J, Martres MP, Protais P, Baudry M. Modulation of receptor mechanisms in the CNS. Hyper- and hyposensitivity in catecholamines. Neuropharmacology 17:665–685, 1978.
140. Schweitzer JW, Schwartz R, Friedhoff AJ. Intact presynaptic terminals required for beta-adrenergic receptor regulation by desipramine. J Neurochem 33:377–379, 1979.
141. Segal DS, Kuczenski R, Mandell AJ. Theoretical implications of drug-induced adaptive regulations for a biogenic amine hypothesis of affective disorder. Biol Psychiatry 9:147, 1974.
142. Siever LJ, Cohen RM, Murphy DL. Antidepressants and α_2-adrenergic autoreceptor desensitization. Am J Psychiatry 138:681–682, 1981.
142a. Siever LJ, Davis KL. Dysregulation of the noradrenergic system in the affective disorders. Psychopharm Bull 20:500–504, 1984.
143. Siever LJ, Insel TR, Jimerson DC, Lake CR, Uhde TW, Aloi J, Murphy DL. Growth hormone response to clonidine in obsessive-compulsive patients. Br J Psychiatry 142:184–187, 1983.
144. Siever LJ, Insel TR, Uhde TW. Noradrenergic challenges in the affective disorders. J Clin Psychopharmacol 1:193–206, 1981.
144a. Siever LJ, Kafka MS, Targum S, Lake CR. Platelet alpha-adrenergic binding and biochemical responsiveness in depressed patients and controls. Psychiatry Res 11:287–302, 1984.

145. Siever LJ, Pickar D, Lake CR, Cohen RM, Uhde TW, Murphy DL. Extreme elevations in plasma norepinephrine associated with decreased α-adrenergic responsivity in major depressive disorder: two case reports. J Clin Psychopharmacol 3:39–41, 1983.

146. Siever LJ, Risch SC, Murphy DL. Central cholinergic-adrenergic imbalance in the regulation of affective state. Psychiatry Res 4:108–109, 1981.

147. Siever LJ, Uhde TW. New studies and perspectives on the noradrenergic receptor system in depression: effects of the alpha-adrenergic agonist clonidine. Biol Psychiatry 19:131–156, 1984.

148. Siever LJ, Uhde TW, Insel TR, Roy BF, Murphy DL. Growth hormone response to clonidine unchanged by chronic clorgyline treatment. Psychiatry Res 6:171–183, 1982.

149. Siever LJ, Uhde TW, Murphy DL. Possible subsensitization of α_2-adrenergic receptors by chronic monoamine oxidase inhibitor treatment in psychiatric patients. Psychiatry Res 6:293–302, 1982.

150. Siever LJ, Uhde TW, Silberman EK, Jimerson DC, Aloi JA, Post RM, Murphy DL. The growth hormone response to clonidine as a probe of noradrenergic receptor responsiveness in affective disorder patients and controls. Psychiatry Res 6:171–183, 1982.

150a. Sitaram N, Jones D, Kelwalta S, Bell J, Stevenson J, Gershon S. Pharmacology of the human iris: development and use of challenge strategies in the study of antidepression response. Prog Neuropsychopharmacol Biol Psych 7:273–286, 1983.

151. Sitaram N, Nurnberger JI, Gershon ES, Gillin JC. Faster cholinergic REM sleep induction in euthymic patients with primary affective illness. Science 208:200–202, 1980.

152. Sitaram N, Ross E, Brown A, Gant C, Jones D, Kelwalla S, Bell J. Changes in pupillary cholinergic and adrenergic sensitivity during antidepressant treatment. Abstracts of the 13th Colleagium International Neuro-Psychopharmacologicum (CINP) Congress, 679, 1982.

153. Slater S, de la Vega CE, Skyler J, Murphy DL. Plasma prolactin stimulation by fenfluramine and amphetamine. Psychopharmacol Bull 12:26–27, 1976.

154. Smith CB, Garcia-Sevilla JA, Hillingsworth PJ. Alpha-$_2$ adrenoceptors in rat brain are decreased after long-term tricyclic antidepressant drug treatment. Brain Res 210:413–418, 1981.

155. Snyder SH. Overview of Neurotransmitter Receptor Binding. In Neurotransmitter Receptor Binding, HI Yamamura, SJ Enna, and MJ Kuhar (eds), 1–11. New York: Raven Press, 1978.

156. Sporn JR, Harden TK, Wolfe BB, Molinoff PB. β-Adrenergic receptor involvement in 6-hydroxydopamine-induced supersensitivity in rat cerebral cortex. Science 194:624–626, 1976.

157. Stein L, Wise CD, Belluzi JD. Neuropharmacology of Reward and Punishment. In Handbook of Psychopharmacology, LL Iverson, SD Iverson, and SJ Snyder (eds), vol 8, 25–53. New York: Plenum Press, 1977.

158. Stjarne L, Brundin J. Dual adrenoceptor–mediated control of noradrenaline secretion from human vasoconstrictor nerves: facilitation by β-receptors and inhibition by α-receptors. Acta Physiol Scand 94: 139–141, 1975.

159. Stone EA. Subsensitivity to norepinephrine as a link between adaption to stress and antidepressant therapy: a hypothesis. Res Commun Psychol Psychiatr Behav 4:241, 1979.

160. Sugrue MF. Current concepts on the mechanisms of action of antidepressant drugs. Pharmacol Ther 13:219–247, 1981.
161. Sugrue MF. Effects of acutely and chronically administered antidepressants on the clonidine-induced decrease in rat brain 3-methyoxy-4-hydroxyphenylethyleneglycol sulphate content. Life Sci 28:377–384, 1981.
162. Sulser F. New perspectives on the mode of action of antidepressant drugs. Trends Pharmacol Sci 1:92–94, 1979.
163. Sulser F, Ventulani J, Mobley P. Mode of action of antidepressant drugs. Biochem Pharmacol 27:257–261, 1978.
164. Svensson TH. Effect of chronic treatment with tricyclic antidepressant drugs on identified brain noradrenergic and serotonergic neurons. Acta Psychiatr Scand 61 [Suppl. 280]: 121–131, 1980.
165. Svensson TH, Bunney BS, Aghajanian GK. Inhibition of both noradrenergic and serotonergic neurons in brain by the α-adrenergic agonist clonidine. Brain Res 92:291–306, 1975.
166. Svensson TH, Usdin T. Feedback inhibition of brain noradrenaline neurons by tricyclic antidepressants: α-Receptor mediation. Science 202:1089–1091, 1978.
167. Tang SW, Helmeste DM, Stancer HC. Interaction of antidepressants with clonidine on rat brain total 3-methoxy-4-hydroxyphenylglycol. Can J Physiol Pharmacol 57:435–437, 1979.
168. Tang SW, Seeman P, Kwan S. Differential effect of chronic desipramine and amitriptyline treatment on rat brain adrenergic and serotonergic receptors. Psychiatry Res 4:129–138, 1981.
169. Tangri KK, Bhargava AK, Bhargava KP. Interrelation between monoaminergic and cholinergic mechanisms in the hypothalamic thermoregulatory centre of rabbits. Neuropharmacology 13:333–346, 1974.
170. Terry LC, Martin JB. Evidence for α-adrenergic regulation of episodic growth hormone and prolactin secretion in the undisturbed male rat. Endocrinology 108:1869–1873, 1981.
171. Tharp MD, Hoffman BB, Lefkowitz RJ. α-Adrenergic receptors in human adipocyte membranes: direct determination by [^{3}H] yohimbine binding. J Clin Endocrinol Metab 52:709–714, 1981.
172. Toivola PTK, Gale CC. Stimulation of growth hormone release by microinjection of norepinephrine into hypothalamus of baboons. Endocrinology 90:895–902, 1972.
173. Toivola PTK, Gale CC, Goodrer CJ, Werrbach JH. Central α-adrenergic regulation of growth hormone and insulin. Hormones 3:193–213, 1972.
174. Uhde TW, Siever LJ, Post RM. Clonidine. Acute Challenge and Clinical Trial Paradigms for the Investigation and Treatment of Anxiety Disorders, Affective Illness, and Pain Syndromes. In The Neurobiology of Mood Disorders, RM Post and JC Ballenger (eds), 554–571. Baltimore: Williams and Wilkins, 1982.
175. U'Prichard DC, Bechtel WD, Rouot B, Snyder SH. Multiple apparent alpha-noradrenergic receptor binding sites in rat brain. Effects of 6-hydroxydopamine. Mol Pharmacol 16:47–60, 1979.
176. U'Prichard DC, Daiguji M, Tong C, Mitrius JC, Meltzer HY. α_2-Adrenergic Receptors: Comparative Biochemistry of Neural and Nonneural Receptors, and In Vivo Analysis in Psychiatric Patients. In Biological Markers in Psychiatry and Neurology, E Usdin and I Hanin (eds), 205–217. Oxford: Pergamon Press, 1982.

177. U'Prichard DC, Snyder SH. ^{3}H-Catecholamine binding to α receptors in rat brain: enhancement by reserpine. Eur J Pharmacol 51:145–155, 1978.
178. van Kammen DP, Docherty JP, Marder SR, Siris SG, Bunney WE, Jr. D-Amphetamine raises serum prolactin in man: evaluations after chronic placebo, lithium and pimozide treatment. Life Sci 23:1478–1492, 1972.
179. van Kammen DP, Murphy DL. Prediction of imipramine antidepressant response by a one-day D-amphetamine trial. Am J Psychiatry 135:1179–1184, 1976.
180. Vetulani J, Stawarz RJ, Dingell JV, Sulser F. A possible common mechanism of action of antidepressant treatments. Naunyn Schmiedebergs Arch Pharmacol 293:109–114, 1976.
181. Vetulani J, Sulser F. Action of various antidepressant treatments reduce reactivity of noradrenergic cyclic AMP–generating system in limbic forebrain. Nature 257:495–496, 1975.
182. Wang RY, Aghajanian GK. Enhanced sensitivity of amygdaloid neurons to serotonin and norepinephrine after chronic antidepressant treatment. Commun Psychopharmacol 4:83–90, 1980.
183. Wang Y-C, Pandey GN, Mendels J, Frazer A. Platelet adenylate cyclase responses on depression: implications for a receptor defect. Psychopharmacologia (Berlin) 36:291–300, 1974.
184. Watkins J, Fitzgerald G, Zamboulis C, Brown MJ, Dollery CT. Absence of opiate and histamine H_2 receptor–mediated effects of clonidine. Clin Pharmacol Ther 28:605–610, 1980.
185. Wehr TA, Goodwin FK. Catecholamines in Depression. In Handbook of Studies on Depression, GD Burrows (ed), 283–303. Amsterdam: Excerpta Medica, 1977.
186. Wehr TA, Muscettola G, Goodwin FK. Urinary 3-methoxy-4-hydroxyphenylglycol circadian rhythm. Arch Gen Psychiatry 37:257–263, 1980.
187. Wiech NL, Ursillo RC. Acceleration of desipramine-induced decrease of rat corticocerebral beta-adrenergic receptors by yohimbine. Commun Psychopharmacol 4:95–100, 1980.
188. Williams LT, Lefkowitz RJ. Regulation of rabbit myometrial alpha-adrenergic receptors by estrogen and progesterone. J Clin Invest 60:815–818, 1977.
189. Williams LT, Snyderman R, Lefkowitz RW. Identification of β-adrenergic receptors in human lymphocytes by (-) [^{3}H] alprenolol binding. J Clin Invest 57:149–155, 1976.
190. Wolfe BB, Harden TK, Sporn JR, Molinoff PB. Presynaptic modulation of beta-adrenergic receptors in rat cerebral cortex after treatment with antidepressants. J Pharmacol Exp Ther 207:446–457, 1978.
191. Wyatt RJ, Portnoy B, Kupfer DJ, Snyder I, Engelman K. Resting plasma concentrations in patients with depression and anxiety. Arch Gen Psychiatry 24:65–70, 1971.
192. Zandburg P, DeJong W, deWied D. Effect of catecholamine-receptor stimulating agents on blood pressure after local application in the nucleus tractus solitarii of the medulla oblongata. Eur J Pharmacol 55:43–56, 1979.
193. Ziegler MG, Lake CR, Wood JH, Brooks BR, Ebert MH. Relationship between norepinephrine in blood and cerebrospinal fluid in the presence of a blood-cerebrospinal fluid barrier for norepinephrine. J Neurochem 28:677–679, 1977.

13

Parkinsonism and Depression: Dopaminergic Mediation of Neuropathologic Processes in Human Beings

Henry H. Holcomb

Four lines of evidence suggest that aspects of Parkinson's disease and depression share common neural mechanisms. First, parkinsonian patients suffer from depressive symptoms more frequently than control groups with matched incapacity [41,76]. Second, autopsy studies of parkinsonian patients reveal brain levels of norepinephrine [NE] [31,43], serotonin (5-hydroxytryptamine; 5-HT) [42], and dopamine (DA) [31,43,70] to be much lower than controls, and metabolites of these neurotransmitters in cerebrospinal fluid (CSF) of depressed patients tend to be lower than in CSF of controls [66,79,80,90]. Third, both parkinsonian [98] and depressed patients [22] benefit from drugs that increase the activity of monoamine neurotransmitters at central receptor sites (i.e., L-dopa in parkinsonian patients and a variety of antidepressants in depressed patients). This chapter explores how parkinsonism, a noncyclic, well-characterized illness, can help us understand depression, a cyclic, reversible, and poorly understood illness, by examining their shared neural mechanisms, related symptomatology, and similar treatments.

MOOD MODULATION BY DRUGS THAT ALTER CENTRAL DOPAMINE ACTIVITY

DA is an important neurotransmitter in neuronal circuits associated with mood modulation. This section discusses several groups of drugs which alter DA neuronal function and mood. These drugs are also potent modulators of motor behavior and markedly improve or worsen the symptoms of parkinsonism depending on their DA agonist or antagonist properties.

DA agonists may act indirectly by increasing levels of synaptic DA or directly by activating DA receptors. Amphetamine and L-dopa increase synaptic DA by promoting transmitter synthesis, release, or reduced reuptake. Apomorphine

(APO), bromocriptine, and piribedil directly stimulate DA receptors. α-methyl-*P*-tyrosine (AMPT) and reserpine reduce DA synthesis and storage respectively and are therefore considered DA antagonists. Neuroleptics are DA antagonists by virtue of their DA receptor–blocking action.

Amphetamine is a potent stimulator of DA [58] and NE [8] release, and it reduces their reuptake. These actions are associated with a dramatic rise in synaptic catecholamine (CA) levels. Because noradrenergic and dopaminergic neurons are electrophysiologically inhibited by their respective neurotransmitters, amphetamine markedly inhibits the firing of NE neurons in the locus coeruleus [37] and DA neurons in the substantia nigra [17,18].

Controlled clinical studies describe the behavioral effects of amphetamine [29]. Van Kammen and Murphy [89] reported a marked enhancement in mood and activation in a group of nine depressed patients who took 30 mg of D-amphetamine. Rapoport et al [73] studied the effects of 0.5 mg/kg of body weight and 0.25 mg/kg D-amphetamine sulfate in normal college-aged men. Using a self-report mood scale, subjects indicated feelings of euphoria and irritability and an increased energy level at both doses. In an effort to determine the chemical basis of amphetamine's excitatory effects, Nurnberger et al [63] administered 0.3 mg/kg intravenous amphetamine to normal subjects. When pretreated with haloperidol, a DA antagonist, (0.014 mg/kg intramuscular), subjects failed to experience behavioral excitement. Propranolol, a β-noradrenergic blocker (0.1 mg/kg intravenously) did not, however, markedly block behavioral arousal. Although this study suggests that amphetamine's behavioral excitatory effects result from increased DA activity, interpretation is complicated by haloperidol's multiple sites of action. A recent electrophysiologic study of neuroleptics demonstrating potent α-adrenoceptor antagonist properties [57] emphasized the multifaceted and confounding nature of drug interactions in the central nervous system (CNS).

Whereas amphetamine enhances DA activity by stimulating its release and blocking its reuptake [8], L-dopa acts by enhancing DA synthesis and release [30, 54,65]. Inhibitors of dopa decarboxylase (the enzyme which forms DA by decarboxylating L-dopa) block the synthesis of DA and consequently prevent L-dopa from suppressing spontaneous DA neuron firing [17]. In contrast, drugs which act by binding directly to DA receptors, for example, APO, are not retarded in their suppressant function by enzyme inhibitors [17].

Clinical investigations of L-dopa's behavioral effects have produced diverse observations. Goodwin's [34] review lists confusion, depression, overactivity, psychosis, and hypomania as the leading behavioral side effects of the drug in parkinsonian patients. The incidence ranged from 4.1 to 1.5% in these five categories of side effects. In a group of 23 depressed patients studied at the National Institute of Mental Health [36], only five showed a consistent improvement in depression while taking L-dopa. In seven of eight trials given to the responders, a relapse occurred following placebo substitution. Of those patients who failed to improve with L-dopa, all exhibited a notable increase in angry feelings and behavior. No increase in anxiety ratings was observed. In a subgroup of patients with a previous history of mania, L-dopa administration was consistently associated with induction of mania or hypomania in all five bipolars in one study and six of seven in another [36,59]. A more recent study [48] found that L-dopa administration markedly shortened the length of phase in manic-depressive cyclic illness. L-dopa's influence on memory and cognition are reviewed in a later section.

Bromocriptine, piribedil, and APO are direct DA agonists by virtue of their tendency to bind to and activate DA receptors located presynaptically and postsynaptically. Roth [77] has exploited the biochemical differences between presynaptic and postsynaptic DA receptors and has demonstrated that bromocriptine [10], piribedil [91], and APO [62] are potent DA agonists at the presynaptic site. When DA agonists activate presynaptic DA receptors, the synthetic activity of tyrosine hydroxylase (TH) is markedly inhibited and the accumulation of dopa is diminished. A drug's capacity to activate this negative feedback loop and reduce DA synthesis is a good indication of its affinity for the presynaptic DA receptor. Clinical studies reviewed here and animal behavior studies [2,3,] indicate that these DA agonists have similarly potent actions at postsynaptic receptors.

Two studies have suggested that bromocriptine may appreciably ameliorate depression or mania, depending on the dose used. Eleven of 12 depressed patients treated with 5 to 15 mg per day of bromocriptine showed some general improvement, but only three had a "good" response [24]. Three manic patients treated with similar doses exhibited a marked reduction in excitement over a 48-hour period [24]. In a second study [61], nine depressed patients treated for 5 weeks with 20 to 60 mg daily showed nearly complete recovery. Bromocriptine's mood-altering potential is also illustrated by the case of a 19-year-old woman being treated with bromocriptine (2.5 mg/day) for neuroleptic-induced galactorrhea. During the treatment, she exhibited an exacerbation of mania that had previously been controlled with chlorpromazine [45]. Discontinuation of the DA agonist resulted in a prompt remission of manic symptoms. In depressed patients, high doses of bromocriptine are probably necessary to activate postsynaptic DA receptors. Low doses of DA agonists are sufficient to act on presynaptic receptors; this will reduce DA activity by activating a negative feedback system [77]. Hence, low doses are likely to ameliorate mania but not alter depression; high doses should relieve depression and exacerbate mania.

Low doses of APO produce sedation in animals [26] and human beings [25]. Neuroleptics in low doses prevent APO-induced sedation in animals [26]. Because of its strong emetic properties, APO is given to humans in low doses which are considered relatively specific for presynaptic receptors [83]. In a particularly interesting but seldom-cited study, Tesarova [87] administered APO (0.5–1.0 mg, subcutaneously, tid) for 12 to 14 days to normal volunteers and patients with "neurotic" disorders. Depression was induced in 64% of the neurotics and in 37.2% of the normal volunteers. Historically unique, this study suggested that long-term administration of a drug known to selectively suppress DA neuron firing, when given in these low doses, can induce melancholia. Were such a study performed today in a clinical research center equipped with modern neurobiologic measurement systems, useful information might be gained regarding the biology of depression. The marked psychomotor retardation produced in these subjects is especially interesting in light of the presumed connection between depression and parkinsonism.

Piribedil studies in normal and psychiatric patients have indicated that this DA agonist has pronounced effects on mood and arousal which are reversed by DA-receptor blockers [5,6]. Angrist et al [5] administered piribedil intravenously to five normal volunteers. Given in low doses it produced marked sedation, motor suppression, and dysphoria. Haloperidol, given in low doses intravenously, reversed this syndrome. In a study with depressed patients, Post et al [68] found that high doses of piribedil (120–220 mg/day) significantly reduced depression ratings in seven of ten patients. Substantial clinical improvement was evident in four of ten. Pretreatment CSF homovanillic acid (HVA) levels correlated significantly ($r = -0.66$) with improvement. This low level of DA metabolite may be an indicator of suppressed central DA activity. Piribedil may be particularly useful in patients who suffer from a depression associated with reduced DA activity. This hypothesis is reviewed in a monograph by Jimerson and Post [44]. In summary, piribedil, bromocriptine, and APO suppress motor and emotional activity when given in low doses, presumably by stimulating presynaptic negative feedback systems. High doses of these drugs enhance emotional and motor activity by stimulating postsynaptic DA receptors.

Research on depression caused by CA depletion and synthesis inhibition was extensively represented in early biologic psychiatry literature [14,19,35,36, 79,80]. The 20-year-old CA theory of depression relies heavily on the effects of reserpine [35] and AMPT, an inhibitor of TH [14]. Because these drugs reduce the availability of NE and DA throughout the entire nervous system it is unclear which of the changes they produce are adequate or necessary to induce or worsen depression. Drugs with relatively specific activities have been used to probe dopaminergic aspects of affective illness with considerable success [61,67,87]. It is, however, unfortunate that these drugs have prominent effects on both presynaptic and postsynaptic DA receptors. A new generation of drugs (e.g., [3-hydroxyphenyl]-N-n-propyl-piperidine) exhibiting specific inhibitory or activating effects on a single class of receptors (DA autoreceptors in the case of this drug) will allow formulation of more meaningful questions in this field.

Thus far, only drugs with relatively well-defined characteristics and mechanisms have been discussed with respect to mood modulation. It is, however, not clear how antidepressants induce mania [71]. Tricyclics and monoamine oxidase inhibitors (MAO-I) are associated with a marked increase in the cycling rate of bipolar patients [20,71,93]. Because mania is rapidly neutralized by relatively specific DA receptor blockers [69], it is reasonable to suspect that antidepressant treatments enhance DA receptor sensitivity or postsynaptic receptor function. This suspicion is reinforced by a recent case report [27] describing enhanced antidepressant efficacy with desipramine when methylphenidate was added to a patient's treatment. Because methylphenidate is particularly effective in promoting DA release and blocking its reuptake [13,32], this strategy may be especially useful for patients with a dopaminergic component to their depression.

PARKINSON'S DISEASE: BIOCHEMISTRY AND TREATMENT

In 1959, the first studies describing a DA deficiency in the substantia nigra and caudate of parkinsonian patients were performed [42]. Since that time, investigators have found deficiencies in CA and their metabolites in multiple brain regions. These deficiencies include marked DA and NE reductions in the ventral tegmentum as well as in the substantia nigra compacta and reticular regions [43]. Metabolites of DA are also reduced in frontal cortex (Brodmann area 9), caudate, and hippocampus [78]. HVA levels are notably reduced in those three regions as well as in cingulate and entorhinal cortex. This extensive cortical disturbance in brains of parkinsonian patients may promote cognitive deficits. Parkinsonian limbic forebrain regions demonstrate deficient DA levels in the lateral hypothalamus, parolfactory gyrus, and nucleus accumbens; DA metabolites are also low in medial and lateral olfactory areas [70]. This extensive limbic involvement may partially account for this group's marked predilection to depression and other mood disturbances [15, 16,41,76].

Depression is commonly reported in parkinsonism. The reviews of Brown et al [15,16] outline the history of this association and Robins [76] carefully fixes the characteristics and prevalence of depression in this group. Parkinsonian patients carefully matched for age and sex with 45 chronically disabled patients (considerably more disabled than the parkinsonian patients) were rated on the Hamilton Rating Scale [76]. Parkinsonian patients were far more depressed than the controls. Specific items on the Hamilton Scale indicated that parkinsonian patients had higher scores on items relating to suicide, work and interests, retardation, psychic anxiety, somatic symptoms, and loss of insight. Severity of disability did not affect depression ratings. Patients with parkinsonism clearly suffer a degree of depression that cannot solely be due to the stress of physical disability.

Whether by acting presynaptically or postsynaptically, drugs which increase central monomine activity alter mood state. Similarly, the movement disorder characteristic of parkinsonism is partially ameliorated by drugs which enhance central monoamine activity. Amphetamine [21], L-dopa [98], piribedil [53], bromocriptine [51–53,88], and APO [21] reduce the motor symptoms of parkinsonism (rigidity, tremor, akinesia). It is not clear why deprenyl (an MAO-I, type B) [47], tricyclic antidepressants (Table 13.1), and ECT frequently reduce the severity of parkinsonian symptoms. In Table 13.1, most of the literature's references describing antidepressant treatment of parkinsonism are listed. An earlier general discussion of DA psychopharmacology as it relates to depression and parkinsonism is provided by Randrup et al [72]. Willner [100,101,102] has recently reviewed the literature pertaining to DA's role in affective illness.

Of 133 parkinsonian patients given tricyclic antidepressants, 74 (54%) gained significant motor improvement (see Table 13.1). In contrast, of the 25 parkinsonian patients receiving ECT, 20 (80%) exhibited marked symptom reduction. This disparity in treatment response between tricyclics and ECT is similar to that reported for the treatment of depression [22,46]. Animal research with antidepressants and locomotor activity suggests that ECT has a stronger facilitating effect than tricyclics

Table 13.1 The Effect of Tricyclic Antidepressants and Electroconvulsive Therapy on the Severity of Parkinsonism

Reference	*Date*	*Treatment*	*No. of Patients*	*Response*
		Tricyclic Treatments		
Anderson et al [4]	1980	Nortriptyline, 50–150 mg/day, long term	19	Reduced depressive symptoms; no effect on neurologic symptoms
Bedard et al [11]	1977	Nomifensine, 150 mg/day, long-term, plus L-dopa	8	No improvement
Laitinen [49]	1969	Desipramine, 100 mg/day, 3 wk	20	Good response in 50%, especially rigidity and gait
Mandell et al [56]	1961	Imipramine, 250 mg/day, 2–3 wk	15	Good to excellent response in 10/15; no response in 5
Park et al [64]	1977	Nomifensine, 200 mg/day, 2 wk	29	Significant improvement in tremor and facial expression in the entire group
Sigwald et al [81]	1959	Imipramine, 100–400 mg/day, treatment duration not given; L-dopa therapy concurrent	12	75% exhibited clinically significant improvement, especially akinesia
Strang [85]	1965	Imipramine, 50–150 mg/day, 4 mo	30	16 patients exhibited significant improvement; rigidity and tremor were best treated
		ECT Treatments and Number of Treatments		
Ananth et al [1]	1979	8 over 2 wk	1	Amelioration of drug-induced parkinsonism and lysis of psychopathology
Asnis [7]	1977	6 over 3 wk	1	Improved neurologic signs; reduction in depression; improved handwriting
Balldin et al [9]	1980	4–8 over 2–4 wk	5	Marked reduction in "on-off" symptoms in entire group
Dysken et al [28]	1976	12 over 4 wk	1	Improved depression, marked improvement in rigidity, bradykine-

Table 13.1 *(continued)*

Reference	*Date*	*Treatment*	*No. of Patients*	*Response*
				sia, facial expression and tremor
Fromm [33]	1959	Not given	8	Marked improvement in rigidity and bradykinesia in 5 patients; equivocal improvement in tremor in 2 patients; 1 patient showed no improvement
Holcomb et al [40]	1983	14 over 40 days followed by 8 over 15 days	1	Marked reduction in depression, bradykinesia, rigidity, posture and tremor; mild worsening of buccolingual dyskinesia
Lebensohn and Jenkins [50]	1975	4 each, all within 1 wk	2	Marked improvement in depressive and parkinsonian symptoms in both
Ward et al [92]	1980	6 over 3 wk	5	No improvement in "on-off" symptoms in any
Yudofsky [99]	1979	Unknown	1	Marked improvement in depressive and parkinsonian symptoms

on motility induced by monoamine agonists [38,55,84]. The biology of this stronger effect is obscure.

COGNITIVE FUNCTION MODIFIED BY DEPRESSION, PARKINSONISM, AND DOPAMINE AGONISTS

In this last section cognitive function is considered in three clinical settings: depression, parkinsonism, and DA agonist drug administration. The third set of studies is further divided: (1) tryptophan and L-dopa administration to depressed patients and normal volunteers, and (2) amphetamine administration to depressed patients and normals.

Depression severely impairs memory and other cognitive functions. In 152 depressed patients with documented extensive memory dysfunction, recovery from depression was associated with marked improvement in memory [86]. In more recent studies, Weingartner et al [23,82,95–97] provided a detailed conceptual outline of the cognitive changes associated with depression [97]. Depressed subjects are far less successful than normal volunteers in recalling words associated by their meaning (semantic). Depressed patients also recalled poorly those words that were randomly grouped, but recalled "organized" word groups normally [95]. Words associated by virtue of acoustic similarity are recalled equally well by normals and depressed persons [95].

The capacity to sustain physical and mental effort is also impaired in depressed patients, and the degree of this incapacity is highly correlated with severity of depression [23]. Again the data suggest that depressed individuals may function normally in psychosocial contexts that are highly organized and coherently clustered. Their performance is likely to diminish rapidly when a task becomes either structurally disorganized or temporally extended (long response delays require constant rehearsal).

Abstract reasoning also suffers deterioration in depressive states. Compared to controls, patients exhibit reduced "focusing" or sorting skills and a tendency to be perseverant or retain false hypotheses [82]. Inasmuch as abstract reasoning requires effort or sustained attention, it is likely to diminish in efficiency with the onset and progression of depression.

Cognitive impairment patterns observed in depressed patients resemble those found in parkinsonian patients [94]. Information-processing tasks that require sustained cognitive activity (attention–demanding or effortful) clearly distinguish normal volunteers from patients with parkinsonism. Using six memory tasks that range in difficulty from the highly automatic to the highly effortful, parkinsonian patients exhibited a progressively poorer performance at effortful tasks [94]. Parkinsonian patients performed well at word-frequency monitoring but scored only 50% as well as normals at a task requiring serial list learning. These results clearly indicate that effortful cognitive processes requiring sustained attention deteriorate in Parkinson's disease, but it is not yet known to what extent this deficit is repaired by therapy.

Cognitive performance improves after L-dopa treatment [12]. Memory improvement with L-dopa also occurs in depressed patients. Free recall improved markedly in eight depressed patients given L-dopa (5.5 gm/day) [60]. A serial learning task also improved notably though mood state was unchanged. In another study, L-dopa and L-tryptophan improved free recall verbal learning [39]. In normal subjects, automatic processes and access to knowledge in long-term memory appear unaffected by L-dopa treatment; those processes requiring effort and extensive cognitive capacity are, however, markedly improved by this DA agonist [96].

Finally, it is instructive to recall amphetamine's cognitive effects on normal prepubertal boys [73,74] and depressed patients [75]. In both groups free recall is considerably enhanced by acute doses of amphetamine. Cued recall, on the other hand, improves in prepubertal boys but not in depressed subjects. Semantic recall is enhanced whereas acoustic recall is not notably improved in depressed subjects receiving oral amphetamine [75]. DA agonists clearly improve effortful cognitive functions. In contrast, Parkinson's disease and depression impair memory tasks requiring sustained mental effort. In both illnesses it appears that this cognitive behavioral disturbance is partially dependent on DA pathway pathology.

CONCLUSIONS

Mood, movement, and memory are impaired in parkinsonian and depressed patients. Whereas DA agonists apparently reduce the severity of these impairments by directly activating DA receptors, it remains unclear how antidepressant treatments improve these neurobehavioral functions. Long-term antidepressant treatment studies in animals consistently implicate enhanced monoamine postsynaptic receptor responsivity, measured electrophysiologically [22] and behaviorally [38, 55,84]. Such studies strongly suggest that antidepressant treatments may be therapeutically useful in treating the neurobehavioral deficits common to depression and parkinsonism by enhancing postsynaptic DA, 5-HT, and NE receptor sensitivity. It remains unclear how enhancement of this group of receptor functions is related to the desensitization of β-adrenergic receptors which apparently accompanies long-term antidepressant treatment.

REFERENCES

1. Ananth J, Samra D, Kolivakis T. Amelioration of drug-induced parkinsonism by ECT. Am J Psychiatry 136:1094, 1979.
2. Anden NE, Rubenson A, Fuxe K, Hökfelt T. Evidence for dopamine receptor stimulation by apomorphine. J Pharm Pharmacol 19:627–629, 1967.
3. Anden NE, Strombom U, Svensson TH. Dopamine and noradrenaline receptor stimulation: reversal of reserpine-induced suppression of motor activity. Psychopharmacologia (Berlin) 29:289–298, 1973.
4. Anderson J, Aabro E, Gulmann N, Hjelmsted A, Pedersen HE. Anti-depressive treatment in Parkinson's disease. Acta Neurol Scand 62:210–219, 1980.
5. Angrist B, Ain M, Rotrosen J, Gershon S, Halpern FS, Sacher EJ. Behavioral and neuroendocrine effects of low dose ET-495: antagonism by haloperidol. J Neural Transm 44:249–262, 1979.
6. Angrist B, Thompson H, Shopsin B, Gershon S. Clinical studies with dopamine receptor stimulants. Psychopharmacologia (Berlin) 44:273–280, 1975.
7. Asnis G. Parkinson's disease, depression, and ECT: a review and case study. Am J Psychiatry 134:191–195, 1977.
8. Axelrod J. Amphetamine: Metabolism, Physiological Disposition and its Effects on Catecholamine Storage. In Amphetamines and Related Compounds, E Costa, S Garattini (eds), 207–216. New York: Raven Press, 1970.
9. Balldin J, Eden S, Granerus AK, Modigh K, Svanborg A, Walinder J, Wallin L. Electroconvulsive therapy in Parkinson's syndrome with "on-off" phenomenon. J Neural Transm 47:11–21, 1980.
10. Bannon MJ, Grace AA, Bunney BS, Roth RH. Evidence for an irreversible interaction

of bromocriptine with central dopamine receptors. Naunyn Schmiedebergs Arch Pharmacol 312:37–41, 1980.

11. Bedard P, Parkes JD, Marsden CD. Nomifensine in Parkinson's disease. Br J Pharmacol 4:187S–190S, 1977.
12. Bowen FP, Kamienny RS, Burns MM, Yahr MD. Parkinsonism: effects of levodopa treatment on concept formation. Neurology (Minneap) 25:701–704, 1975.
13. Braestrup C, Scheel-Kruger J. Methylphenidate-like effects of the new antidepressant drug nomifensine. Eur J Pharmacol 38:305–312, 1976.
14. Brodie HKH, Murphy DL, Goodwin FK, Bunney WE, Jr. Catecholamines and mania: the effect of alpha-methyl-para-tyrosine on manic behavior and catecholamine metabolism. Clin Pharmacol Ther 12:218–224, 1971.
15. Brown GL, Wilson WP. Parkinsonism and depression. South Med J 65:540–545, 1972.
16. Brown GL, Wilson WP, Green RL. Mental Aspects of Parkinsonism and Their Management. In Parkinson's Disease-Rigidity, Akinesia, Behavior, Selected Communications on the Topic, S Siegfried (ed), 265–278. Vienna: Verlag Hans Hube, 1973.
17. Bunney BS, Aghajanian GK, Roth RH. Comparison of effects of L-dopa, amphetamine and apomorphine on firing rate of rat dopaminergic neurons. Nature New Biol 245:123–125, 1973.
18. Bunney BS, Walters JR, Roth RH, Aghajanian GK. Dopaminergic neurons: effect of antipsychotic drugs and amphetamine on single cell activity. J Pharmacol Exp Ther 185:560–571, 1973.
19. Bunney WE, Jr, Davis JM. Norepinephrine in depressive reactions. Arch Gen Psychiatry 13:483–494, 1965.
20. Bunney WE Jr, Wehr TR, Gillin JC, Post RM, Goodwin FK, van Kammen DP. The switch process in manic depressive psychosis. Ann Intern Med 87:319–335, 1977.
21. Calne B. Parkinsonism: Physiology, Pharmacology and Treatment. London: Edward Arnold, 1970.
22. Charney DS, Menkes DB, Heninger GR. Receptor sensitivity and the mechanism of action of antidepressant treatment. Arch Gen Psychiatry 38:1160–1180, 1981.
23. Cohen RM, Weingartner H, Smallberg SA, Pickar D, Murphy DL. Effort and cognition in depression. Arch Gen Psychiatry 39:593–597, 1982.
24. Colonna L, Petit M, Lepine JP. Bromocriptine in affective disorders: a pilot study. J Affect Disorders 1:173–177, 1979.
25. Corsini GU, Del Zompo M, Manconi S, Onali PL, Mangoni A, Gessa GL. Evidence for dopamine receptors in the human brain mediating sedation and sleep. Life Sci 20:1613–1618, 1977.
26. Di Chiara G, Porceddu ML, Vargiu L, Argiolas A, Gessa GL. Evidence for dopamine receptors mediating sedation in the mouse brain. Nature 264:564–567, 1976.
27. Drimmer EJ, Gitlin MJ, Gwirtsman HE. Desipramine and methylphenidate combination treatment for depression: case report. Am J Psychiatry 140:241–242, 1983.
28. Dysken M, Evans HM, Chan CH, Davis JM. Improvement of depression and Parkinsonism during ECT (a case study). Neuropsychobiology 2:81–86, 1976.
29. Ebert MH, van Kammen DP, Murphy DL. Plasma Levels of Amphetamine and Behavioral Response. In Pharmacokinetics of Psychoactive Drugs: Blood Levels and Clinical Response, LA Gottschalk, S Merlis (eds), 157–169. New York: Spectrum Publications, 1976.
30. Everett GM, Borcherding JW. L-dopa: effect on concentrations of dopamine, norepinephrine, and serotonin in brains of mice. Science 168:849–850, 1970.

31. Farley IJ, Hornykiewicz O. Noradrenaline in Subcortical Brain Regions of Patients with Parkinson's Disease and Control Subjects. In Advances in Parkinsonism, W. Birkmayer and O. Hornykiewicz (eds), 178–185. Basel: Editions Roche, 1976.
32. Ferris RM, Tang FL. Comparison of the effects of the isomers of amphetamine, methylphenidate, and deoxypepradrol on the uptake of 1-[^{3}H] norepinephrine and [^{3}H]dopamine by synaptic vesicles from rat whole brain, striatum and hypothalamus. J Pharmacol Exp Ther 210:422–428, 1979.
33. Fromm GH. Observations on the effect of electroshock treatment on patients with Parkinsonism. Bull Tulane Med Faculty 18:71–73, 1959.
34. Goodwin FK. Behavioral effects of L-dopa in man. Semin Psychiatry 3:477–492, 1971.
35. Goodwin FK, Bunney WE, Jr. Depressions following reserpine: a reevaluation. Semin Psychiatry 3:435–448, 1971.
36. Goodwin FK, Murphy DL, Brodie HK. L-dopa, catecholamines, and behavior: a clinical and biochemical study in depressed patients. Biol Psychiatry 2:341–366, 1970.
37. Graham AW, Aghajanian GK. Effects of amphetamine on single cell activity in a catecholamine nucleus, the locus coeruleus. Nature 234:100–102, 1971.
38. Grahame-Smith DG, Green AR, Costain DW. Mechanism of the anti-depressant action of electroconvulsive therapy. Lancet 1:254–256, 1978.
39. Henry GM, Weingartner H, Murphy DL. Influence of affective states and psychoactive drugs on verbal learning and memory. Am J Psychiatry 130:966–971, 1973.
40. Holcomb HH, Sternberg DE, Heninger GR. Effects of electroconvulsive therapy on mood, Parkinsonism and tardive dyskinesia in a depressed patient: ECT and dopamine systems. Biol Psychiatry 18:865–873, 1983.
41. Horn S. Some psychological factors in Parkinsonism. J Neurol Neurosurg Psychiatry 37:27–31, 1974.
42. Hornykiewicz O. Parkinson's disease: from brain homogenate to treatment. Fed Proc 32:183–190, 1973.
43. Javoy-Agid F, Taquet H, Ploska A, Cherif-Zahar C, Ruberg M, Agid Y. Distribution of catecholamines in the ventral mesencephalon of human brain, with special reference to Parkinson's disease. J Neurochem 36:2101–2105, 1981.
44. Jimerson DC, Post RM. Psychomotor Stimulants and Dopamine Agonists in Depression. In The Neurobiology of Mood Disorders, RM Post and JC Ballenger (eds), 619–628. Baltimore: Williams and Wilkins, 1984.
45. Johnson JM. Treated mania exacerbated by bromocriptine. Am J Psychiatry 138:980–982, 1981.
46. Kessler KA. Tricyclic Antidepressants: Mode of Action and Clinical Use. In Psychopharmacology: A Generation of Progress, MA Lipton, A DiMascio, and KF Killam (eds), 1289–1302. New York: Raven Press, 1978.
47. Knoll J. The possible mechanisms of action of (−) deprenyl in Parkinson's disease. J Neural Transm 43:177–198, 1978.
48. Ko GN, Leckman JF, Heninger GR. Induction of rapid mood cycling during L-dopa treatment in a bipolar patient. Am J Psychiatry 138:1624–1625, 1981.
49. Laitinen L. Desipramine in treatment of Parkinson's disease. Acta Neurol Scand 45:109–113, 1969.
50. Lebensohn ZM, Jenkins RB. Improvement of Parkinsonism in depressed patients treated with ECT. Am J Psychiatry 132:283–285, 1975.
51. Lees AJ, Haddad S, Shaw KM, Kohout L, Stern GM. Bromocriptine in Parkinsonism: a long-term study. Arch Neurol 35:503–505, 1978.

52. Lieberman A, Zolfaghari M, Boal D. The antiparkinsonian efficacy of bromocriptine. Neurology (Minneap) 26:405–409, 1976.
53. Lieberman A, Zolfaghari M, Boal D, Hassouri H, Vogel B. The Use of Dopamine Receptor Agonists in Parkinson's Disease. In Advances in Parkinsonism, W Birkmayer and O Hornykiewicz (eds), 507–512. Basel: F Hoffman La Roche and Co. Ltd., 1976.
54. Lytle LD, Hurko O, Romero JA, Cottman K, Leehey D, Wurtman RJ. The effects of 6-hydroxydopamine pretreatment on the accumulation of dopa and dopamine in brain and peripheral organs following L-dopa administration. J Neural Transm 33:63–71, 1972.
55. Maj J, Mogilnicka E, Klimek V. The effect of repeated administration of antidepressant drugs on the responsiveness of rats to catecholamine agonists. J Neural Transm 44:221–235, 1979.
56. Mandell AJ, Markham CH, Fowler W. Parkinson's syndrome, depression and imipramine: a preliminary report. Calif Med 95:12–14, 1961.
57. Marwaha J, Aghajanian GK. Typical and atypical neuroleptics are potent antagonists of α_1-adrenoceptors of the dorsal lateral geniculate nucleus: an electrophysiological study. Naunyn Schmiedebergs Arch Pharmacol 321:32–37, 1982.
58. Meyerhoff JL, Kant GJ. Release of endogenous dopamine from corpus striatum. Life Sci 23:1481–1486, 1978.
59. Murphy DL, Brodie HKH, Goodwin FK, Bunney WE, Jr. Regular induction of hypomania by L-dopa in "bipolar" manic-depressive patients. Nature 229:135–136, 1971.
60. Murphy DL, Henry GM, Weingartner H. Catecholamines and memory: enhanced verbal learning during L-dopa administration. Psychopharmacologia (Berlin) 27:319–326, 1972.
61. Nordin C, Siwers B, Bertilsson L. Bromocriptine treatment of depressive disorders: clinical and biochemical effects. Acta Psychiatr Scand 64:25–33, 1981.
62. Nowycky MC, Roth RH. Dopaminergic neurons: role of presynaptic receptors in the regulation of transmitter biosynthesis. Prog Neuropsychopharmacol 2:139–158, 1978.
63. Nurnberger JI, Gershon ES, Simmons-Alling S, Nadi NS, Tamminga C, Goldstein D. Neurochemical characterization of responses to dextroamphetamine. Soc Biol Psychiatry Abstracts, p. 138, 1983.
64. Park DM, Findley LJ, Teychenne PF. Nomifensine in Parkinsonism. Br J Clin Pharmacol 4:185S–186S, 1977.
65. Ponzio F, Achilli G, Perego C, Rinaldi G, Algeri S. Does acute L-dopa increase release of dopamine from dopaminergic neurons. Brain Res 273:45–51, 1983.
66. Post RM, Ballenger JC, Goodwin FK. Cerebrospinal Fluid Studies of Neurotransmitter Function in Manic and Depressive Illness. In Neurobiology of Cerebrospinal Fluid, vol. 1, JH Wood (ed), 685–717. New York: Plenum Press, 1980.
67. Post RM, Gerner RH, Carman JS, Bunney WE, Jr. Effects of low doses of a dopamine receptor stimulator in mania. Lancet 1:203–204, 1976.
68. Post RM, Gerner RH, Carman JS, Gillin JC, Jimerson DC, Goodwin FK, Bunney WE, Jr. Effects of a dopamine agonist piribedil in depressed patients. Arch Gen Psychiatry 35:609–615, 1978.
69. Post RM, Jimerson DC, Bunney WE, Jr, Goodwin FK. Dopamine and mania: behavioral and biochemical effects of the dopamine receptor blocker pimozide. Psychopharmacology (Berlin) 67:297–305, 1980.

70. Price KS, Farley IJ, Hornykiewicz O. Neurochemistry of Parkinson's disease: relation between striatal and limbic dopamine. Adv Biochem Psychopharmacol 19:293–300, 1978.
71. Prien RF, Klett CJ, Caffey EM. Lithium carbonate and imipramine in prevention of affective episodes: a comparison in recurrent affective illness. Arch Gen Psychiatry 29:420–425, 1973.
72. Randrup A, Munkvad I, Fog R, Gerlach J, Molander L, Kjellberg B, Scheel-Kruger J. Mania, Depression, and Brain Dopamine. In Current Developments in Psychopharmacology (vol. 2), WB Essman and L Valzelli (eds), 207–248. New York: Spectrum Publications, 1975.
73. Rapoport JL, Buchsbaum MS, Weingartner H, Zahn TP, Ludlow C, Mikkelsen EJ. Dextroamphetamine: its cognitive and behavioral effects in normal and hyperactive boys and normal men. Arch Gen Psychiatry 37:933–943, 1980.
74. Rapoport JL, Buchsbaum MS, Zahn TP, Weingartner H, Ludlow C, Mikkelsen EJ. Dextroamphetamine: cognitive and behavioral effects in normal prepubertal boys. Science 199:560–563, 1978.
75. Reus VI, Silberman E, Post RM, Weingartner H. D-amphetamine: effects on memory in a depressed population. Biol Psychiatry 14:345–356, 1979.
76. Robins AH. Depression in patients with Parkinsonism. Br J Psychiatry 128:141–145, 1976.
77. Roth RH. Dopamine autoreceptors: pharmacology, function and comparison with post-synaptic dopamine receptors. Commun Psychopharmacol 3:429–445, 1979.
78. Scatton B, Rouquier L, Javoy-Agid F, Agid Y. Dopamine deficiency in the cerebral cortex in Parkinson's disease. Neurology (NY) 32:1039–1040, 1982.
79. Schildkraut JJ. The catecholamine hypothesis of affective disorders: a review of supporting evidence. Am J Psychiatry 122:509–522, 1965.
80. Schildkraut JJ. Depression and Biogenic Amines. In American Handbook of Psychiatry. DA Hamburg and KH Brodie (eds), 460–487. New York: Basic Books, 1975.
81. Sigwald J, Bouttier D, Raymondeaud CI, Marquez M, Gal JC. Etude de l'action sur l'akinésie parkinsonienne de deux dérivés de l'iminodibenzyle: ou imipramine ou 8307 RP. Presse Med 67:1697–1698, 1959.
82. Silberman EK, Weingartner H, Post RM. Thinking disorder in depression: logic and strategy in an abstract reasoning task. Arch Gen Psychiatry 40:775–780, 1983.
83. Skirboll LR, Grace AA, Bunney BS. Dopamine auto- and postsynaptic receptors: electrophysiological evidence for differential sensitivity to dopamine agonists. Science 206:80–82, 1979.
84. Spyraki C, Fibiger HC. Behavioral evidence for supersensitivity of postsynaptic dopamine receptors in the mesolimbic system after chronic administration of desipramine. Eur J Pharmacol 74:195–206, 1981.
85. Strang RR. Imipramine in treatment of Parkinsonism: a double-blind placebo study. Br Med J 2:33–34, 1965.
86. Stromgren LS. The influence of depression on memory. Acta Psychiatr Scand 56:109–128, 1977.
87. Tesarova O. Experimental depression caused by apomorphine and phenoharmane. Pharmakopsychiatrie 5:13–19, 1972.
88. Thorner MO, Fluckiger E, Calne DB. Bromocriptine Therapy for Parkinsonism. In Bromocriptine, A Clinical and Pharmacological Review, MO Thorner et al (eds), 124–141. New York: Raven Press, 1980.
89. van Kammen DP, Murphy DL. Attenuation of the euphoriant and activating effects

of D- and L-amphetamine by lithium carbonate treatment. Psychopharmacologia (Berlin) 44:215–224, 1975.

90. van Pragg HM, Korf J. Cerebral monoamines and depression: an investigation with the probenecid technique. Arch Gen Psychiatry 28:827–831, 1973.
91. Walters JR, Roth RH. Dopaminergic neurons: an in vivo system for measuring drug interactions with presynaptic receptors. Naunyn Schmiedebergs Arch Pharmacol 296:5–14, 1976.
92. Ward C, Stern GM, Pratt RTC, McKenna P. Electroconvulsive therapy in Parkinsonian patients with the "on-off" syndrome. J Neural Transm 49:133–135, 1980.
93. Wehr TA, Goodwin FK. Rapid cycling in manic-depressives induced by tricyclic antidepressants. Arch Gen Psychiatry 36:555–559, 1979.
94. Weingartner H, Burns S, Diebel R, LeWitt PA. Cognitive impairments in Parkinson's disease: distinguishing between effort demanding and automatic cognitive processes. Psychiatry Res 11:223–235, 1984.
95. Weingartner H, Cohen RM, Murphy DL, Martello J, Gerdt C. Cognitive processes in depression. Arch Gen Psychiatry 38:42–47, 1981.
96. Newman RP, Weingartner H, Smallberg SA, Calne DB. Effortful and automatic memory processes: effects of dopamine. Neurology 34:805–807, 1984.
97. Weingartner H, Silberman E. Cognitive Changes in Depression. In Frontiers of Clinical Neuroscience, vol. 1, Neurobiology of Mood Disorders, RM Post and JC Ballenger (eds), 121–135. Baltimore: Williams and Wilkins, 1984.
98. Yahr MD. Overview of present day treatment of Parkinson's disease. J Neural Transm 43:227–238, 1978.
99. Yudofsky SC. Parkinson's disease, depression, and electroconvulsive therapy: a clinical and neurobiologic synthesis. Compr Psychiatry 20:579–581, 1979.
100. Willner P. Dopamine and depression: a review of recent evidence. I. Empirical studies. Brain Res Reviews 6:211–224, 1983.
101. Willner P. Dopamine and depression: a review of recent evidence. II. Theoretical Approaches. Brain Res Reviews 6:225–236, 1983.
102. Willner P. Dopamine and depression: a review of recent evidence. III. The effects of antidepressant treatments. Brain Res Reviews 6:237–243, 1983.

V

Schizophrenia and the Catecholamines

14

Studies of Norepinephrine in Schizophrenia

Joel E. Kleinman
Audrey Reid
C. Raymond Lake
Richard Jed Wyatt

The norepinephrine (NE) hypothesis of schizophrenia in its most general form holds that a relationship exists between NE and schizophrenic psychopathology. Evidence supports both increased and decreased noradrenergic activity in the schizophrenic syndrome. Given the diversity of the schizophrenic syndrome and the numerous approaches to measuring noradrenergic activity, this is not surprising. Nevertheless, the majority of the more recent data favors the notion of increased noradrenergic activity in schizophrenia. For the purpose of this review, measurements of noradrenergic activity in schizophrenia are divided into two general categories: biochemistry and pharmacology. The biochemistry category includes measurements of NE, its metabolites, its enzymes of synthesis and degradation, its receptors, and its uptake. The pharmacology category includes drugs known to perturb the noradrenergic system and their effects on the psychopathology of control subjects and schizophrenic patients.

BIOCHEMISTRY

Norepinephrine Measurements

One of the simplest and most direct approaches to measurement of noradrenergic activity involves the analysis of NE levels in urine, plasma, brain tissue, and cerebrospinal fluid (CSF) (Table 14.1). No NE abnormalities have been reported in urine from schizophrenic patients. Early reports found normal urinary NE concentrations using spectrofluorometric techniques [14,95]. Schizophrenic patients in these studies were predominantly of the chronic undifferentiated subtype, if they were subtyped at all. A more recent study which subtyped the schizophrenic patients

Table 14.1 Norepinephrine Levels in Schizophrenia

Author (Reference No.)	*Date*	*Type of Sample*	*Control (n)*	*Schizophrenia (n)*	*Findings*
Ackenheil et al [1]	1979	Plasma	211 pg/ml (29)	361 pg/ml (11)	↑ NE in acute S patients with P hallucinatoric syndromes
Naber et al [97]	1980	Serum	210 pg/ml	770 pg/ml (23) male 900 (35) female	↑ NE in male and female chronic S treated with neuroleptics; n for C not cited
Kemali et al [76]	1982	Plasma	228 pg/ml (55)	262 pg/ml (46) S 265 (37) P 249 (9) H 265 (27) acute 260 (19) chronic	↑ NE in S as well as P and acute subtypes
Castellani et al [27]	1982	Plasma	201 pg/ml (24)	208 pg/ml (23) S 212 (10) SA 197 (17) UND 238 (6) P	Supine NE in C similar to S and S subtypes
		Plasma	365 pg/ml (24)	541 pg/ml (23) S 561 (10) SA 555 (17) UND 501 (6) P	Greater ↑ in NE on standing in all S groups than C; no difference among P, UND, and SA subtypes
Gomes et al [53]	1980	CSF	207 pg/ml (18)	259 pg/ml (11) chronic 216 (10) acute	↑ NE in chronic S

Lake et al [82]	1980	CSF	91 pg/ml (29)	125 pg/ml (35) S 144 (14) P 101 (10) UND 122 (11) SA	↑ NE in S as well as P subtype
Kemali et al [76]	1982	CSF	125 pg/ml (10)	151 pg/ml (8) S 160 (5) P 138 (3) H 159 (3) acute 147 (5) chronic	↑ NE in S as well as P subtype
Bergsman [14]	1959	Urine	22.03 ng/min (18)	41.08 ng/min (6) acute 28.31 (18) chronic	No difference between S groups and C
Kemali et al [76]	1982	Urine	36.5 μg/24 hr (20)	35.9 μg/24 hr (16) S 35.0 (12) P 38.6 (4) H 35.4 (12) acute 38.7 (4) chronic	No difference between S groups and C
Farley et al [44]	1978	Nucleus accumbens	1.58 μg/gm tissue (8)	2.40 μg/gm tissue (4)	↑ NE in S
		Bed nucleus of stria terminalis	1.23 (54)	2.72 (4)	↑ NE in S
		Ventral septum	0.53 (4)	1.59 (4)	↑ NE in S
		Mammillary body	0.45 (12)	0.69 (4)	↑ NE in S
		Hypothalamus total	1.83 (12)	1.86 (4)	No difference between S and C
		Medial olfactory (pre-optic) area	1.49 (8)	1.69 (4)	No difference between S and C
		Paramedian thalamic nuclei	0.48 (4)	0.53 (4)	No difference between S and C

Table 14.1 *(continued)*

Author (Reference No.)	*Date*	*Type of Sample*	*Control (n)*	*Schizophrenia (n)*	*Findings*
Bird et al [18]	1979	Nucleus accumbens	1.3 μg/gm protein (40)	1.8 μg/gm protein (47)	No difference between S and C
		Anterior perforated substance	0.7 (25)	1.5 (35)	No difference between S and C
		Caudate	0.7 (47)	0.5 (44)	No difference between S and C
		Septal nuclei	4.2 (35)	4.2 (32)	No difference between S and C
		Amygdala center nucleus	1.9 (12)	2.1 (19)	No difference between S and C
Carlsson [23]	1979	Mesencephalon	1.49 nmol/gm tissue (26)	2.65 nmol/gm tissue (4)	↑ NE in S
Crow et al [34]	1979	Nucleus accumbens	132 ng/gm tissue (10)	131 ng/gm tissue (9)	No difference between S and C
		Putamen	65 (10)	119 (9)	↑ NE in S
		Caudate	75 (10)	104 (9)	No difference between S and C
Winblad et al [144]	1979	Hypothalamus	0.86 μg/gm tissue (10)	0.95 μg/gm tissue (10)	No difference between S and C
		Caudate nucleus	0.02 (16)	0.03 (10)	No difference between S and C
		Putamen	0.05 (16)	0.05 (10)	No difference between S and C
		Thalamus	0.08 (14)	0.08 (9)	No difference between S and C
		Mesencephalon	0.12 (14)	0.14 (8)	No difference between S and C

		Pons	0.06 (14)	0.02 (9)	No difference between S and C
		Hippocampus	0.01 (13)	0.02 (9)	No difference between S and C
		Cortex gyrus hippocampus	0.01 (8)	0.01 (10)	No difference between S and C
		Cortex gyrus cinguli	0.02 (8)	0.02 (9)	No difference between S and C
		Cortex lobus frontalis	0.02 (14)	0.01 (8)	No difference between S and C
Kleinman et al [77]	1979	Hypothalamus	8.7 ng/mg protein (10)	14.2 ng/mg protein (11)	No difference between S and C; 4 of the S group are psychotics other than S; 2 of 3 P had high NE levels in the nucleus accumbens
		Nucleus accumbens	1.65 (7)	1.54 (6)	
		Substantia nigra	1.25 (8)	1.29 (8)	
Kleinman et al [78]	1982	Nucleus accumbens	0.82 ng/mg protein (12)	2.54 ng/mg protein (10) chronic P 0.99 (8) chronic UND	↑ NE in chronic P in nucleus accumbens and hypothalamus; ↑ NE in chronic UND in hypothalamus
		Hypothalamus	9.3 (16)	36.0 (11) chronic P 28.4 (10) chronic UND	

C = control; CSF = cerebrospinal fluid; H = hebephrenic; n = number of subjects; NE = norepinephrine; P = paranoid; S = schizophrenic; SA = schizoaffective; UND = undifferentiated; ↑ = increased.

found no difference in NE levels in urine from schizophrenic and control subjects using a radioenzymatic technique, although this group reported increased NE in plasma and CSF from schizophrenic patients as noted below [76]. The obvious problem with this type of study is the questionable relevance of urine measurements to a syndrome that most probably involves the brain.

Studies of plasma NE concentrations in schizophrenia are somewhat more promising. Plasma NE concentrations in sitting, drug-free (at least 4 weeks) acute schizophrenic patients were increased relative to control subjects [1]. These patients had predominantly "paranoid hallucinatoric syndromes." Chronic unsubtyped schizophrenic patients treated with neuroleptics also had increased supine serum NE concentrations [97]. A recent report found plasma NE levels of schizophrenic patients increased in response to some neuroleptics such as chlorpromazine but not to others such as haloperidol [27]. This same report found normal supine plasma NE concentrations in drug-free chronic schizophrenic and schizoaffective patients [27]. Further, they discovered that, upon standing, plasma NE concentrations increased to a greater degree in chronic schizophrenic and schizoaffective patients than in control subjects [27]. No significant differences were seen among paranoid, undifferentiated, and schizoaffective subtypes [27].

CSF NE concentrations were also increased in schizophrenic patients, especially those with paranoid features [82]. These patients were drug-free for at least 2 weeks and for an average of 4 weeks [81]. Neuroleptic-treated chronic schizophrenic patients also had increased CSF NE concentrations relative to acute schizophrenic patients and several other psychiatric and nonpsychiatric control subjects [53]. A recent study found increased CSF NE, in addition to increased plasma NE, in schizophrenics, particularly in paranoids [76].

Surprisingly, there have been more reported postmortem studies of brain tissue NE concentrations than of NE levels in the CSF, blood, or urine of schizophrenics (Table 14.1). Several studies have demonstrated increases in NE concentrations in some areas of paranoid schizophrenic brains [23,44,77,78]. Two of the studies [44,78] noted increases in the nucleus accumbens, a structure with connections to the limbic system. Reports that failed to demonstrate increases in NE concentrations in the nucleus accumbens [17,18,34] or elsewhere [17,18,144] did not subtype the schizophrenic patients. One of these studies [17,18] with a large number of subjects found significant increases with parametric statistics, but not with nonparametric tests.

Norepinephrine Metabolites

If NE increases in the plasma, CSF, and brain are of any functional significance, then NE metabolites should be increased as well. One of the major NE metabolites, 3-methoxy-4-hydroxyphenylglycol (MHPG), has been studied in urine, blood, CSF, and brain tissue (Table 14.2). Urinary MHPG has been consistently normal in several studies [70,71,133]. Joseph et al [70] reported normal 24-hour total, glucuronide-conjugated and sulfate-conjugated MHPG urine levels in 18 drug-free chronic

Table 14.2 Norepinephrine Metabolite Levels in Schizophrenia

Author (Reference No.)	*Date*	*Metabolite*	*Type of Sample*	*Control (n)*	*Schizophrenia (n)*	*Findings*
Joseph et al [70]	1976	MHPG, total	Urine	2.74 mg/24 hr (13)	2.89 mg/24 hr (18)	No difference between S and C
		MHPG, glucuronide	Urine	1.49 mg/24 hr (13)	1.55 mg/24 hr (18)	No difference between S and C
		MHPG-sulfate	Urine	1.02 mg/24 hr (13)	1.17 mg/24 hr (18)	No difference between S and C
Taube et al [133]	1978	MHPG	Urine	1029 μg/24 hr (10)	931 μg/24 hr (11)	No difference between S and C
Sweeney et al [131]	1980	MHPG, free	Plasma	3.4 ng/ml (8) AM 2.9 (8) PM	3.0 ng/ml (2) AM 2.4 (2) PM	No difference between S and C; C = A and 1 SA patient(s); SA patient in D state
Sternberg et al [127]	1982	MHPG	Plasma	3.8 ng/ml (11)	4.0 ng/ml (11)	No difference between S and C
Shopsin et al [122]	1973	MHPG	CSF	10–23 ng/ml (20)	7–30 ng/ml (26)	S falls within range of C
Post et al [110]	1975	MHPG	CSF	16 ng/ml (10)	16 ng/ml (17)	No difference between S and C
Van Praag and Korf [137]	1975	MHPG	CSF	9 ng/ml	11 ng/ml (5)	No difference between S and C
Rimon et al [113]	1979	MHPG	CSF	—	12.3 ng/ml (67) lobotomy 15.7 (30) no lobotomy	No effect of lobotomy on CSF MHPG in S patients
Berger et al [13]	1980	MHPG, free	CSF	8.8 ng/ml (23)	8.2 ng/ml (9) S 9.3 (13) D	No difference among S, C and D
		MHPG, total	CSF	9.2 ng/ml (23)	8.1 ng/ml (9) S 9.9 (13) D	No difference among S, C and D

Table 14.2 *(continued)*

Author (Reference No.)	*Date*	*Metabolite*	*Type of Sample*	*Control (n)*	*Schizophrenia (n)*	*Findings*
Sedvall and Wode-Helgodt [119]	1980	MHPG	CSF	—	39 pmol/ml (18) no family history of S 42 (9) family history of S	No difference in CSF MHPG between S patients with family history of S and those with negative histories
McDonald and Weise [90]	1962	VMA	Urine	Ambulatory		Chronic S tend to have ↑ VMA; significant ↑ in VMA when subjects are on bed rest for 24 hr
			8 AM–4 PM	2.4 μg/kg/hr (10)	2.8 μg/kg/hr (9)	
			4 PM–12 M	2.3 (10)	2.5 (9)	
			12 M–8 AM	1.8 (10)	2.3 (9)	
				Bed rest		
			8 AM–4 PM	2.0 (10)	3.0 (9)	
			4 PM–12 M	2.2 (10)	2.7 (9)	
			12 M–8 AM	1.8 (10)	2.3 (9)	
Joseph et al [70]	1976	VMA	Urine	4.09 mg/24 hr (13)	4.65 mg/24 hr (18)	No difference between S and C
Kleinman et al [77]	1979	MHPG, free	Hypothalamus	658.1 pg/mg protein (10)	1171.8 pg/mg protein (11)	Free MHPG ↑ in S in hypothalamus; ↓ conjugated MHPG in hypothalamus in S; 4 of the S group are psychotics other than S
			Nucleus accumbens	327.0 (7)	311.8 (6)	
			Substantia nigra	378.7 (8)	310.4 (8)	
		MHPG, conjugated	Hypothalamus	677.0 (10)	444.7 (11)	
			Nucleus accumbens	505.2 (7)	603.0 (6)	
			Substantia nigra	757.4 (8)	639.1 (8)	

		MHPG, total	Hypothalamus	1335.0 (10)	1616.1 (11)	
			Nucleus accumbens	832.2 (7)	914.8 (6)	
			Substantia nigra	1136.0 (8)	949.5 (8)	
Kleinman et al [78]	1982	MHPG, free	Nucleus accumbens	0.30 ng/mg protein (14)	0.46 ng/mg protein (10) chronic P 0.40 (8) chronic UND	↑ Total and conjugated MHPG in chronic P in nucleus accumbens; ↑ free MHPG in chronic P in hypothalamus
		MHPG, conjugated	Nucleus accumbens	0.47 (13)	1.15 (10) chronic P 0.75 (7) chronic UND	
		MHPG, total	Nucleus accumbens	0.71 (13)	1.61 (10) chronic P 1.06 (8) chronic UND	
		MHPG, free	Hypothalamus	1.13 (16)	4.55 (11) chronic P 2.75 (10) chronic UND	

A = affective disorder; C = controls; CSF = cerebrospinal fluid; D = depressed; M = midnight; MHPG = 3-methoxy-4-hydroxyphenylglycol; n = number of subjects; P = paranoid; S = schizophrenic; SA = schizoaffective; UND = undifferentiated; VMA = vanillylmandelic acid; ↑ = increase; ↓ = decrease; AM = 7:30 A.M. fasting sample; PM = 3:30 P.M. nonfasting sample.

schizophrenic patients. The major finding in this study was that an inverse relationship existed between psychopathology and 24-hour urinary MHPG-sulfate. The obvious explanation is that the sicker the patient, the lower his or her NE turnover. An alternate interpretation is that sicker patients have less complete urine collections. Although 24-hour urinary creatinine concentrations were normal, suggesting complete collections, sicker patients excreted approximately 25 percent less urine than the healthiest patients [70]. Moreover, the 24-hour urine volumes for the schizophrenic patients in this study (1710 ml) were much less than those reported for schizophrenic subjects in general, who have been reported to excrete abnormally high volumes of urine [60,61]. When this same group did a similar study of acutely schizophrenic patients, MHPG excretion was not found to be related to severity of illness [71]. Nevertheless, male schizophrenic patients who had relatively high MHPG urine levels at the start of the study had better outcomes 1 year later. Moreover, decreases in urinary MHPG while patients were on placebo were associated with more favorable outcomes. Once again, however, 24-hour urine volumes and creatinine concentrations were considerably less than one might expect, suggesting incomplete collections. Finally, subtype diagnoses were not mentioned.

Although vanillylmandelic acid (VMA) is not thought to be the major metabolite of central nervous system (CNS) NE, it has been measured in the urine of chronic schizophrenic patients and controls (see Table 14.2). Urinary VMA was initially reported to be increased in male patients [90], but a subsequent report did not confirm this finding [70]. Once again, subtypes were not mentioned. Regardless, neither urinary MHPG nor VMA concentrations in schizophrenic patients lend support to the notion of increased noradrenergic activity in the schizophrenic syndrome.

Surprisingly, plasma MHPG has been measured in only two studies involving schizophrenic patients [127,131]. Neither study found any difference in unconjugated MHPG between chronic schizophrenic patients and controls. Only two schizophrenic patients were studied in the first report [131] and seven schizophrenic and four schizoaffective patients were studied in the second [127].

The studies of MHPG in CSF of schizophrenic patients have been consistently negative [13,110,113,119,122,137]. Unfortunately, none of the studies were able to conclusively rule out the possibility of increased noradrenergic activity in chronic schizophrenia. The first of these studies involved 13 acute schizophrenic and four acute schizoaffective patients who had normal free MHPG in CSF relative to 29 control subjects (10 normal and 19 neurologic patients) [110]. A second study of five acute schizophrenic patients was also negative with regard to CSF MHPG [137]. Patients were drug-free for 1 week, and little is known of their psychopathology or the nature or number of control subjects [137]. A third study showed that CSF MHPG values for schizophrenics fell within the range for control subjects [122]. The remaining three reports appeared to study chronic schizophrenics. Unfortunately, two of these were without control subjects [113,119]. One study [119] compared schizophrenic patients with and without a family history of schizophrenia and found no difference in CSF MHPG. This study involved schizophrenics with acute exacerbations, 42 percent of whom were first-break patients and 58% of whom were experiencing recurrences. Patients were drug-free for at least 1 week.

The second study compared 67 lobotomized schizophrenic patients with 30 non-lobotomized schizophrenic controls and found no difference in CSF MHPG [113]. These subjects were clearly chronic schizophrenics, and were drug-free only 4 days. The third study found that nine schizophrenic patients, drug-free for at least 2 weeks, had normal free and total CSF MHPG levels relative to normal controls and depressed patients [13]. In none of the six reports were patients divided according to phenomenologic subtypes.

The only group which examined MHPG in the brains of chronic schizophrenic patients found increased total and conjugated MHPG in the nucleus accumbens and increased free MHPG in the hypothalamus relative to normal controls [77,78]. Because these patients also had increased NE concentrations, there did not appear to be an increase in turnover. Regardless, further studies need to be done to confirm this finding.

Enzyme Studies

Studies of the enzymes of NE synthesis and degradation in schizophrenics include dopamine β-hydroxylase (DBH), which converts dopamine (DA) to NE (Table 14.3), monoamine oxidase (MAO), which catabolizes monoamines, catechol-O-methyltransferase (COMT) which catabolizes catechols, tyrosine hydroxylase (TH), which converts tyrosine to dihydroxyphenlylalanine (DOPA), and dopa decarboxylase (DDC), which converts dopa to DA. At least 15 studies of plasma or serum DBH activity and approximately 4 dozen studies of platelet MAO activity are in the literature.

The majority of studies of plasma or serum DBH found no difference between schizophrenic patients and control subjects [22,27,37,39,52,83,93,102,120,142,158]. Only two of these studies involved drug-free patients [27,158]. Four of the negative studies examined levels among subtypes and found no differences [27,37,39,93]. In contrast, four studies reported decreased DBH activity in serum or plasma of schizophrenic patients [20,47,94,157], and one study noted increased DBH activity [87]. In two of these studies, subjects were drug-free [47,94], and in one the decrease was confined to chronic paranoid schizophrenic patients [94]. Book et al [20] reported a unique genetic isolate study in which low serum DBH and low platelet MAO activities "defined" schizophrenic members of a large family. Finally, Yu et al [157] found decreased DBH activity in schizophrenic patients as compared to normal controls when samples were analyzed without copper ions (Cu^{++}) and N-ethylmaleimide, two "antiinhibitors" of plasma DBH activity.

CSF DBH activity was normal in schizophrenic and schizoaffective patients [85,128]. In another study [129], high CSF DBH activity was noted in process schizophrenics and low activity in reactive schizophrenics.

Finally, brain DBH activity was measured in 3 postmortem studies [33, 147,150]. The first of these studies reported decreased DBH activity in the diencephalon, hippocampus, and pons-medulla in schizophrenic patients compared with control subjects [147]. This finding was not confirmed by two other studies [33,150], but differences in these studies may be explained by subtyping. Paranoid schizo-

Table 14.3 Dopamine-β-Hydroxylase Activity in Schizophrenia

Author (Reference No.)	*Date*	*Type of Sample*	*Control (n)*	*Schizophrenia (n)*	*Units*	*Findings*
Shopsin et al [120]	1972	Serum	15–75 (33)	5–65 (12)	nmol/ml/20 min	Values for S fall within range for C
Wetterberg et al [142]	1972	Plasma	92 (106)	96 (52)	nmol/ml/20 min	No difference between S and C
Dunner et al [39]	1973	Plasma	335 (41)	383 (22) S 373 (10) CAT 409 (3) P 385 (9) chronic UND	nmol/ml/hr	No difference between S and C or between subtypes and C
Lamprecht et al [83]	1973	Plasma	498 (34)	673 (24) S twins 663 (24) non-S twins	nmol/ml/hr	No difference in S twins, non-S twins, and C
Markianos et al [87]	1976	Plasma	62.8 (142)	90.2 (73)	nmol/ml/hr	↑ DBH in S
Meltzer et al [93]	1976	Serum	26.4 (73)	23.0 (35) S 22.6 (25) acute 24.2 (10) chronic 23.3 (20) P 21.7 (15) non-P	μmol/L/min	No difference between S and C or between subtypes and C
Okada et al [102]	1976	Serum	—	21.13 (8)	μmol/L/min	24-hr diurnal rhythm of DBH of S similar to C
Fujita et al [47]	1978	Serum	42.53 (153)	16.17 (149)	μmol/L/min	↓ DBH in S
Book et al [20]	1978	Plasma	331 (26)	186 (9)	nmol/ml/20 min	↓ DBH in S
Zizolfi et al [158]	1979	Serum	10.4 (10)	4.9 (29) psychotic 4.2 (5) neurotic	μmol/L/min	No difference between C and psychotics or neurotics; 27 of the psychotics are S

Delisi et al [37]	1980	Plasma	37.23 (11)	29.83 (44) S 25.00 (12) chronic UND with P 30.60 (8) chronic UND without P 35.58 (7) P 30.51 (17) SA	μmol/L/min	Study done at St. Elizabeth's; no difference between S and C; chronic UND with P features tend to have ↓ DBH than any group including C but not significantly
			61.78 (12)	48.18 (56) S 44.46 (19) chronic UND with P 50.81 (28) chronic UND without P 49.79 (9) P	μmol/L/min	Study done at NIH; no difference between S and C; chronic UND with P features tend to have ↓ DBH than any group including C but not significantly
Meltzer et al [94]	1980	Serum	20.0 (90)	18.1 (78) S 21.2 (17) acute non-P 16.8 (14) acute P 17.0 (37) chronic non-P 15.2 (10) chronic P	μmol/L/min	No difference between S and C; ↓ DBH in chronic P than C; other groups no different from C
Yu et al [157]	1980	Plasma	732 (20) 182 (20)	808 (24) 112 (24)	nmol/ml/hr	No difference between S and C; S DBH ↓ when assayed in absence of anti-inhibitors = values 182 and 112
Castellani et al [27]	1982	Serum	573 (24)	552 (23) S 487 (6) P 575 (17) UND 672 (10) SA	nmol/ml/hr	No difference between S and C; ↓ DBH in P but not significantly; no difference between UND and SA subtypes and C

Table 14.3 *(continued)*

Author (Reference No.)	*Date*	*Type of Sample*	*Control (n)*	*Schizophrenia (n)*	*Units*	*Findings*
Okada et al [102]	1976	CSF	—	14 (2)	nμmol/ml/hr	Low but detectable amount of DBH in S
Lerner et al [85]	1978	CSF	—	0.52 (11) S and SA 0.57 (16) alcoholism 0.51 (5) personality disorders 0.71 (16) A	nmol/ml/hr	No difference between S and SA and the other groups
Sternberg et al [128]	1978	CSF	0.0232	0.0228	nmol/ml/hr/mg protein	No difference between S and C
Wise and Stein [147]	1973	Pons-medulla Diencephalon Hippocampus	8.86 (12) 5.83 (12) 2.87 (12)	6.09 (18) 3.38 (18) 1.42 (18)	nmol/gm/20 min	Larger ↓ in DBH in diencephalon and hippocampus than in pons-medulla but ↓ in all 3 areas
Wyatt et al [150]	1975	Pons-mesencephalon Hypothalamus Hippocampus	77.3 (9) 140.8 (9) 39.8 (9)	65 (9) 118.3 (9) 35.5 (9)	nmol/gm/hr	No difference between S and C
Cross et al [33]	1978	Hypothalamus Hippocampus Parietal cortex Frontal cortex Occipital cortex Temporal cortex	131 (12) 24.1 (12) 25.2 (12) 24.1 (12) 26.9 (12) 24.2 (12)	156.4 (12) 24.8 (12) 21.2 (12) 26.8 (12) 23.9 (12) 25.2 (12)	nmol/gm/hr	No difference between S and C

A = affective; C = controls; CAT = catatonic; DBH = dopamine-β-hydroxylase; n = number of subjects; P = paranoid; S = schizophrenic; SA = schizoaffective; UND = undifferentiated; ↑ = increase; ↓ = decrease.

phrenics apparently have normal brain DBH activity in contrast to decreased activity in undifferentiated schizophrenic patients [148]. It seems that the low values in the initial report [147] are also attributable to undifferentiated schizophrenic patients [148]. Unfortunately, the patients were not subtyped in the remaining study [33].

Perhaps the most frequently studied enzyme in schizophrenia research is MAO. In the periphery, MAO has been measured in platelets, lymphocytes, skeletal muscle, and skin fibroblasts (for a review see reference 36). Initial findings of decreased platelet MAO activity in chronic schizophrenic patients [96] have been confirmed by numerous studies [36]. More recent studies have suggested that this finding is a result of a neuroleptic-induced decrease in platelet MAO activity rather than the schizophrenic state itself [36,63,103].

Regarding the brain, initial reports of decreased MAO activity in the hypothalamus and basal ganglia [19,138] were not confirmed by numerous subsequent studies involving the same brain regions as well as others [34,38,40,45,100,112 117,118,134,146]. For that matter one study reported increased MAO-type B in the pons of chronic schizophrenic patients [45], and others found increases in the ratios of MAO-type B relative to MAO-type A in various brain regions of chronic schizophrenic patients [40,118]. The latter finding, however, is not supported by another research group [34]. Although these differences in ratios of types of MAO were not examined according to subtype of schizophrenia, both drugs and degenerative brain processes were hypothesized as causes [45].

One other enzyme involved in the degradation of NE is COMT, which is measured in erythrocytes [89,122]. COMT activity in erythrocytes may be decreased in chronic paranoid schizophrenic patients [122]. Other reports have shown increased or normal COMT activity in chronic schizophrenic patients [29,89]. Regardless, this finding has not been confirmed in several brain regions [34,149].

Both of the remaining enzymes essential to the synthesis of NE, TH and DDC, have been measured in the brains of schizophrenic patients. In three studies [34,91,149] that examined as many as 50 brain regions [91], only two statistically significant findings emerged. Decreased TH activity in the olfactory area and DDC activity in the globus pallidus were reported in chronic schizophrenic patients, most of whom were of the paranoid subtype [91]. Because of the large number of regions studied, these findings are discounted by the investigators [91]. Moreover, DDC activity in the globus pallidus of chronic schizophrenic patients was normal in another study [149].

Norepinephrine Receptors and Uptake

Noradrenergic binding sites or receptors have been studied on both lymphocytes and platelets. α-adrenergic receptors in platelets seem to be increased in drug-free chronic schizophrenic patients [72,73]. β-receptors on the lymphocytes of schizophrenic patients were not altered [132].

In the brain, α-adrenergic binding as determined by binding of ^{3}H-WB4101 was normal [35]. This binding was thought to be an α_1 type as opposed to the α_2 type found on platelets. α_1-adrenergic binding in the frontal cortex [12] and basal ganglia [35] appeared to be normal in schizophrenic patients. No studies of α_2-adrenergic binding in human brains have been reported.

Because the major termination of noradrenergic action in neurons is a function of reuptake, this process was studied in platelets and plasma. NE uptake in platelets of drug-free acute schizophrenic patients was normal [115]. A relatively new technique reportedly measures neuronal uptake of NE from plasma [42]. As yet only two drug-free schizophrenic patients have been studied, and both had normal uptake [42].

PHARMACOLOGY

Another strategy for studying the role of NE in schizophrenia is to examine drugs that affect NE (Table 14.4). Perturbations of the noradrenergic system can be accomplished by giving (1) metabolic precursors (tyrosine or levodopa [L-dopa]); (2) stimulators of release (amphetamines); (3) blockers of enzymes of synthesis (α-methyl-*p*-tyrosine [AMPT], methyldopa, or DBH inhibitors such as disulfiram) or degradation (MAO inhibitors [MAO-I]); (4) blockers of α-receptors (phenoxybenzamine, clonidine, or neuroleptics) or β receptors (propranolol); and (5) inhibitors of storage (reserpine).

Table 14.4 Pharmacologic Evidence Compatible with a Norepinephrine Hypothesis of Schizophrenia*

NE Metabolism	*Amount of NE at Receptor*	*Induces or Exacerbates Schizophrenic Symptoms*	*Improves Schizophrenic Symptoms*
Precursor	Increased	L-Dopa	—
Synthesis inhibitor	Decreased	—	AMPT** (plus phenothiazine)
	? Increased	Fusaric Acid†	—
		Disulfiram†	—
Releaser	Increased	Amphetamine	—
		Methylphenidate	—
Receptor blocker	Decreased	—	Neuroleptics
Depletor	Decreased	—	Reserpine
Reuptake blocker	Increased	Amphetamine	—

NE = norepinephrine; AMPT = α-methyl-*p*-tyrosine.

* These data can equally support the dopamine hypothesis of schizophrenia.

** AMPT is ineffective alone; it allows phenothiazine dosage to be decreased.

† Even though these drugs should theoretically decrease NE, as they are dopamine-β-hydroxylase inhibitors, it has been reported that they may actually increase NE levels [75,80].

Administration of L-tyrosine, a metabolic precursor of NE, to schizophrenic patients produced no aggravation of symptomatology [109,143]. Neither were control subjects adversely affected by oral doses of L-tyrosine [143]. On the other hand, administration of a second metabolic precursor, L-dopa, exacerbated symptoms in schizophrenic subjects [5,116,151] and caused psychotic symptoms in some nonschizophrenic subjects [54,68]. Other reports found that low doses of L-dopa reduced psychotic symptoms in schizophrenic subjects at [49,62,74], especially if they had been symptomatic for less than 5 years [62]. Because these metabolic precursors increase both DA and NE, it is unclear which monoamine is responsible for their effects.

A second strategy for perturbing the NE system is to stimulate release, which can be accomplished with amphetamine or methylphenidate. In control subjects, high doses of amphetamine [2,10,30,41,56,156] induced psychosis. Similarly, amphetamine or methylphenidate intensified psychotic symptoms in schizophrenic subjects [3,4,6,64–67,135,136]. Although most investigators interpret the increased psychotic symptomology as a DA-mediated phenomenon, the actions of NE have not been ruled out.

In theory, the exacerbation of psychotic symptoms can also be accomplished by agents that block NE's degradation, such as MAO-I. Surprisingly, most nonpsychotic subjects did not become psychotic on MAO-I, and most schizophrenic subjects did not experience worsening of their symptoms [21,26]. Again, the mechanism of action is debatable because MAO-I should have increased not only NE but DA and serotonin (5-hydroxytryptamine; 5-HT) as well. One MAO-I, clorgyline, lowered plasma NE levels in depressed patients [108].

According to the NE hypothesis of schizophrenia, drugs which decrease noradrenergic activity should lead to clinical improvement (see Table 14.4). One of the first drugs found which lessened NE activity and reduced symptoms in psychotic subjects was reserpine [59,79,84,101,145]. Reserpine is of particular interest because its antipsychotic actions are not confined to schizophrenic subjects [59,79,84,101,145] and it not only depletes NE, but also DA and 5-HT.

A similar lack of specificity is characteristic of AMPT, a TH inhibitor. TH is the rate-limiting enzyme in the synthesis of both DA and NE [98,126]. Initial reports indicated that AMPT was not effective in the treatment of acute or chronic schizophrenia [28,50]. Subsequent reports have shown that AMPT allows smaller phenothiazine doses to be used in the treatment of chronic schizophrenic patients [24,25,41]. In other studies of chronic schizophrenic patients, AMPT has been shown to have limited, if any, benefits [51,99].

The next step in the synthesis of NE from tyrosine involves decarboxylation of dopa (see Chapter 1). α-methyl-3,4-dihydroxy-L-phenylalanine (methyldopa) inhibits the decarboxylase enzyme that catalyzes the conversion of dopa to DA [125]. However, a clinical trial of methyldopa in chronic schizophrenic patients was not a therapeutic success [104].

The last step in the synthesis of NE involves the hydroxylation of DA to NE by DBH. DBH can be inhibited by disulfiram and fusaric acid. If increased noradrenergic activity is related to psychotic symptoms, inhibition of DBH should decrease synaptic NE levels leading to clinical improvement. However, the opposite clinical effects were found: nonschizophrenic patients developed psychotic symptoms [11,43,86,88,124] and schizophrenic patients [58,124] became more symptomatic. Moreover, fusaric acid, when given to manic patients, shifted manic symptoms to psychotic symptoms [55]. This dilemma has perhaps been resolved by recent studies reporting increased rather than decreased plasma NE levels after the administration of either disulfiram [80] or fusaric acid [75]. The mechanisms by which these DBH inhibitors actually increased plasma NE levels are unknown.

Reduction of noradrenergic activity can also be accomplished by receptor blockade. Three major types of NE receptors include α_1, α_2, and β receptors. Blockers or agonists of each of these receptors have been administered to schizophrenic patients. Neuroleptics, the mainstay of treatment of schizophrenia, probably have α_1-blocking properties in addition to DA-blocking properties [31,107]. Unfortunately, α_1-blocking potency did not correlate with antipsychotic clinical efficacy in commonly used neuroleptics [32]. Although early reports of the potential of α-blocking compounds to treat schizophrenia were promising [92,114], a more recent report found phenoxybenzamine, an α-blocker, to be ineffective [15].

Considerably greater success in the treatment of schizophrenia was achieved using β-blockers such as propranolol [7–9,57,139,140,152–155]. Enormous doses of propranolol were necessary to successfully treat psychotic symptoms, and not all studies were positive [16,48,111,121]. It appears that propranolol works by increasing serum neuroleptic concentrations [105,106], and that propranolol's antipsychotic actions have little to do with its β-blocking property.

A promising new approach involves stimulation of α_2-receptors, which are inhibitors of noradrenergic activity. Initial trials of clonidine, an α_2-agonist, in schizophrenic subjects were negative [69,123,130]. A more recent report found clonidine as effective as a conventional neuroleptic (trifluoperazine) in the treatment of chronic schizophrenia [46]. Finally, clonidine's failure to affect plasma MHPG in schizophrenic patients as compared to controls was interpreted as evidence of impaired regulation of NE turnover [127]. In this last study, the major difference between controls and patients appeared to be that placebo increased plasma MHPG in the controls, but not in the patients.

CONCLUSIONS

A considerable body of evidence implicates NE in the pathogenesis of schizophrenic symptoms. More specificially, biochemical findings suggest that schizophrenic patients with paranoid features are more likely to have abnormalities of the NE system. Pharmacologic investigations have not as yet focused on the paranoid schizophrenia paradigm. Although evidence is incomplete and somewhat inconsistent, it is compelling enough to warrant further studies of NE in the schizophrenic syndrome. Several directions of research should probably be taken to test these hypotheses. Studies of NE levels in urine and blood should focus on comparisons of paranoid and undifferentiated schizophrenic patients. This strategy should also be useful when studying CSF, brain, and pharmacologic perturbations of the NE system. Further study of the association between increased NE and/or MHPG in CSF and limbic structures of paranoid schizophrenic patients is necessary. Premorbid studies should be followed by postmortem studies whenever possible. One postmortem study which is clearly required involves measurements of α_2-receptors in the brain. Increased α_2 binding in platelets and some indications of the therapeutic benefits of clonidine, an α_2-agonist, indicate the relevance of this study. Finally, infusions of radioactive metabolic precursors and/or radioactive ligands such as clonidine, propranolol, or phenoxybenzamine should be studied with positron-emission tomography.

REFERENCES

1. Ackenheil M, Albus M, Muller F, Muller T, Welter D, Zander K, Engel R. Catecholamine Response to Short-Time Stress in Schizophrenic and Depressive Patients. In Catecholamines: Basic and Clinical Frontiers, E Usdin, I Kopin, J Barchas (eds), vol 2, 1937–1939. New York: Pergamon Press, 1979.
2. Angrist B, Gershon S. The phenomenology of experimentally induced amphetamine psychosis—preliminary observations. Biol Psychiatry 2: 95–107, 1970.
3. Angrist B, Gershon S. Clinical Response to Several Dopaminergic Agonists in Schizophrenic and Nonschizophrenic Subjects. In Advances in Biochemical Psychopharmacology, E Costa and GL Gessa (eds), vol. 16, 677–680. New York: Raven Press, 1977.
4. Angrist B, Rotrosen J, Gershon S. Responses to apomorphine, amphetamine and neuroleptics in schizophrenic subjects. Psychopharmacology (Berlin) 67:31–38, 1980.
5. Angrist B, Sathanathan G, Gershon S. Behavioral effects of L-DOPA in schizophrenic patients. Psychopharmacologia (Berlin) 31:1–12, 1973.
6. Angrist B, Thompson H, Shopsin B. Clinical studies with dopamine receptor stimulants. Psychopharmacologia (Berlin) 44:273–280, 1975.
7. Atsmon A. Early observations of the effect of propranolol on psychotic patients. Adv Clin Pharmacol 12:86–90, 1976.
8. Atsmon A, Blum I, Steiner M, Latz A, Wijsenbeek LT. Further studies with propranolol in psychotic patients. Relation to initial psychiatric state, urinary catecholamines and 3-methoxy-4-hydroxyphenylglycol excretion. Psychopharmacologia (Berlin) 27:249–254, 1972.
9. Atsmon A, Blum I, Wijsenbeek LT, Maoz B, Steiner M, Ziegelman G. The short-term effects of adrenergic-blocking agents in a small group of psychotic patients. Preliminary clinical observations. Psychiatr Neurol Neurochir 74:251–258, 1971.
10. Bell DS. The experimental reproduction of amphetamine psychosis. Arch Gen Psychiatry 29:35–40, 1973.
11. Bennett A, McKeever L, Turk H. Psychotic reactions during tetraethythiuram disulfide (Antabuse) therapy. JAMA 145:483–484, 1951.
12. Bennett JP, Enna SJ, Bylund DB, Gillin JC, Wyatt RJ, Snyder SH. Neurotransmitter receptors in frontal cortex of schizophrenics. Arch Gen Psychiatry 36:927–933, 1979.
13. Berger PA, Faull KF, Kilkowski J, Anderson PJ, Kraemer H, Davis KL, Barchas JD. CSF monoamine metabolites in depression and schizophrenia. Am J Psychiatry 137:174–180, 1980.

14. Bergsman A. The urinary excretion of adrenalin and noradrenalin in some mental diseases. Acta Psychiatr Neurol Scand (Suppl 34): 133:1–107, 1959.
15. Bigelow LB. Unpublished observations, 1978.
16. Bigelow LB, Zalcman S, Kleinman JE, Weinberger D, Luchins D, Tallman J, Karoum F, Wyatt RJ. Propranolol Treatment of Chronic Schizophrenia: Clinical Response, Catecholamine Metabolism and Lymphocyte β-Receptors. In Catecholamines: Basic and Clinical Frontiers, E Usdin, IJ Kopin, and JD Barchas (eds), 1851–1853. New York: Pergamon Press, 1979.
17. Bird ED, Spokes EG, Iversen LL. Brain norepinephrine and dopamine in schizophrenia. Science 204:93–94, 1979.
18. Bird ED, Spokes EG, Iversen LL. Increased dopamine concentration in limbic areas of brain from patients dying with schizophrenia. Brain 102:347–360, 1979.
19. Birkhauser H. Cholinesterase und mono-aminoxydase in zentralen nervensystem. Schweiz Med Wochenschr 71:750–752, 1941.
20. Book JA, Wetterberg L, Modrzewska S. Schizophrenia in North Swedish geographical isolate, 1900–1977. Epidemiology, genetics and biochemistry. Clin Genet 14:373–394, 1978.
21. Brenner R, Shopsin B. The use of monoamine oxidase inhibitors in schizophrenia. Biol Psychiatry 15:633–647, 1980.
22. Brown F, Coleman JH. Dopamine-β-hydroxylase in nerve function and mental illness. Dis Nerv Syst 36:383–385, 1975.
23. Carlsson A. The Impact of Catecholamine Research on Medical Science and Practice. In Catecholamines: Basic and Clinical Frontiers, E Usdin, I Kopin, and J Barchas (eds), vol. 1, 4–19. New York: Pergamon Press, 1979.
24. Carlsson A, Persson T, Roos BE, Walinder J. Potentiation of phenothiazines by α-methyltyrosine in treatment of chronic schizophrenia. J Neural Transm 33:83–90, 1972.
25. Carlsson A, Roos BE, Walinder J, Skoot A. Further studies on the mechanism of anti-psychotic action: potentiation by α-methyltyrosine of thioridazine effects in chronic schizophrenics. J Neural Transm 34:125–132, 1973.
26. Carman JS, Gillin JC, Murphy DL, Weinberger DR, Kleinman JE, Bigelow LB, Wyatt RJ. Effects of a selective inhibitor of type A monoamine oxidase—Lilly 51641—on behavior, sleep and circadian rhythms in depressed and schizophrenic patients. Commun Psychopharmacol 2:513–523, 1978.
27. Castellani S, Ziegler MG, van Kammen DP, Lake CR. Plasma norepinephrine and serum dopamine-β-hydroxylase activity in schizophrenia. Arch Gen Psychiatry 39:1145–1149, 1982.
28. Charalampous KD, Brown S. A clinical trial of alpha-methyl-paratyrosine in mentally ill patients. Psychopharmacologia (Berlin) 11:422–425, 1967.
29. Cohn CK, Dunner DL, Axelrod J. Reduced catechol-O-methyl transferase activity in red blood cells of women with primary affective disorder. Science 170:1323–1324, 1970.
30. Connell PH. Amphetamine Psychosis. Chapman and Hell, London, 1958.
31. Courvoisier S, Fournel J, Ducrot R, Kolsky M, Koetschet P. Propriétés pharmacodynamiques du chlorhydrate de chloro-3 (dimethylamino-3-propyl)-10-phenothiazine, (4,560 R.P.): étude experimentale d'un nouveau corps utilisé dans l'anesthésie potentialisée et dans l'hibernation artificielle. Arch Int Pharmacodyn 92:305–361, 1953.
32. Creese I, Burt DR, Snyder SH. Dopamine receptor binding predicts clinical and pharmacological potencies of anti-schizophrenic drugs. Science 192:481–483, 1976.

33. Cross AJ, Crow TJ, Killpack WS, Longden A, Owen F, Riley GJ. The activities of brain dopamine-β-hydroxylase and catechol-O-methyltransferase in schizophrenics and controls. Psychopharmacology (Berlin) 59:117–121, 1978.
34. Crow TJ, Baker HF, Cross AJ, Joseph MH, Lofthouse R, Longden A, Owen F, Riley GJ, Glover V, Killpack WS. Monoamine mechanisms in chronic schizophrenia: Postmortem neurochemical findings. Br J Psychiatry 132:249–256, 1979.
35. Crow TJ, Cross AJ, Owen D, Ferrier N, Johnstone EC, MaCreadie RM, Owens DGC. Neurochemical studies in postmortem brains in schizophrenia: changes in the dopamine receptor in relation to psychiatric and neurological symptoms. American Psychiatric Association Abstracts, p. 39, 1981.
36. DeLisi LE, Wise CD, Bridge TP, Phelps BH, Potkin SG, Wyatt RJ. Monoamine Oxidase and Schizophrenia. In Biological Markers in Psychiatry and Neurology, E Usdin and I Hanin (eds), 79–96. Oxford and New York: Pergamon Press, 1982.
37. DeLisi LE, Wise CD, Potkin SG, Zalcman S, Phelps BH, Lovenberg W, Wyatt RJ. Dopamine-β-hydroxylase, monoamine oxidase and schizophrenia. Biol Psychiatry 15:899–907, 1980.
38. Domino EF, Krause RR, Bowers J. Various enzymes involved with putative neurotransmitters. Arch Gen Psychiatry 29:195–201, 1973.
39. Dunner DL, Cohn CK, Weinshilboum RM, Wyatt RJ. The activity of dopamine-β-hydroxylase and methionine-activating enzyme in blood of schizophrenic patients. Biol Psychiatry 6:215–219, 1973.
40. Eckert B, Gottfries CG, von Knorring L, Oreland L, Wiberg A, Winblad B. Brain and platelet monoamine oxidase in schizophrenics and cycloid psychotics. Prog Neuropsychopharmacol 4:57–68, 1980.
41. Ellinwood EH. Amphetamine Psychosis: Individuals, Settings and Sequences. In Current Concepts on Amphetamine Abuse, EH Ellinwood and S Cohen (eds), p. 143. Washington, DC: U.S. Government Printing Office, 1969.
42. Esler M, Turbott J, Schwarz R, Leonard P, Bobik A, Skews H, Jackman G. The peripheral kinetics of norepinephrine in depressive illness. Arch Gen Psychiatry 39:295–300, 1982.
43. Ewing JA, Mueller RA, Rouse BA, Silver D. Low levels of dopamine-β-hydroxylase and psychosis. Am J Psychiatry 134:927–928, 1977.
44. Farley IJ, Price KS, McCullough E, Deck JHN, Hordynski W, Hornykiewicz O. Norepinephrine in chronic paranoid schizophrenia: above-normal levels in limbic forebrain. Science 200:456–458, 1978.
45. Fowler CJ, Carlsson A, Winblad A. Monoamine oxidase-A and -B activities in the brain stem of schizophrenics and non-schizophrenic psychotics. J Neural Transm 52:23–32, 1981.
46. Freedman R, Kirch D, Bell J, Adler LE, Pecevich M, Pachtman E, Denver P. Clonidine treatment of schizophrenia: double-blind comparison to placebo and neuroleptic drugs. Acta Psychiatr Scand 65:35–45, 1982.
47. Fujita K, Ito T, Maruta K, Teradaira R, Beppu H, Nakagami Y, Kato Y. Serum dopamine-β-hydroxylase in schizophrenic patients. J Neurochem 30:1569–1572, 1978.
48. Gardos G, Cole JO, Volicer L, Orzack MH, Oliff AC. A dose-response study of propranolol in chronic schizophrenics. Curr Ther Res 15:314–323, 1973.
49. Gerlack J, Luhdorf K. The effect of L-dopa on young patients with simple schizophrenia, treated with neuroleptic drugs. Psychopharmacologia (Berlin) 44:105–110, 1975.
50. Gershon S, Hekimian LJ, Floyd A, Jr., Hollister LE. Alpha-methyl-*p*-tyrosine (AMPT) in schizophrenia. Psychopharmacologia (Berlin) 11:189–194, 1967.

51. Gillin JC, Kleinman JE, Nasrallah HA, Bigelow LB, Rogol A, Luchins D, Carman J, Weinberger D, Wyatt RJ. Inhibition of Dopamine Synthesis in Chronic Schizophrenia: A Follow-up Study. In Catecholamines: Basic and Clinical Frontiers, E Usdin, IJ Kopin, and JD Barchas (eds), 1845–1847. New York: Pergamon Press, 1979.
52. Goldstein M, Freedman LS, Epstein RP, Pask DH. Studies on dopamine-β-hydroxylase in mental disorders. J Psychiatr Res 11:205–210, 1974.
53. Gomes UCR, Shanley BC, Potgieter L, Roux JT. Noradrenergic overactivity in chronic schizophrenia: evidence based on cerebrospinal fluid noradrenaline and cyclic nucleotide concentrations. Br J Psychiatry 137:346–351, 1980.
54. Goodwin FK, Murphy DL, Brodie HKH, Bunney WE, Jr. L-DOPA, catecholamines and behavior: A clinical and biochemical study in depressed patients. Biol Psychiatry 2:341–366, 1970.
55. Goodwin FK, Sack RL. Behavioral effects on a new dopamine-β-hydroxylase inhibitor (fusaric acid) in man. J Psychiatr Res 11:211–217, 1974.
56. Griffith JD, Cavanaugh J, Held J, Oates JA. Dextroamphetamine. Evaluation of psychomimetic properties in man. Arch Gen Psychiatry 26:97–100, 1972.
57. Hanssen T, Heyden T, Sundberg I, Alfredsson G, Nyback H, Wetterberg L. Propranolol in schizophrenia. Clinical, metabolic, and pharmacological findings. Arch Gen Psychiatry 37:685–690, 1980.
58. Heath RG, Nesselhov W, Bishop MP, Byers LW. Behavioral and metabolic changes associated with administration of tetraethylthiuram disulfide (Antabuse). Dis Nerv Syst 26:99–105, 1965.
59. Hollister LE, Traub L, Beckman WG. Psychiatric Use of Reserpine and Chlorpromazine: Results of Double-Blind Studies. In Psychopharmacology, NS Kline (ed), 65–74. Washington, DC: American Association for the Advancement of Science, 1956.
60. Hoskins RG. Schizophrenia from the physiological point of view. Ann Intern Med 7:445–456, 1933.
61. Hoskins RG, Sleeper FH. Organic functions in schizophrenia. Arch Neurol Psychiatry 30:123–140, 1933.
62. Inanaga K, Tanaka M. Effects of L-DOPA on Schizophrenia. In Psychopharmacology, Sexual Disorders and Drug Abuse, TA Ban, JR Boissier, GJ Gessa, H Heimann, L Hollister, HE Lehmann, I Munkvad, H Steinberg, F Fulser, A Sundwall, and O. Vinar (eds), 229–233. Amsterdam: North-Holland, 1973.
63. Jackman HL, Meltzer HY. Factors affecting determination of platelet monoamine oxidase activity. Schiz Bull 6:259–266, 1980.
64. Janowsky DS, Davis JM. Dopamine, psychomotor stimulants, and schizophrenia: effects of methylphenidate and the stereoisomers of amphetamine in schizophrenics. Adv Biochem Psychopharmacol 12:317–323, 1974.
65. Janowsky DS, Davis JM. Methylphenidate, dextroamphetamine and l-amphetamine: effects on schizophrenic symptoms. Arch Gen Psychiatry 33:304–308, 1976.
66. Janowsky DS, El-Yousef K, Davis JM, Sekerke HJ. Provocation of schizophrenic symptoms of intravenous administration of methylphenidate. Arch Gen Psychiatry 28:185–191, 1973.
67. Janowsky DS, Storms L, Judd LL. Methylphenidate hydrochloride effects on psychological tests in acute schizophrenic and nonpsychotic patients. Arch Gen Psychiatry 34:189–194, 1977.
68. Jenkins RB, Groh RH. Mental symptoms in parkinsonian patients treated with L-DOPA. Lancet 2:177–179, 1970.

69. Jimerson DC, Post RM, Stoddard FJ, Gillin JC, Bunney WE, Jr. Preliminary trial of the noradrenergic agonist clonidine in psychiatric patients. Biol Psychiatry 15:45–57, 1980.
70. Joseph MH, Baker HF, Johnstone EC, Crow TJ. Determination of 3-methoxy-4-hydroxyphenylglycol conjugates in urine. Application to the study of central noradrenaline metabolism in unmedicated schizophrenic patients. Psychopharmacology (Berlin) 51:47–51, 1976.
71. Joseph MH, Baker HF, Johnstone EC, Crow TJ. 3-Methoxy-4-hydroxyphenylglycol excretion in acutely schizophrenic patients during a controlled clinical trial of the isomers of flupenthixol. Psychopharmacology (Berlin) 64:35–40, 1979.
72. Kafka MS, van Kammen DP, Kleinman JE. The Alpha-Adrenergic Receptor in Man: Normal Function and Pathology. In Neuroreceptors Basic and Clinical Aspects, E Usdin, WE Bunney, Jr. and JM Davis (eds), 129–139. New York: Wiley and Sons, 1981.
73. Kafka MS, van Kammen DP, Kleinman JE, Nurnberger JI, Siever LJ, Uhde TW, Polinsky RJ. Alpha-adrenergic receptor function in schizophrenia, affective disorders and some neurological disease. Commun Psychopharmacol 4:477–486, 1980.
74. Kai Y. The effect of L-dopa and vitamin B_6 in schizophrenia. Folia Psychiatr Neurol Jpn 30:19–26, 1976.
75. Kato T, Hashimoto Y, Nagatsu T, Shinoda T, Okada T, Takeuchi T, Umezawa H. 24-hour rhythm of human plasma noradrenaline and the effect of fusaric acid, a dopamine-beta-hydroxylase inhibitor. Neuropsychobiology 6:61–65, 1980.
76. Kemali O, Del Vecchio M, Maj M. Increased noradrenaline levels in CSF and plasma of schizophrenic patients. Biol Psychiatry 17:711–717, 1982.
77. Kleinman JE, Bridge P, Karoum F, Speciale S, Staub R, Zalcman S, Gillin JC, Wyatt RJ. Catecholamines and Metabolites in the Brains of Psychotics and Normals: Postmortem Studies. In Catecholamines: Basic and Clinical Frontiers, E Usdin, IJ Kopin, and JD Barchas (eds), 1845–1847. New York: Pergamon Press, 1979.
78. Kleinman JE, Karoum F, Rosenblatt JE, Gillin JC, Hong J, Bridge TP, Zalcman S, Storch F, Carman R, Wyatt RJ. Postmortem Neurochemical Studies in Chronic Schizophrenia. In Biological Markers in Psychiatry and Neurology, E Usdin and I Hanin (eds), 67–76. New York: Pergamon Press, 1982.
79. Kline NS. Use of Rauwolfia serpentina benth in neuropsychiatric conditions. Ann NY Acad Sci 59:107–132, 1954.
80. Lake CR, Major LF, Ziegler MG, Kopin IJ. Increased sympathetic nervous system activity in alcoholic patients treated with disulfiram. Am J Psychiatry 134:1411–1414, 1977.
81. Lake CR, Sternberg DE, van Kammen DP, Ballenger JC, Ziegler MG, Post RM, Kopin IJ, Bunney WE, Jr. Elevated cerebrospinal fluid norepinephrine in schizophrenics: confounding effects of treatment drugs. Science 210:97, 1980.
82. Lake CR, Sternberg DE, van Kammen DP, Ballenger JC, Ziegler MG, Post RM, Kopin IJ, Bunney WE, Jr. Schizophrenia: elevated cerebrospinal fluid norepinephrine. Science 207:331–333, 1980.
83. Lamprecht F, Wyatt RJ, Belmaker R, Murphy DL, Pollin W. Plasma Dopamine-Beta-Hydroxylase in Identical Twins Discordant for Schizophrenia. In Frontiers in Catecholamine Research, E Usdin and SH Snyder (eds), 1123–1126. New York: Pergamon Press, 1973.
84. Lehmann HE, Hanrahan GE. Chlorpromazine: new inhibiting agent for psychomotor excitement and manic states. Arch Neurol Psychiatry 71:227–237, 1954.

85. Lerner P, Goodwin FK, van Kammen DP, Post RM, Major LF, Ballenger JC, Lovenberg W. Dopamine-beta-hydroxylase in cerebrospinal fluid of psychiatric patients. Biol Psychiatry 13:685–694, 1978.
86. Major LF, Lerner P, Ballenger JC, Brown GL, Goodwin FK, Lovenberg W. Dopamine-β-hydroxylase in the cerebrospinal fluid: relationship to disulfiram-induced psychosis. Biol Psychiatry 14:337–344, 1979.
87. Markianos ES, Nystrom K, Reichel H. Serum dopamine-β-hydroxylase in psychiatric patients and normals. Effects of D-amphetamine and haloperidol. Psychopharmacology (Berlin) 50:259–267, 1976.
88. Martensen-Larsen D. Psychotic phenomenon provoked by tetraethylthiuram disulfide. Q J Stud Alc 12:206–216, 1951.
89. Matthysse S, Baldessarini RJ. S-adenosylmethionine and catechol-O-methyltransferase in schizophrenia. Am J Psychiatry 128:1310–1312, 1972.
90. McDonald RK, Weise VK. The excretion of 3-methoxy-4-hydroxymandelic acid in normal and in chronic schizophrenic male subjects. J Psychiatry Res 1:173–184, 1962.
91. McGeer PL, McGeer EG. Possible changes in striatal and limbic cholinergic systems in schizophrenia. Arch Gen Psychiatry 34:1319–1323, 1977.
92. Medinets HE, Kline NS, Mettler FA. Effect of N,N-dibenzyl-B-chloroethylamine hydrochloride (Dibenamine) on autonomic functions and catatonia in schizophrenic subjects. Proc Soc Exp Biol Med 69:238–246, 1948.
93. Meltzer HY, Cho HW, Carroll BJ, Russo P. Serum dopamine-β-hydroxylase activity in the affective psychoses and schizophrenia. Decreased activity in unipolar psychotically depressed patients. Arch Gen Psychiatry 33:585–591, 1976.
94. Meltzer HY, Nasr SJ, Tong C. Serum dopamine-β-hydroxylase activity in schizophrenia. Biol Psychiatry 15:781–788, 1980.
95. Mileikovskii YA. Excretion of catecholamines and tryptophan derivatives in schizophrenia. Zh Nevropatol Psikhiatr 76:710–714, 1976.
96. Murphy DL, Wyatt RJ. Reduced monoamine oxidase activity in blood platelets from schizophrenic patients. Nature 253:659–660, 1972.
97. Naber D, Finkbeiner C, Fischer H, Zander K-J, Achkenheil M. Effect of long-term neuroleptic treatment on prolactin and norepinephrine levels in serum of chronic schizophrenics: relations to psychopathology and extrapyramidal symptoms. Neuropsychobiology 6:181–189, 1980.
98. Nagatsu T, Levitt M, Undenfriend S. Tyrosine hydroxylase, the initial step in norepinephrine biosynthesis. J Biol Chem 239:2910–2917, 1964.
99. Nasrallah HA, Donnelly EF, Bigelow LB, Rivera-Calimlin L, Rogol AB, Potkin S, Rauscher FP, Wyatt RJ, Gillin JC. Inhibition of dopamine synthesis in chronic schizophrenia: clinical ineffectiveness of metyrosine. Arch Gen Psychiatry 34:649–655, 1977.
100. Nies A, Robinson DS, Harris LS, Lamborn KR. Comparison of Monoamine Oxidase Substrate Activities in Twins, Schizophrenics, Depressives and Controls. In Neuropsychopharmacology of Monoamines and Their Regulatory Enzymes, E Usdin (ed), 59–70. New York: Raven Press, 1974.
101. Noce RH, Williams DB, Rappaport W. Reserpine (Serpasil) in the management of the mentally ill and mentally retarded. JAMA 156:821–824, 1954.
102. Okada T, Ohta T, Shinoda T, Kato T, Ikuta T, Nagatsu T. Dopamine-β-hydroxylase activity in serum and cerebrospinal fluid in neuropsychiatric disease. Neuropsychobiology 2:139–144, 1976.

103. Owen F, Bourne RC, Crowe TJ, Fadhl AA, Johnstone EC. Platelet monoamine oxidase activity in acute schizophrenia: relationship to symptomatology and neuroleptic medication. Br J Psychiatry 139:16–22, 1981.
104. Pecknold JC, Ananth JV, Ban TA, Lehmann HE. The use of methyldopa in schizophrenia: a review and comparative study. Am J Psychiatry 128:1207–1211, 1972.
105. Peet M, Middlemiss DN, Yates RA. Pharmacokinetic interaction between propranolol and chlorpromazine in schizophrenic patients. Lancet 2:978, 1980.
106. Peet M, Middlemiss DN, Yates RA. Propranolol in schizophrenia. II. Clinical and biochemical aspects of combining propranolol with chlorpromazine. Br J Psychiatry 138:112–117, 1981.
107. Peroutka SJ, U'Prichard DC, Greenberg DA, Snyder SH. Neuroleptic drug interactions with norepinephrine alpha-receptor binding sites in rat brain. Neuropharmacology 16:549–556, 1977.
108. Pickar D, Lake CR, Cohen RM, Jimerson DC, Murphy DL. Alterations in noradrenergic function during clorgyline treatment. Commun Psychopharmacol 4:379–386, 1980.
109. Pollin W, Caron PV, Jr, Ketz SS. Effects of amino acid feedings in schizophrenic patients treated with iproniazid. Science 133:104–105, 1961.
110. Post RM, Fink E, Carpenter WT, Goodwin FK. Cerebrospinal fluid amine metabolites in acute schizophrenia. Arch Gen Psychiatry 32:1063–1069, 1975.
111. Rackensperger W, Gaupp R, Mattke DJ, Schwartz D, Stulte KH. Behandlung von akuten schizophrenen psychosen mit beta-receptoren-blockern. Arch Psychiatr Nervenkr 219:29–36, 1974.
112. Reveley MA, Glover V, Sandler M, Spokes EG. Brain monoamine oxidase activity in schizophrenics and controls. Arch Gen Psychiatry 38:663–665, 1981.
113. Rimon R, Roos BE, Kampman R, Hyyppa S, Ranta P, Myllyla V. Monoamine metabolite levels in cerebrospinal fluid and brain atrophy in lobotomized schizophrenic patients. Ann Clin Res 11:25–29, 1979.
114. Rockwell FV. Dibenamine therapy in certain psychopathological syndromes. Psychosomatics 10:230–237, 1948.
115. Rotman A, Munitz H, Modai I, Tjano S, Wijsenbeek LT. A comparative uptake study of serotonin, dopamine and norepinephrine by platelets of acute schizophrenic patients. Psychiatry Res 3: 239–246, 1980.
116. Sathanathan G, Angrist BM, Gershon S. Response threshold to L-DOPA in psychiatric patients. Biol Psychiatry 7:139–146, 1973.
117. Schwartz MA, Aikens AM, Wyatt RJ. Monoamine oxidase activity in brains from schizophrenic and mentally normal individuals. Psychopharmacologia (Berlin) 38:319–328, 1974.
118. Schwartz MA, Wyatt RJ, Yang H-YT, Neff NH. Multiple forms of brain monoamine oxidase in schizophrenic and normal individuals. Arch Gen Psychiatry 31:557–560, 1974.
119. Sedvall GC, Wode-Helgodt B. Aberrant monoamine metabolite levels in CSF and family history of schizophrenia. Arch Gen Psychiatry 37:1113–1116, 1980.
120. Shopsin B, Freedman LS, Goldstein M, Gershon S. Serum dopamine-β-hydroxylase (DBH) in affective states. Psychopharmacologia (Berlin) 25:11–16, 1972.
121. Shopsin B, Hirsch H, Gershon S. Visual hallucinations and propranolol. Biol Psychiatry 10:105–107, 1975.
122. Shopsin B, Wilk S, Gershon S, Roffman M, Goldstein M. Collaborative Psychopharmacologic Studies Exploring Catecholamine Metabolism in Psychiatric Disorders.

In Frontiers in Catecholamine Research, E Usdin and S Snyder (eds), 1173–1179. New York: Pergamon Press, 1973.

123. Simpson GM, Kunz-Bartholini E, Watts TP. A preliminary evaluation of the sedative effects of Catapres, a new antihypertensive agent, in chronic schizophrenic patients. J Clin Pharmacol 7:221–225, 1967.

124. Smilde J. Risks and unexpected reactions in disulfiram therapy of alcoholism. Q J Stud Alc 24:489, 1963.

125. Sourkes TL. Inhibition of dihydroxyphenylalanine decarboxylase by derivatives of phenylalanine. Arch Biochem 51:444–456, 1954.

126. Spector S, Sjoerdsma A, Undenfriend S. Blockade of endogeneous norepinephrine synthesis by alpha-methyltyrosine, an inhibitor of tyrosine hydroxylase. J Pharmacol Exp Ther 147:86–95, 1965.

127. Sternberg DE, Charney DS, Heninger GR, Leckman JF, Hafstad KM, Landis DH. Impaired presynaptic regulation of norepinephrine in schizophrenia. Effects of clonidine in schizophrenic patients and normal controls. Arch Gen Psychiatry 39:285–289, 1982.

128. Sternberg DE, van Kammen DP, Ballenger JC, Lerner P, Marder SR, Post RM. Cerebrospinal fluid dopamine-beta-hydroxylase and schizophrenia. American Psychiatric Association New Research Abstracts, p. 32, 1978.

129. Sternberg DE, van Kammen DP, Lerner P, Bunney WE, Jr. DBH and reactive schizophrenia. Annual Meeting of the Society of Biological Psychiatry Abstracts No. 34, p. 66, 1980.

130. Sugarman AA. A pilot study of ST-155 (Catapres) in chronic schizophrenia. J Clin Pharmacol 7:226–230, 1967.

131. Sweeney DR, Leckman JF, Maas JW, Hattox S, Heninger GR. Plasma free and conjugated MHPG in psychiatric patients: A pilot study. Arch Gen Psychiatry 37:1100–1103, 1980.

132. Tallman J. Unpublished observations. 1979.

133. Taube SL, Kirstein LS, Sweeney DR, Heninger GR, Maas JW. Urinary 3-methoxy-4-hydroxyphenylglycol and psychiatric diagnosis. Am J Psychiatry 135:78–82, 1978.

134. Utena H, Kanamura H, Suda S, Nakamura R, Machiyama Y, Takahashi R. Studies on the regional distribution of the monoamine oxidase activity in the brains of schizophrenic patients. Proc Jpn Acad 44:1078–1083, 1968.

135. van Kammen DP, Bunney WE, Jr., Docherty JP, Jimerson DC, Post RM, Siris S, Ebert M, Gillin JC. Amphetamine-Induced Catecholamine Activation in Schizophrenia and Depression: Behavioral and Physiological Effects. In Advances in Biochemical Psychopharmacology, E Costa and GL Gessa (eds), vol. 16, 655–659. New York: Raven Press, 1977.

136. van Kammen DP, Docherty JP, Marder SR, Rayner JN, Bunney WE, Jr. Long-term pimozide pretreatment differentially affects behavioral responses to dextroamphetamine in schizophrenia. Arch Gen Psychiatry 39:275–281, 1982.

137. Van Praag HM, Korf J. The Dopamine Hypothesis of Schizophrenia: Some Direct Observations. In On the Origin of Schizophrenic Psychoses, HM Van Praag (ed), 81–98. Amsterdam: De Erven Bohn BV, 1975.

138. Vogel WH, Orfei V, Century B. Activities of enzymes involved in the formation and destruction of biogenic amines and in various areas of human brains. J Pharmacol Exp Ther 165:195–203, 1969.

139. Volk W, Bier W, Braum JP, Gruter W, Spiegelberg U. Behandlung von erregten

psychosen mit einem beta-receptoren-blocker (oxprenolol) in hoher dosierung. Nervenarzt 43:491–492, 1972.

140. von Zerssen D. Beta-adrenergic blocking agents in the treatment of psychoses. A report on 17 cases. Adv Clin Pharmacol 12:105–114, 1976.

141. Walinder J, Skott A, Carlsson A, Roos BE. Potentiation by metyrosine of thioridazine effects in chronic schizophrenics. Arch Gen Psychiatry 33:501–505, 1976.

142. Wetterberg L, Aberg H, Ross SB, Froden O. Plasma dopamine-β-hydroxylase activity in hypertension and various neuropsychiatric disorders. Scand J Clin Lab Invest 30:283–289, 1972.

143. Williams CH. Aspects of tyrosine metabolism in schizophrenia. Psychosom Med 1:286–291, 1971.

144. Winblad B, Bucht G, Gottfries CG, Roos BE. Monoamines and monoamine metabolites in brains from demented schizophrenics. Acta Psychiatr Scand 60:17–28, 1979.

145. Winkelman NW, Jr. Chlorpromazine in treatment of neuropsychiatric disorders. JAMA 155:18–21, 1954.

146. Wise CD, Baden MH, Stein L. Postmortem measurements of enzymes in human brain: evidence of a central noradrenergic deficit in schizophrenia. J Psychiatr Res 11:185–198, 1974.

147. Wise CD, Stein L. Dopamine-β-hydroxylase deficits in the brains of schizophrenic patients. Science 181:344–347, 1973.

148. Wise CD, Stein L. Dopamine-β-hydroxylase activity in brains of chronic schizophrenic patients. Science 187:370, 1975.

149. Wyatt RJ, Erdelyi W, Schwartz M, Herman M, Barchas JD. Difficulties in comparing catecholamine-related enzymes from the brains of schizophrenics and controls. Biol Psychiatry 13:317–333, 1978.

150. Wyatt RJ, Schwartz MA, Erdelyi E, Barchas JD. Dopamine-β-hydroxylase activity in brains of chronic schizophrenic patients. Science 187:368–370, 1975.

151. Yaryura-Tobias JA, Diamond B, Merlis S. The action of L-DOPA on schizophrenic patients (a preliminary report). Curr Ther Res 12:528–581, 1970.

152. Yorkston NJ, Zaki SA, Malik MKU, Morrison RC, Harvard CWH. Propranolol in the control of schizophrenic symptoms. Br Med J 4:633–635, 1974.

153. Yorkston NJ, Zaki SA, Pitcher DR, Gruzelier JH, Hollander D, Serjeant HGS. Propranolol as an adjunct to the treatment of schizophrenia. Lancet 2:575–578, 1977.

154. Yorkston NJ, Zaki SA, Themen JFA, Harvard CWH. Propranolol to control schizophrenic symptoms. Adv Clin Pharmacol 12:91–104, 1976.

155. Yorkston NJ, Zaki SA, Themen JFA, Harvard CWH. Safeguards in the treatment of schizophrenia with propranolol. Postgrad Med J 52:175–180, 1976.

156. Young D, Scoville WB. Paranoid psychosis in narcolepsy and the possible danger of benzedrine treatment. Med Clin North Am (Boston) 22:637–646, 1938.

157. Yu PH, O'Sullivan KS, Keegan D, Boulton AA. Dopamine-beta-hydroxylase and its apparent endogenous inhibitory activity in the plasma of some psychiatric patients. Psychiatry Res 3:205–210, 1980.

158. Zizolfi S, Famiglietti LA, Del Vecchio M, Kemali D. Platelet monoamine oxidase and serum dopamine-β-hydroxylase activities in psychotic patients. Acta Neurol (Napoli) 34:142–149, 1979.

15

Studies of the Dopamine Hypothesis of Schizophrenia

David E. Sternberg
Irl Extein

The group of disorders known collectively as schizophrenia continues to be a critical problem for modern psychiatry and accounts for large expenditures by society and tragedy for many families. Different patterns of behavior connected by some common features have come to be recognized and diagnosed as schizophrenia. It remains uncertain whether these patterns of behavior are variations of one illness or are, in fact, several different illnesses. Although the work of Rosenthal and Kety [67] indicates some genetic contribution to the etiology underlying the symptomatic disruptions of cognition, perception, and, presumably, brain function noted in schizophrenia, the pathophysiology remains obscure. The heterogeneity of symptomatology and clinical course makes the pursuit of a single etiologic factor in this group of disorders questionable and suggests, rather, that an underlying biochemical heterogeneity is responsible.

Many hypotheses about the etiology of schizophrenia have focused on alterations in central catecholamine metabolism. The predominant hypothesis for a neurochemical defect in schizophrenia is the "dopamine (DA) hypothesis of schizophrenia," which suggests that there is an excess of DA neuronal activity in specific brain areas in schizophrenic patients. Such excess DA activity could occur through increased presynaptic DA release via increased DA synthesis and/or faulty negative feedback regulation, or through supersensitive postsynaptic DA receptors.

The DA hypothesis of schizophrenia is supported by indirect pharmacologic evidence. Drugs such as amphetamine and methylphenidate, which increase central DA function, can, in high and long-term doses, produce a paranoid schizophrenic-like syndrome in normal subjects [6,80]. These drugs also exacerbate positive symptoms (i.e., hallucinations, delusions) in schizophrenic patients [4,36,37,38, 86,93]. On the other hand, drugs that deplete (such as reserpine) or block (such as the neuroleptics) central DA transmission produce a therapeutic effect [3,9,60]. Furthermore, recent support of the DA hypothesis derives from studies of the neuroleptic compounds which have shown that the drugs' clinical antipsychotic potencies are closely correlated with various measures of their anti-DA potency, such as their in vitro inhibition of DA receptor binding [23,79], their reversal of DA-related animal behaviors [23], and their elevation of human plasma prolactin [77].

This chapter reviews the biologic studies that test the DA hypothesis using schizophrenic patients. Studies are divided into two categories: (1) presynaptic DA mechanisms and (2) postsynaptic DA mechanisms. The presynaptic category includes measurements of DA, its metabolites, and its enzymes of synthesis and degradation. The postsynaptic category includes measurement of DA receptor binding and neuroendocrinologic studies.

PRESYNAPTIC DOPAMINERGIC MECHANISMS

The simplest notion of the DA hypothesis is that excessive DA is synthesized and released from presynaptic DA neurons. DA and/or its primary metabolite, homovanillic acid (HVA), have been measured in the cerebrospinal fluid (CSF), urine, and postmortem brains of schizophrenic patients.

Cerebrospinal Fluid Studies

In some studies, CSF HVA levels have been measured in schizophrenic patients and are presumed to reflect the amount of activity of central DA neurons. The increase in DA turnover that occurs when DA receptors are blocked by neuroleptic drugs is reflected in an increase in lumbar CSF HVA levels [32,58]. Because the major source of CSF HVA appears to be the nigrostriatal DA system, specifically the caudate nucleus which borders directly on the lateral ventricles and thus provides its metabolites with direct access to CSF [80], many investigators criticize studies such as these. They argue that the mesolimbic and mesocortical DA tracts, which are more likely to be etiologically important in schizophrenia, probably do not contribute much to CSF HVA [51]. However, there is some evidence that these limbic and cortical DA systems may be functionally and anatomically linked to the corpus striatum [53].

If schizophrenia is associated with a generalized increase in brain DA turnover, then HVA should be increased in unmedicated schizophrenic patients. As noted in Table 15.1, almost all reports indicate that baseline levels of HVA in patients with a variety of schizophrenic diagnoses do not differ from those of comparison groups. Rimon et al [66] reported that although there are no notable differences in the groups as a whole, patients with paranoid schizophrenia have significantly higher CSF HVA levels than both nonparanoid patients and controls. Sedvall and Wode-Helgodt [76] found that patients with a family history of schizophrenia have significantly higher mean CSF HVA levels than schizophrenics without such a family history.

Most recent CSF studies use the probenecid technique to inhibit egress of HVA from the CSF and thereby diminish the marked HVA concentration gradient that exists from ventricular to lumbar CSF. Overall, the studies of lumbar CSF

Table 15.1 Cerebrospinal Fluid Studies of Dopamine Systems in Schizophrenia

Author (Reference No.)	*Date*	*Results*	*Diagnosis*	*Controls*	*Comment*
Baseline Studies					
Persson et al [58]	1969	HVA–N	CS	PSY, NORM	Patients receiving neuroleptics
Bowers et al [12]	1969	HVA–N	?	PSY, NORM	
Chase et al [21]	1970	HVA–N	AS, CS	NEUROL	
Rimon et al [66]	1971	HVA–N	AS	PSY	↑ HVA in paranoids vs. controls or nonparanoids
Fyro et al [32]	1974	HVA–N	CS	PSY	
Sedvall et al [75]	1974	HVA–N	CS	PSY	
Post et al [59]	1975	HVA–N	AS	PSY, NORM, NEUROL	
Sedvall et al [76]	1980	HVA–N	AS, CS	PSY, NORM	↑ HVA in patients with family history of schizophrenia
Probenecid Studies					
Bowers [9]	1972	HVA–N	AS	NORM	Low-dose probenecid
Bowers [10]	1973	HVA–N	AS, CS	PSY, NORM	↓ HVA in schneiderian-positive patients
Bowers [11]	1974	HVA–↓	AS, CS	PSY	Lowest HVA in poor-prognosis patients
Sedvall et al [75]	1974	HVA–N	CS	PSY	HVA higher in women and manic patients
Post et al [59]	1975	HVA–N	AS	PSY	All good prognosis patients; lower HVA in schneiderian-positive patients; not higher in paranoids; HVA lower on recovery than before or compared with manics
Berger et al [7]	1980	HVA–N DOPAC–N	AS, CS	PSY, NORM	Analysis also performed using probenecid levels
Gattaz et al [33]	1983	DA–N	CS	PSY, NORM	↑ DA levels appear related to neuroleptic treatment

HVA = homovanillic acid; N = no statistical difference; CS = chronic schizophrenia; PSY = psychiatric nonschizophrenic controls; NORM = normal controls; AS = acute schizophrenia; NEUROL = neurologic controls; ↑ = increased; ↓ = decreased; DOPAC = 3,4 dihydroxyphenylacetic acid; DA = dopamine.

HVA in unmedicated schizophrenic patients using probenecid report normal HVA levels (see Table 15.1). However, some differences are seen in patient subgroups. Bowers [10] noted that schizophrenic patients with schneiderian first-rank symptoms [74] have lower HVA accumulations than both patients without such symptoms and depressed patients or controls. In the only study which showed a marked difference (i.e., low) between the patients and controls, Bowers [11] reported that when the patients were divided on the basis of a prognostic scale, the poor-prognosis group had significantly *lower* mean HVA levels than either the good-prognosis group or patients with affective psychosis. In agreement with Bowers [10], Post et al [59] reported a similar decrease in HVA accumulations in good-prognosis schizophrenic patients with more schneiderian first-rank symptoms. In addition, they noted that, following recovery from the acute psychosis, the accumulations of HVA were reduced compared to those measured in the acute stage. The findings of Bowers [11] and Post et al [59] of decreased DA turnover in remitted and chronic patients may be interpreted as a reflection of a trait-related increase in DA receptor sensitivity in schizophrenic patients.

DA receptor supersensitivity could produce, via feedback inhibition, the lower DA turnover observed in chronic patients and in patients in remission from psychosis. Increased DA turnover might then occur only during the initial period of acute psychosis through an impairment of normal regulatory mechanisms. Both Bowers [11] and Curzon [29] pointed out that if brain DA receptors are supersensitive in schizophrenic patients, then there could be increased functional DA activity in the face of low or normal HVA levels.

Another assessment of DA activity in CSF can be provided by measurement of 3,4 dihydroxyphenylacetic acid (DOPAC), an intermediate DA metabolite which may be a better index of DA neuronal firing than is HVA [68,69]. Berger et al [7] reported normal concentrations of CSF DOPAC in schizophrenic patients in both baseline and probenecid studies.

Only recently has the concentration of DA itself in the CSF of schizophrenic patients been compared to controls [33]. Unmedicated patients and controls show no significant differences.

Postmortem Brain Dopamine and Metabolite Studies

Another test of the DA hypothesis, more direct than measuring neurotransmitter or metabolite levels in CSF but with its own inherent complications, is examination of DA, HVA, and DOPAC levels in specific areas of postmortem schizophrenic brains (Table 15.2). Although investigations have reported increased levels in some areas of schizophrenic brain, the effects are small and are not obtained in all studies.

Bird et al [8] reported that DA levels are elevated in a group of psychotic patients in the limbic nucleus accumbens. After enlarging their study and dividing the patients into schizophrenic and schizophrenic-like patients, Mackay et al [46] noted elevated DA concentrations in the nucleus accumbens and caudate of the

Table 15.2 Postmortem Brain Levels of Dopamine and Homovanillic Acid in Schizophrenics and Controls

Author (Reference No.)	Date	Caudate		Nucleus Accumbens		Putamen		Cingulate Gyrus		Frontal Lobe		Septal Region		Comments
		DA	HVA	DA	HVA	DA	HVA	DA	HVA	DA	HVA	DA	HVA	
Bird et al [8]	1977	N	—	↑	—	N	—	—	—	—	—	N	—	Psychotic patients (including schizophrenics) vs. controls
Crow et al [27,28]	1978 1980	↑	↓	N	N	N	N	—	—	—	—	—	—	DOPAC—N in all regions examined
Crow et al [26]	1979	↑	N	N	N	↑	N	—	—	—	—	—	—	
Winblad et al [91]	1979	N	N	—	—	N	N	N	—	N	—	—	—	All patients on neuroleptics prior to death; 6 of 12 patients lobotomized
Bacopoulos et al [5]	1979	—	—	—	N	—	N	—	↑	—	↑	—	—	All patients on neuroleptics; no tolerance to neuroleptics in cortex
Farley et al [31]	1980	N	N	N	N	N	N	—	—	—	—	↑	N	Chronic paranoid patients
Wyatt et al [92]	1981	—	—	N	N	—	—	—	—	—	—	—	—	DOPAC—N in nucleus accumbens
Mackay et al [46]	1982	↑	—	↑	—	—	—	—	—	—	—	—	—	↑ especially in patients with early onset of illness; no relationship noted to prior neuroleptic treatment

DA = dopamine; HVA = homovanillic acid; N = no significant difference between schizophrenics and controls; ↑ or ↓ = significantly ($p < 0.05$) increased or decreased in schizophrenics compared with controls; — = levels not reported; DOPAC = 3,4 dihydroxyphenylacetic acid.

schizophrenic group and reported that this elevated DA concentration is especially marked in those patients who had an early onset of psychosis and died at a young age. The increases in DA levels did not seem related to treatment with neuroleptic medication.

As seen in Table 15.2, these results are not widely replicated. Because the majority of the patients investigated received neuroleptics shortly before death, drug effects must be considered in the interpretation of the results. Furthermore, such factors as the length of time between death and autopsy, age of the subjects, manner of death, and different dissection techniques for defining anatomic areas may have influenced the data.

The investigation of Bacopoulos et al [5] is especially interesting with regard to the site of action of antipsychotic medications. When the brains of schizophrenic patients who had been receiving neuroleptic medication were compared to those from age-matched controls, elevations in HVA were found in the cingulate gyrus and frontal cortex only. HVA concentrations were in the normal range in all areas from three patients who had never received neuroleptic treatment. The authors suggested that the elevated HVA in the cortical regions indicates an absence in the cortex of a neurochemical tolerance similar to the absence of a clinical tolerance to the antipsychotic effects of neuroleptics. They thus proposed a cortical site for the clinical action of neuroleptics.

Studies of Enzyme Activity

Most of the enzymes involved in the synthesis and degradation of DA are the same as those for norepinephrine (NE). A review of investigations into the enzymes of synthesis (i.e., tyrosine hydroxylase [TH] and dopa decarboxylase) and degradation (i.e., monoamine oxidase [MAO] and catechol-O-methyltransferase [COMT]) in schizophrenic patients is found in Chapter 14.

Dopamine β-hydroxylase (DBH), the enzyme which converts DA to NE, is present in brain NE neurons but not in brain DA neurons. Discussion of studies of DBH activity in schizophrenia is also found in Chapter 14. Recently, we reported that CSF DBH activity is in the normal range in schizophrenic patients [82]. However, when this measure, which is markedly constant over time in individuals and which is under appreciable genetic control, was examined within the schizophrenic group, significant differences were noted. CSF DBH activity levels were significantly lower in those schizophrenic patients who became nonpsychotic during neuroleptic treatment than in those who remained psychotic [81]. Furthermore, the patients with better premorbid socialization, better prognosis, and less psychopathology between psychotic episodes also tended to have lower levels of CSF DBH activity [81]. Low CSF DBH activity thus appears to delineate a subgroup of schizophrenic patients with an acute "reactive" syndrome (characterized by episodic psychotic behavior in response to stress), which is very responsive to neuroleptic treatment. One may hypothesize that genetically determined low levels of DBH activity may lead DBH, under stressful stimulation, to become a rate-limiting enzyme in NE synthesis, thus leading to increased levels of DA in NE neurons. When released from NE neurons, DA may act directly on adrenergic systems as a "false" neurotransmitter or may act on anatomically nearby DA systems. Low DBH may thus be characteristic of a schizophrenic subgroup whose members, as evidenced by their responsiveness to neuroleptic treatment, may have a hyper-dopaminergic disorder, as distinguished from patients who are not responsive to neuroleptic treatment and may thus have different or additional pathophysiology.

POSTSYNAPTIC DOPAMINERGIC MECHANISMS

Because most studies have not demonstrated increased DA turnover in schizophrenic patients, there is a recent trend in research to focus on a postsynaptic DA pathophysiology in schizophrenia. Such investigations have included measurement of DA receptor binding in postmortem schizophrenic brains as well as neuroendocrine strategies.

Studies of Dopamine Receptor Binding in Postmortem Brain Tissue

With four of five laboratories reporting postsynaptic DA receptor supersensitivity [43–45,56,62–65], the most reproducible finding in postmortem schizophrenic brain tissue is an increase in the number of DA receptor binding sites of the D2 type found in the caudate, nucleus accumbens, and olfactory tubercle (Table 15.3). Because of the potential importance of these observations toward understanding etiology, it is essential to evaluate whether such differences reflect an intrinsic aspect of the disease process or are secondary to neuroleptic treatment, which can itself augment the number of DA receptor binding sites.

Lee et al [43] first described increased binding of tritiated neuroleptic drugs in postmortem schizophrenic brain tissue using a single concentration of tritiated haloperidol or spiperone. Such increases in tritiated spiperone binding in the caudate and putamen from schizophrenic brain tissue were replicated by Lee and Seeman [42], Reisine et al [63]. These studies were extended by Owen et al [56], who were the first to carry out a full-saturation analysis of the binding sites, which revealed that the increased binding was due to increases in the number of the receptors rather than any increase in receptor affinity. Indeed, receptor affinity is reduced, probably secondary to the presence of residual neuroleptic drugs in the schizophrenic brain tissues. The work of Mackay et al [44] replicated the findings of Owen and colleagues. Only Reynolds et al [64, 65] did not find a difference in DA receptor number in postmortem schizophrenic brain tissue.

Although some of the studies [41,42,62,63] included a few apparently neuroleptic-free patients (total number of patients = 21), and such patients also had increased numbers of DA receptors (albeit less marked), more investigation is needed to resolve the role of prior neuroleptic treatment in increasing DA receptor

Table 15.3 Postmortem Dopamine Receptor Binding Studies in Schizophrenia

Author (Reference No.)	*Date*	*Ligand*	*Results*	*Comment*
Lee et al [43]	1978	Haloperidol Spiperone	↑ Binding in caudate and putamen	Ligand used in single concentration
Owen et al [56]	1978	Spiroperidol ADTN (a DA agonist)	↑ Receptor number via spiroperidol in caudate, putamen, and nucleus accumbens; ↓ receptor affinity (secondary to residual neuroleptic); ADTN binding normal	First full-saturation analysis; 5 patients had no neuroleptic treatment 1 year prior to death; they had ↑ receptor number (less than neuroleptic-treated patients) and normal affinity
Lee and Seeman [41,42]	1980a 1980b	Haloperidol Spiperone Apomorphine	↑ Haloperidol and spiroperidol binding in caudate and putamen; normal apomorphine binding	11 patients who had no long-term neuroleptic treatment had same results
Cross et al [24]	1981	Flupenthixol	↑ Receptor number in caudate	7 patients without long-term neuroleptic treatment; Flupenthixol is a selective D2 DA receptor antagonist

Reisine et al [62,63]	1980	Spiroperidol	↑ Binding in caudate and putamen N Binding in cortex	3 patients not receiving neuroleptic prior to death had ↑ binding in caudate
Mackay et al [44,45]	1980	Spiperone	↑ Receptor number in caudate and nucleus accumbens; ↓ receptor affinity (secondary to residual neuroleptic)	
Reynolds et al [64,65]	1980	Spiperone	N Receptor number and ↓ receptor affinity in putamen	4 drug-free patients had N receptor number and affinity
Mackay et al [46]	1982	Spiperone	↑ Receptor number in caudate and nucleus accumbens; ↓ receptor affinity	Patients who were drug-free more than 1 month prior to death did not differ from controls

ADTN = 2-amino-6,7-dihydroxy-1,2,3,4-tetrahydronaphthalene; DA = dopamine; ↑ or ↓ = significantly ($p < 0.05$) increased or decreased in schizophrenics compared with controls; N = no significant difference in schizophrenics compared with controls.

binding sites. Because chronic neuroleptic blockade of DA receptors produces an increase in the number of tritiated neuroleptic–labeled D2 but not of the tritiated apomorphine–labeled D3 DA receptors [17], the finding of no increase in D3 receptor binding in the patients [41–43,78] suggests that the increase in D2 receptors may have been secondary to neuroleptic treatment. Furthermore, the report of Mackay et al [46] that an increased D2 receptor number was found only in patients who received neuroleptic medication up to the time of death, whereas patients whose neuroleptic treatment stopped at least 1 month prior to death showed no receptor number increases, supports the suspicion that the reported receptor increases may have been entirely drug related.

Neuroendocrine Studies of Dopamine Function

Neuroendocrinologic methods are extensively used to test the DA hypothesis by examining DA activity in the hypothalamic-pituitary system as a reflection of generalized DA activity in the schizophrenic brain. DA regulates pituitary-mediated hormonal activity, specifically through stimulatory control of growth hormone (GH) secretion by DA acting at the hypothalamic level [47,53,89] and inhibitory control of prolactin (PRL) release through primarily direct DA action on the pituitary [15]. Investigations of DA activity in this system in schizophrenic patients have studied basal plasma PRL and GH levels as well as the effects of DA agonists and antagonists on PRL and GH levels.

If schizophrenic patients have increased central DA activity, they might also have decreased levels of serum PRL. However, most studies of baseline PRL levels in unmedicated acute and chronic schizophrenics found no differences compared to controls [13,14,35,48,50,55]. However, in one study, severity of formal thought disorder related inversely to plasma PRL in unmedicated chronic patients [39], and Kleinman et al [40] recently reported that patients with normal cerebral ventricular size have reduced plasma PRL levels (compared to patients with enlarged ventricles) and that a significant inverse correlation exists between PRL levels and the degree of psychotic symptomatology. These studies suggest a relationship between DA activity and psychopathology, at least in some schizophrenic patients.

Administration of chlorpromazine to both schizophrenic patients and controls produces similar elevations of PRL [48]. After challenge with apomorphine, a direct DA agonist, Rotrosen et al [71] found less PRL suppression in 17 chronic schizophrenics compared with 10 controls, but the authors report that the apomorphine-induced PRL suppression is not a reliable measurement. Meltzer and Stahl [51] found no difference in this PRL nadir.

No differences have been documented in baseline GH levels between unmedicated schizophrenic patients and controls [30,48,57,72]. Rotrosen et al [70, 73], studying the GH response to apomorphine in a group of floridly psychotic schizophrenic patients, showed that although the mean GH peak did not differ between the patients and controls, the distribution of responses in the two groups differed significantly, with the schizophrenic patients tending toward a bimodal distribution. Whereas the GH response to indirect DA agonists such as L-dopa and amphetamine produces highly variable results, the GH response to apomorphine appears to be very reliable [71]. Four separate investigations [30,57,73,85] demonstrated, in comparison with controls, an exaggerated GH response to apomorphine in acute schizophrenics and a small number of chronic patients with little or no previous neuroleptic treatment. On the other hand, most chronic schizophrenics showed a blunting of the GH response to apomorphine. The degree of blunting of the GH response may be related to the duration of previous neuroleptic treatment [30,73].

One possible explanation for these findings is that the exaggerated GH responses in the acute patients may represent evidence of DA receptor supersensitivity that is characteristic of their disease process whereas the blunted responses in the chronic patients are either secondary to neuroleptic treatment or are evidence that the more chronically ill schizophrenics have subsensitive DA receptors. This hypothesis is supported by the reports of different effects of DA agonist drugs on the clinical state of acute compared with chronic schizophrenic patients [2,4,14,18,22,34,37].

CONCLUSIONS

The DA hypothesis of schizophrenia has been a useful paradigm for investigation as evidenced by the many studies reported here. However, the available biochemical approaches have not confirmed a DA disturbance as the primary etiology in schizophrenia. Indeed, indirect pharmacologic studies are still the major support for the hypothesis despite the extensive biochemical investigation of schizophrenic patients. Furthermore, pharmacologic evidence does not necessarily indicate the primary locus of the defect. Nearly all pharmacologic agents active on DA systems also notably affect other neurotransmitter systems. The relationships between central NE [83], serotonin (5-hydroxytryptamine; 5-HT) [61], γ-aminobutyric acid (GABA) [88], substance P [19], endorphins [1], and other neurotransmitter systems and DA activity in schizophrenia require further study.

The hypothesis that schizophrenics have supersensitive brain DA receptors is supported by the postmortem brain DA receptor binding studies of four of five laboratories and the neuroendocrine reports of an exaggerated GH response to apomorphine in acute patients. However, the hypothesized DA receptor supersensitivity is challenged by the suggestions that the elevated receptor binding is related to neuroleptic treatment [46] and by the reported lack of an enhanced sensitivity in schizophrenics to amphetamine-induced psychosis following abrupt withdrawal of neuroleptic treatment [87].

Modifications in the hypothesis which might lead to further understanding of the syndrome's pathogenesis include (1) the DA abnormality may only occur in a very specific brain area (e.g., prefrontal cortex) and (2) the primary disturbance in schizophrenia may occur in another neurotransmitter system that interacts with DA neurons. Neuroleptics may thus be operating on a "secondary" DA system.

Similarly, although anticholinergic drugs are of clinical benefit in Parkinson's disease, the primary defect in parkinsonism lies in the nigrostriatal DA system rather than in a cholinergic system. Furthermore, although neuroleptics rapidly produce DA receptor blockade, as evidenced by the rapid neuroleptic-induced rise in plasma PRL [49], the full clinical antipsychotic response to them requires a number of weeks. Thus, whereas DA receptor blockade does appear necessary for the antipsychotic effects of neuroleptic medication, that blockade may allow other slower processes to take place which are more directly responsible for the therapeutic change. (3) Several biochemical factors involved in central DA function (e.g., low MAO, low DBH, DA receptor supersensitivity) may each be a vulnerability factor toward the illness. That is, each abnormality may be a necessary but not sufficient element for the development of schizophrenia. (4) The heterogeneity of the clinical syndrome of schizophrenia itself may be responsible for the inconclusive results. As stated earlier, schizophrenia probably represents a variety of disease entities, each having a different biologic dysfunction [16]. Some or all of these may entail a defect in DA systems. Thus, Crow [25] has attempted to draw a neurobiologic distinction between schizophrenic patients who have good antipsychotic responses to neuroleptic treatment and patients who remain psychotic during such treatment. He proposed that there are two syndromes with distinct disease processes: (1) an acute episodic schizophrenic syndrome with positive symptoms reversed by neuroleptic treatment, the illness thus being associated with increased DA neurotransmission (type I syndrome); and (2) a chronic deteriorating syndrome with negative symptoms not reversed by neuroleptic treatment, the illness thus being unrelated to DA transmission, but possibly related to structural brain changes (type II syndrome). Recent pharmacologic [54], neuroendocrinologic [40], and neuroradiologic [90] reports have provided preliminary support for this hypothesized distinction. The DA hypothesis may then only apply to the type I subgroup.

Because of the clinical heterogeneity of people diagnosed as schizophrenic and the complex relationships among neurobiologic systems, rather than attempting to find a single "cause" for the entire spectrum of schizophrenia, we suggest that studies concentrate on two more modest goals.

First, a finer delineation of diagnostic and biologic heterogeneity would be obtained by identifying the following: (1) clinical (paranoid versus catatonic, early versus late onset); (2) pharmacologic (neuroleptic responders versus partial responders versus nonresponders); and (3) biochemical (high versus low CSF substance levels) subgroups in large populations of schizophrenic patients. The next step would be to identify patterns in these subgroups. The presumed heterogeneity of the disorder poses special problems for the clinical investigator. Statistically significant findings in a large group of patients are very likely to be secondary to the previously discussed nonspecific factors and to artifacts such as drug treatment (past or present). On the other hand, studies with a small patient sample are not likely to recognize an abnormality that may occur in only a small proportion of patients diagnosed as schizophrenic. A fruitful approach to finding this subgroup would be to focus on those patients with extremely aberrant values, even though they may not affect the statistical significance of the entire study population. In this way, the biologic value can be used as an independent variable to identify a subgroup of schizophrenic patients with consequences for etiology, course, and treatment response.

The second goal should be to relate biologic factors to specific component behaviors that make up the schizophrenic disorders: one can classify the behavioral components into separate groups to examine whether specific biologic variables relate more to one of these component groups than to the variety of behavioral disorders grouped under the diagnosis schizophrenia. A distinction that we think especially useful in conceptualizing schizophrenia is that of "state components" and "trait components." State components refer to aspects of the psychotic state itself, such as behavioral disorganization, hallucinations, and delusions. Specific state-related biologic concomitants may relate primarily to the psychotic state and would be less evident during periods of remission. Trait components would be those aspects evident in the prepsychotic or postpsychotic period, such as social isolation, affective blunting, impaired role functioning, impaired eye tracking, CAT scan abnormalities, or other as yet unknown behaviors. Trait-related biologic concomitants would relate to behaviors of the nonpsychotic state, would not change over time, and thus could reflect a genetic vulnerability to psychotic decompensation. Further delineation of biologic measures that are state-related or trait-related would provide an approach to understanding those aspects of the illness that are present in a range of people, including nonschizophrenics, as well as to understanding those aspects that are illness specific.

REFERENCES

1. Ahtee L, Attila LMH. Opioid Mechanism in Regulation of Cerebral Monoamines in Vivo. In Histochemistry and Cell Biology of Autonomic Neurons. O Eranko (ed), 361–365. New York: Raven Press, 1980.
2. Alpert M, Friedhoff AJ, Marcos LR, Diamond F. Paradoxical reaction to L-dopa in schizophrenic patients. Am J Psychiatry 135:1329–1332, 1978.
3. Anden NW, Butcher SG, Corrodi H. Receptor activity and turnover of dopamine and noradrenaline after neuroleptics. Eur J Pharmacol 11:303–314, 1970.
4. Angrist BM, Sathanathan GS, Gershon S. Behavioral effects of L-dopa in schizophrenic patients. Psychopharmacologia (Berlin) 31:1–12, 1973.
5. Bacopoulos N, Spokes EG, Bird ED, Roth RH. Anti-psychotic drug action in schizophrenic patients: Effect on cortical dopamine metabolism after long-term treatment. Science 205:1405–1407, 1979.
6. Bell DS. Comparison of amphetamine psychosis and schizophrenia. Br J Psychiatry 111:701–707, 1965.
7. Berger PA, Faull KF, Kilkowski J, Anderson PH, Kraemer H, David KL, Barchas JD. CSF monoamine metabolites in depression and schizophrenia. Am J Psychiatry 137:174–180, 1980.
8. Bird ED, Barnes J, Iversen LL, Spokes EG, Mackay AVP, Shepherd M. Increased brain dopamine and reduced glutamic acid decarboxylase and choline acetyl transferase activity in schizophrenics and related psychoses. Lancet ii:1157–1159, 1977.

9. Bowers MB. Acute psychosis induced by psychotomimetic drug abuse. II. Neurochemical findings. Arch Gen Psychiatry 27:440–442, 1972.
10. Bowers MB. 5-Hydroxyindoleacetic acid (5-HIAA) and homovanillic acid (HVA) following probenecid in acute psychotic patients treated with phenothiazines. Psychopharmacology (Berlin) 28:309–318, 1973.
11. Bowers MB. Central dopamine turnover in schizophrenic syndromes. Arch Gen Psychiatry 31:50–54, 1974.
12. Bowers MB, Heninger GR, Gerbode FA. Cerebrospinal fluid, 5-hydroxyindoleacetic acid and homovanillic acid in psychiatric patients. Int J Neuropharmacol 8:255–262, 1969.
13. Brambilla F, Guastalla A, Guerini A, Rovere C, Legnani G, Sarno M, Riggi F. Prolactin secretion in chronic schizophrenia. Acta Psychiatr Scand 54:275–286, 1976.
14. Brambilla F, Scarone S, Ponzano M, Maffei C, Nobile P, Rovere C, Guastalla A. Catecholaminergic drugs in chronic schizophrenia. Neuropsychobiology 5:185–200, 1979.
15. Brown GM, Friend WC, Chambers JW. Neuropharmacology of Hypothalamic Pituitary Regulation. In Clinical Neuroendocrinology: a Pathophysiological Approach, G Tollis, F Labrie, and JB Martin (eds), 47–81. New York: Raven Press, 1979.
16. Buchsbaum MS, Haier RJ. Biological homogeneity, symptom heterogeneity, and the diagnosis of schizophrenia. Schiz Bull 4:473–475, 1978.
17. Burt DR, Creese J, Snyder SH. Antischizophrenic drugs. Chronic treatment elevates dopamine receptor binding in brain. Science 196:326–328, 1977.
18. Calil HM, Yesavage JA, Hollister LE. Low-dose levodopa in schizophrenia. Commun Psychopharmacol 1:593–596, 1977.
19. Carlsson A. Comments on Dopamine and Substance P. In Neuro-Regulators and Psychiatric Disorders, E Usdin, D Hamburg, J Barchas (eds), 14–18. London: Oxford University Press, 1977.
20. Carlsson A, Lindqvist M. Effect of chlorpromazine and haloperidol on formation of 3-methoxytyramine and normetanephrine in mouse brain. Acta Pharmacol Toxicol 20:140–144, 1963.
21. Chase TN, Schnur JA, Gordon EK. Cerebrospinal fluid monoamine catabolites in drug-induced extrapyramidal disorders. Neuropharmacology 9:265–268, 1970.
22. Chouinard G, Jones BD. Schizophrenia as dopamine deficiency disease. Lancet 2:99–100, 1978.
23. Creese I, Burt DR, Snyder SH. Dopamine receptor binding predicts clinical and pharmacological potencies of antischizophrenic drugs. Science 192:481–483, 1976.
24. Cross AJ, Crow TJ, Owen F. ^{3}H-Flupenthixol binding in post-mortem brains of schizophrenics: Evidence for a selective increase in dopamine D2 receptors. Psychopharmacology (Berlin) 74:122–124, 1981.
25. Crow TJ. Molecular pathology of schizophrenia: More than one disease process? Br Med J 280:66–68, 1980.
26. Crow TJ, Baker HF, Cross AJ, Joseph MH, Lofthouse R, Longden A, Owen F, Riley GJ, Glover V, Killpack WS. Monoamine mechanisms in chronic schizophrenia: Post-mortem neurochemical findings. Br J Psychiatry 134:249–256, 1979.
27. Crow TJ, Cross AJ, Johnstone EC, Longden A, Owen F, Ridley RM. Time course of the antipsychotic effect in schizophrenia and some changes in post-mortem brain and their relation to neuroleptic medication. Adv Biochem Psychopharmacol 24:495–503, 1980.
28. Crow TJ, Johnstone EC, Longden AJ, Owen F. Dopaminergic mechanisms in schizophrenia: The antipsychotic effect and the disease process. Life Sci 23:563–568, 1978.

29. Curzon G. CSF homovanillic acid: An index of dopaminergic hyperactivity. Adv Neurol 9:349–357, 1975.
30. Ettigi P, Nair NP, Lal S, Cervantes P, Guyda H. Effect of apomorphine on growth hormone and prolactin secretion in schizophrenic patients with or without oral dyskinesia, withdrawn from chronic neuroleptic therapy. J Neurol Neurosurg Psychiatry 39:870, 1976.
31. Farley IJ, Price KS, Hornykiewicz O. Dopamine in the limbic regions of the human brain: Normal and abnormal. Adv Biochem Psychopharmacol 16:57–64, 1977.
32. Fryo B, Wode-Helgodt B, Borg S, Sedvall G. The effect of chlorpromazine on homovanillic acid levels in cerebrospinal fluid of schizophrenic patients. Psychopharmacologia (Berlin) 35:287–294, 1974.
33. Gattaz WF, Riederer P, Reynolds GP, Gattaz D, Beckman H. Dopamine and noradrenalin in the cerebrospinal fluid of schizophrenic patients. Psychiatr Res 8:243–250, 1983.
34. Gerlach J, Luhdorf D. The effect of L-DOPA on young patients with simple schizophrenia, treated with neuroleptic drugs. Psychopharmacologia (Berlin) 44:105–110, 1975.
35. Gruen PH, Sachar EJ, Langer G, Altman N, Leifer M, Frantz A, Halpern FS. Prolactin responses to neuroleptics in normal and schizophrenic subjects. Arch Gen Psychiatry 35:105–116, 1978.
36. Janowsky DS, Davis JM. Dopamine, psychomotor stimulants, and schizophrenia: Effects of methylphenidate and the stereoisomers of amphetamine in schizophrenics. Adv Biochem Psychopharmacol 12:317–323, 1974.
37. Janowsky DS, Davis JM. Methylphenidate, dextro-amphetamine and lev-amphetamine: Effects on schizophrenic symptoms. Arch Gen Psychiatry 33:304–308, 1976.
38. Janowsky DS, El-Yousef MK, David JM, Sekerke HJ. Provocation of schizophrenia symptoms by intravenous administration of methylphenidate. Arch Gen Psychiatry 28:185–191, 1973.
39. Johnstone EC, Crow TJ, Mashiter K. Anterior pituitary hormone secretion in chronic schizophrenia—An approach to neurohumoral mechanisms. Psychol Med 7:223–228, 1977.
40. Kleinman JE, Weinberger DR, Rogol AD, Bigelow LB, Klein ST, Gillin JC, Wyatt RJ. Plasma prolactin concentrations and psychopathology in chronic schizophrenia. Arch Gen Psychiatry 39:655–657, 1982.
41. Lee T, Seeman P. Abnormal neuroleptic/dopamine receptors in schizophrenia. Adv Biochem Psychopharmacol 21:435–442, 1980.
42. Lee T, Seeman P. Elevation of brain neuroleptic/dopamine receptors in schizophrenia. Am J Psychiatry 137:191–197, 1980.
43. Lee T, Seeman P, Tourtellotte WW, Farley IJ, Hornykiewicz O. Binding of ^{3}H-neuroleptics and ^{3}H-apomorphine in schizophrenic brains. Nature 274:897–900, 1978.
44. Mackay AVP, Bird ED, Iversen LL, Spokes EG, Creese I, Snyder SH. Dopaminergic abnormalities in post-mortem schizophrenic brain. Adv Biochem Psychopharmacol 24:325–333, 1980.
45. Mackay AVP, Bird ED, Spokes EG, Rossor M, Iversen LL, Creese I, Snyder SH. Dopamine receptors and schizophrenia: Drug effect or illness? Lancet 2:915–916, 1980.
46. Mackay AVP, Iversen LL, Rossor M, Spokes E, Bird E, Arregui A, Creese I, Snyder SH. Increased brain dopamine and dopamine receptors in schizophrenia. Arch Gen Psychiatry 39:991–997, 1982.
47. Martin JB. Neural regulation of growth hormone secretion: Medical progress report. N Engl J Med 288:1384–1393, 1973.

48. Meltzer H, Fang V. The effect of neuroleptics on serum prolactin in schizophrenic patients. Arch Gen Psychiatry 33:279, 1976.
49. Meltzer HY, Goode DJ, Fang YS. The Effect of Psychotropic Drugs on Endocrine Function. I. Neuroleptics, Precursors and Agonists. In Psychopharmacology: A Generation of Progress, MA Lipton, A DiMascio, and KF Killam (eds), 509–529. New York: Raven Press, 1978.
50. Meltzer HY, Sachar EJ, Frantz AG. Serum prolactin levels in unmedicated schizophrenic patients. Arch Gen Psychiatry 31:564–569, 1974.
51. Meltzer HY, Stahl SM. The dopamine hypothesis of schizophrenia: A review. Schiz Bull 2:19–76, 1976.
52. Mettler FA. Perceptual capacity, functions of the corpus striatum and schizophrenia. Psychiatr Q 29:89–111, 1955.
53. Muller EE, Luizzi A, Coci D, Panerai AE, Oppizzi G, Locatelli V, Mantegazza R, Silvestrini F, Chiodini PG. Role of Dopaminergic Receptors in the Regulation of Growth Hormone Secretion. In Nonstriatal Dopaminergic Neurons, E Contain, GL Gessa (eds), 127–138. New York: Raven Press, 1977.
54. Nasrallah HA, Kleinman JE, Weinberger DR, Gillin JC, Wyatt RJ. Cerebral ventricular enlargement and dopamine synthesis inhibition in chronic schizophrenia. Arch Gen Psychiatry 37:1427, 1980.
55. Ohman R, Axelsson R. Relationship between prolactin response and antipsychotic effect of thioridazine in psychiatric patients. Eur J Clin Pharmacol 14:111–116, 1978.
56. Owen E, Cross AJ, Crow TJ, Longden A, Poulter M, Riley GJ. Increased dopamine receptor sensitivity in schizophrenia. Lancet 2:223–226, 1978.
57. Pandey GN, Garver DL, Tamminga C, Ericksen S, Ali SI, David JM. Postsynaptic supersensitivity in schizophrenia. Am J Psychiatry 134:518–522, 1977.
58. Persson T, Roos BE. Acid metabolites from monoamines in cerebrospinal fluid of chronic schizophrenics. Br J Psychiatry 115:95–98, 1969.
59. Post RM, Fink E, Carpenter WT, Goodwin FK. Cerebrospinal fluid amine metabolites in acute schizophrenia. Arch Gen Psychiatry 32:1063–1069, 1975.
60. Randrup A, Munkvad I. Evidence indicating an association between schizophrenia and dopaminergic hyperactivity in the brain. Ortho Psychiatry 1:2–7, 1972.
61. Rastogi RB, Singhal RL, Lapierre YD. Effect of short- and long-term neuroleptic treatment on brain serotonin synthesis and turnover: focus on the serotonin hypothesis of schizophrenia. Life Sci 29:735–741, 1981.
62. Reisine TD, Pedigo NW, Regan P, Ling N, Yamamura HI. Abnormal Brain Opiate Mechanisms in Schizophrenia. In Endogenous and Exogenous Opiate Agonists and Antagonists, Way EL (ed), 117–120. New York: Pergamon Press, 1980.
63. Reisine TD, Rossor M, Spokes E, Iversen LL, Yamamura HI. Opiate and neuroleptic receptor alterations in human schizophrenic brain tissue. Adv Biochem Psychopharmacol 21:443–450, 1980.
64. Reynolds GP, Reynolds LM, Riederer P, Jellinger K, Gabriel E. Dopamine receptors and schizophrenia: Drug effect or illness? Lancet ii:1251, 1980.
65. Reynolds GP, Riederer P, Jellinger K, Gabriel E. Dopamine receptors and schizophrenia: The neuroleptic drug problem. Neuropharmacology 20:1319–1320, 1981.
66. Rimon R, Roos, BE, Rakkolainen V, Alanen Y. The content of 5-hydroxyindoleacetic acid and homovanillic acid in the cerebrospinal fluid of patients with acute schizophrenia. J Psychosom Res 15:375–378, 1971.
67. Rosenthal D, Kety SS (eds). The Transmission of Schizophrenia. London: Pergamon Press, 1968.

68. Roth RH, Murrin LC, Walters JR. Central dopaminergic neurons: Effects of alterations in impulse flow on the accumulation of dihydroxyphenylacetic acid. Eur J Pharmacol 36:163–171, 1976.
69. Roth RH, Walters JR, Aghajanian GK. Effect of Impulse Flow on the Release and Synthesis of Dopamine in the Rat Striatum. In Frontiers in Catecholamine Research, E Usdin and SH Snyder (eds), 567–574. London: Pergamon Press, 1973.
70. Rotrosen J, Angrist B, Clark C, Gershon S, Halpern FS, Sachar EJ. Suppression of prolactin by dopamine agonists in schizophrenics and controls. Am J Psychiatry 135:949–951, 1978.
71. Rotrosen J, Angrist B, Gershon S, Paquin J, Branchey L, Oleshansky M, Halpern F, Sachar EJ. Neuroendocrine effects of apomorphine: Characterization of response patterns and application to schizophrenia research. Br J Psychiatry 135:444–456, 1979.
72. Rotrosen J, Angrist BM, Gershon S, Sachar EJ, Halpern FS. Dopamine receptor alteration in schizophrenia: Neuroendocrine evidence. Psychopharmacology (Berlin) 51:1–7, 1976.
73. Rotrosen J, Angrist B, Paquin J. Neuroendocrine studies with dopamine agonists in schizophrenia. Psychopharmacol Bull 14:14–16, 1978.
74. Schneider K. Clinical Psychopathology. Translated by WM Hamilton. New York: Grune & Stratton, 1959.
75. Sedvall G, Fyro B, Nyback H, Wiesel FA, Wode-Helgodt B. Mass fragmentometric determination of homovanillic acid in lumbar cerebrospinal fluid of schizophrenic patients during treatment with antipsychotic drugs. J Psychiatr Res 11:75–80, 1974.
76. Sedvall GC, Wode-Helgodt B. Aberrant monoamine metabolite levels in CSF and family history of schizophrenia: Their relationships in schizophrenic patients. Arch Gen Psychiatry 37:1113–1116, 1980.
77. Seeman P, Lee T. Antipsychotic drugs: Direct correlation between clinical potency and presynaptic action on dopamine neurons. Science 188:1217–1219, 1975.
78. Seeman P, Lee T, Bird ED, Tourtellotte WW. Elevation of Brain Neuroleptic/Dopamine Receptors in Schizophrenia. In Perspectives in Schizophrenia Research, C Baxter, and T Melnechuk (eds), 195–207. New York: Raven Press, 1980.
79. Seeman P, Lee T, Chau-Wong M, Wong K. Antipsychotic drug doses and neuroleptic/dopamine receptors. Nature 261:717–719, 1976.
80. Snyder SH. Catecholamines in the brain as mediators of amphetamine psychosis. Arch Gen Psychiatry 27:169–179, 1972.
81. Sourkes TL. On the origin of homovanillic acid (HVA) in the cerebrospinal fluid. J Neural Transm 34:153–157, 1973.
82. Sternberg DE, van Kammen DP, Ballenger JC, Lerner P, Marder SR, Post RM, Bunney WE, Jr. CSF dopamine-beta-hydroxylase in schizophrenia: low activity associated with good prognosis and good response to neuroleptic treatment. Arch Gen Psychiatry 40:743–747, 1983.
83. Sternberg DE, van Kammen DP, Lake CR, Ballenger JD, Post RM, Bunney WE, Jr. The effect of pimozide on cerebrospinal norepinephrine in schizophrenia. Am J Psychiatry 188:1045–1051, 1981.
84. Sternberg DE, van Kammen DP, Lerner P, Bunney WE, Jr. Schizophrenia: Dopamine-beta-hydroxylase activity and treatment response. Science 216:1423–1425, 1982.
85. Tamminga CA, Smith RC, Pandey G, Frohman LA, Davis JM. A neuroendocrine study of supersensitivity in tardive dyskinesia. Arch Gen Psychiatry 34:1199–1203, 1977.
86. van Kammen DP, Bunney WE, Jr. Heterogeneity in Response to Amphetamine in

Schizophrenia: Effects of Placebo, Chronic Pimozide and Pimozide Withdrawal. In Catecholamines: Basic and Clinical Frontiers, E Usdin, IJ Kopin, and J Barchas (eds), 1896–1898. Oxford: Pergamon Press, 1979.

87. van Kammen DP, Docherty JP, Marder SR, Schulz SC, Bunney WE, Jr. Lack of behavioral supersensitivity to D-amphetamine after pimozide withdrawal: a trial with schizophrenic patients. Arch Gen Psychiatry 37:287–290, 1980.

88. van Kammen DP, Sternberg DE, Hare TA, Waters RN, Bunney WE, Jr. CSF levels of gamma-aminobutyric acid in schizophrenia. Arch Gen Psychiatry 39:91–97, 1982.

89. Verde G, Oppizzi G, Colussi G, Gremascoli G, Botalla L, Muller EE, Silvestrini F, Chiodine PG, Liuzzi A. Effect of dopamine infusion on plasma levels of growth hormone in normal subjects and in acromegalic patients. Clin Endocrinol 5:419–423, 1976.

90. Weinberger DR, Cannon-Spoor E, Potkin SG, Wyatt RJ. Poor premorbid adjustment and CT scan abnormalities in chronic schizophrenia. Am J Psychiatry 137:1410–1413, 1980.

91. Winblad B, Bucht G, Gottfries CG, Roos BE. Monoamines and monoamine metabolites in brains from demented schizophrenics. Acta Psychiatr Scand 60:17–28, 1979.

92. Wyatt RJ, Potkin SG, Kleinman JE, Weinberger DR, Luchins DJ, Jeste DV. The schizophrenia syndrome: Examples of biological tools for subclassification. J Nerv Ment Dis 169:110–112, 1981.

93. Yaryura-Tobias JA, Diamond B, Merlis S. The action of L-DOPA on schizophrenic patients (a preliminary report). Curr Ther Res 12:528–531, 1970.

Glossary

ABCTRS	Abbreviated Conners Teacher Rating Scale
ALDH	aldehyde dehydrogenase
ALS	amyotrophic lateral sclerosis
AMPT	α-methyl-*p*-tyrosine
APO	apomorphine
ATPase	adenosine triphosphatase
CA	catecholamine
cAMP	cyclic adenosine 3′,5′-monophosphate
CCK	cholecystokinin
COMT	catechol-O-methyltransferase
CNS	central nervous system
CSF	cerebrospinal fluid
CV	coefficient of variation
ChAT	choline acetyltransferase
DA	dopamine
DBH	dopamine-β-hydroxylase
DDC	dopa decarboxylase
DHPG	3,4-dihydroxyphenylglycol
5,6-DHT	5,6 dihydroxytryptamine (serotonergic neurotoxin)
DMI	desmethylimipramine
Dopa	3,4-dihydroxyphenylalanine
DOPAC	3,4 dihydroxyphenylacetic acid
DSM-III	*Diagnostic and Statistical Manual of Mental Disorders* (3rd edition)
E	epinephrine
ECT	electroconvulsive therapy
EDTA	disodium-ethylenediaminetetraacetic acid
GABA	γ-aminobutyric acid
GCMS	gas chromatography with mass spectroscopy
GH	growth hormone

GAD	glutamic acid decarboxylase
DHE	dehydroergocriptine
5-HIAA	5-hydroxyindoleacetic acid
5-HT	5-hydroxytryptamine (serotonin)
HVA	homovanillic acid
ICC	intraclass correlation coefficients
ICV	intracerebroventricular
LADH	liver alcohol dehydrogenase
LC	locus coeruleus
M	metanephrine
MAO	monoamine oxidase
MAO-I	monoamine oxidase inhibitor
MHPG	3-methoxy-4-hydroxyphenylglycol
3-MT	3-methoxytyramine
NE	norepinephrine
NM	normetanephrine
NTS	nucleus tractus solitarius
17-OHCS	17-hydroxycorticosteroids
6-OHDA	6-hydroxydopamine
PAA	phenylacetic acid
PEA	phenylethylamine
PHPA	*p*-hydroxyphenylacetic acid
PNMT	phenylethanolamine-N-methyltransferase
PRL	prolactin
REM	rapid eye movement
SAM	S-adenosylmethionine
SNS	sympathetic nervous system
TH	tyrosine hydroxylase
TRM	tyramine
TRH	thyrotropin-releasing hormone
TSH	thyroid-stimulating hormone
VMA	vanillylmandelic acid
VTA	ventral tegmental area

Index